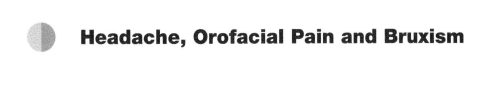# Headache, Orofacial Pain and Bruxism

Publisher: Sarena Wolfaard
Development Editor: Lulu Stader
Project Manager: Nancy Arnott
Designer: Kirsteen Wright
Illustration Manager: Gillian Richards
Illustrator: Jennifer Rose

Headache, Orofacial Pain and Bruxism

Edited by

Peter Selvaratnam PhD(Anatomy), BAppSc(Physio), GradDipManip Therapy, DipAcupuncture, FACP
Specialist Musculoskeletal Physiotherapist, Anatomist. Director, Headache Centre of Victoria; Clinical Associate Professor, Faculty of Medicine, Dentistry and Health Sciences, The University of Melbourne; Adjunct Senior Lecturer, Dept of Anatomy, Faculty of Medicine, Monash University, Australia.

Ken Niere BAppSc(Physio), GradDip(Manip Ther), MManipPhysio, FACP
Specialist Musculoskeletal Physiotherapist, Senior Lecturer
School of Physiotherapy, La Trobe University; Principal, Auburn Spinal Therapy Centre, Australia.

Maria Zuluaga BAppSc(Physio), GradDip(Manip Ther), MWomen's Hlth
Musculoskeletal Physiotherapist. Clinician, Headache Centre of Victoria, Australia.

Content advisers

Stephen Friedmann BDSc (Dental)
Dental Practitioner. Director, Dental Imaging Group of Australia Pty Ltd, Australia

Cathy Sloan MBBS, Dip RANZCOG (Medical)
General Practitioner. Clinician, Brighton Family and Women's Clinic; Surgical Assistant in Ophthalmology, Australia

Foreword by

Ed Byrne AO DSc MD MBA FRCP FRACP
Vice Provost (Health), Head of the UCL Medical School & Executive, Dean of Biomedical Sciences, University College, London, UK

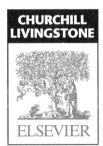

Edinburgh London New York Oxford Philadelphia St Louis Sydney Toronto 2009

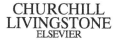

First published 2009, © Elsevier Limited. All rights reserved.

First edition 2009

ISBN 9780443103100

British Library Cataloguing in Publication Data
A catalogue record for this book is available from the British Library

Library of Congress Cataloging in Publication Data
A catalog record for this book is available from the Library of Congress

Notice
Knowledge and best practice in this field are constantly changing. As new research and experience broaden our knowledge, changes in practice, treatment and drug therapy may become necessary or appropriate. Readers are advised to check the most current information provided (i) on procedures featured or (ii) by the manufacturer of each product to be administered, to verify the recommended dose or formula, the method and duration of administration, and contraindications. It is the responsibility of the practitioner, relying on their own experience and knowledge of the patient, to make diagnoses, to determine dosages and the best treatment for each individual patient, and to take all appropriate safety precautions. To the fullest extent of the law, neither the Publisher nor the Editors assume any liability for any injury and/or damage to persons or property arising out of or related to any use of the material contained in this book.

The Publisher

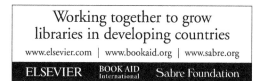

Printed and bound by CPI Group (UK) Ltd, Croydon, CR0 4YY

Transferred to Digital Print 2011

Contents

Section One Diagnosis

Contributors

Ramesh Balasubramaniam BSc, BDSc, MS, Cert Orofacial Pain(UKy), Cert Oral Medicine (UPenn)
Consultant in Orofacial Pain and Oral Medicine. Clinical Associate Professor, School of Dentistry, University of Western Australia. Co-director, Perth Orofacial Pain and Oral Medicine Centre, St John of God Hospital, Perth, Australia.

Richard Bittar MBBS, PhD, FRACS
Neurosurgeon. Consultant Neurosurgeon, Royal Melbourne Hospital; Consultant Neurosurgeon, The Alfred Hospital; Director, Precision Neurosurgery, Australia.

Kerrie Bolton Advanced DipAppSc(Myotherapy)
Myotherapist. Clinician, The Headache Centre of Victoria, Australia.

Lisa Campbell BAppSc(Physio), Certified Feldenkrais Practitioner
Senior Clinician Physiotherapist, Caulfield Pain Management and Research Centre, Australia.

George Chalkiadis MBBS, DA, FANZCA, FFPMANZCA
Anaesthetist and Pain Management Specialist. Head, Children's Pain Management Service, Royal Children's Hospital, Melbourne, Australia. Murdoch Children's Research Institute, Clinical Associate Professor, University Department of Paediatrics, University of Melbourne, Australia.

Karol Connors BAppSc(Physio), Grad Dip Geron, MPhysio, Accredited Feldenkrais Practitioner
Neurophysiotherapist, Physiotherapy Manager, Calvary Health Care Bethlehem; Sessional Lecturer, School of Physiotherapy, La Trobe University, Australia.

Robert Delcanho BDSc, MS, Certificate in Orofacial Pain and Dysfunction, FFPMANZCA
Consultant in Orofacial Pain and Oral Medicine. Clinical Associate Professor, School of Medicine and Dentistry, University of Western Australia. Co-Director, Perth Orofacial Pain and Oral Medicine Centre, St John of God Hospital, Perth, Australia.

Ian Devlin MBBS, FRACGP
General Practitioner. St Kilda Road Medical Centre, Australia.

Mark W Faragher BMedSc, MBBS, FRACP
Neurologist. Consulting Neurologist, Alfred Hospital, Consulting Neurologist, Peter McCallum Cancer Institute. Hon. Senior Lecturer, Faculty of Medicine, Monash University; Clinical Adjunct Associate Professor, Faculty of Medicine, University of Notre Dame, Australia.

Stephen Friedmann BDSc
Dental Practitioner. Director, Dental Imaging Group of Australia, Australia.

Philip Gabel BAppSc(Physio), MSc(Research)
Sports and Spinal Physiotherapist. Researcher, Centre for Health and Sports Excellence, University of the Sunshine Coast, Australia.

Jack A Gerschman BDSc, LDS, PhD, GradDipMentHlthSc(ClinHyp), FFPMANZCA, FIBA FACLM, FACB
Oral Medicine Specialist. Associate Professor, Faculty of Medicine, Alfred Hospital and Monash University, Australia.

Peter Gibbons MBBS, DO, DM-SMed, MHSc
Osteopath and Medical Practitioner. Adjunct Associate Professor, Department of Rehabilitation Sciences, College of Allied Health, Oklahoma University Science Center, USA. Clinical Instructor, Division of Biokinesiology and Physical Therapy, University of S. California, USA. Director, Spinal Education Group, Australia.

Jayantilal Govind MBChB, DPH, MMed, FAFOEM
Director and Senior Staff Specialist, Occupational and Pain Medicine, Canberra Hospital, Australia. Senior Lecturer, Australian National University, ACT, Australia and University of Otago, New Zealand.

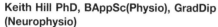

Keith Hill PhD, BAppSc(Physio), GradDip (Neurophysio)
Neurophysiotherapist. Senior Researcher, National Ageing Research Institute; Professor of Allied Health, La Trobe University and Northern Health, Australia.

Gwendolen Jull MPhty, PhD, FACP
Specialist Musculoskeletal Physiotherapist. Professor, Division of Physiotherapy, The University of Queensland, Australia.

Pablo M Kimos MSc, DDS
Specialist Dental Practitioner (Orthodontist). Former resident, TMD/Orofacial Pain Clinic. Clinical instructor, Faculty of Medicine and Dentistry, University of Alberta, Canada.

Andrew Kornberg MBBS FRACP
Neurologist. Director of Neurology, Royal Children's Hospital, Melbourne, Australia. Associate Professor, University Department of Paediatrics, University of Melbourne, Australia. Murdoch Children's Research Institute.

Gilles J Lavigne DMD, PhD
Specialist Dental Practitioner. Professor and Dean, Faculty of Medicine and Dentistry, Université de Montréal; Canada Research Chair in pain, sleep and trauma; Sleep Study Center, Trauma Research Unit, Hopital du Sacré-Coeur, Canada.

Paul W Major BSc, MSc, DDS
Specialist Dental Practitioner. Professor and Director, Orthodontic Graduate Program, Faculty of Medicine and Dentistry, University of Alberta, Canada.

Paul R Martin BSc(Hons), DipClinPsych, Dphil, FBPS, HonFAPS
Director of Psychology, Southern Health, Victoria; Professor of Clinical Psychology, Monash University, Australia.

Russell Mottram BAppSc(Chiro), MACC
Chiropractor. Clinician; Sessional Lecturer, School of Chiropractic, RMIT University, Australia.

Kate Murray PhD, MSc, BAppSc(Physio)
Neurophysiotherapist. Researcher, School of Physiotherapy, The University of Melbourne; Principal, DizzyDay Clinic, Australia.

Ken Niere BAppSc(Physio), GradDip(ManipTher), MManipPhysio, FACP
Specialist Musculoskeletal Physiotherapist. Senior Lecturer, School of Physiotherapy, La Trobe University; Principal, Auburn Spinal Therapy Centre, Australia.

Stephen O'Leary MBBS, BMedSc, PhD, FRACS
ENT Surgeon. Principal Otolaryngologist, Royal Victorian Eye and Ear Hospital; Professor of Otolaryngology, The University of Melbourne, Australia.

Harry JM von Piekartz PhD
Manual Therapist specializing in orofacial pain, Physiotherapist, International lecturer in neuromusculoskeletal therapy. Professor of Physiotherapy, University of Applied Science Osnabrück, Germany; Director, Clinic for Physical Therapy and Applied Neurobiomedical Science, The Netherlands.

Julian L Rait MBBS, FRANZCO, FRACS, FAICD
Ophthalmologist. Associate Professor, Department of Ophthalmology, University of Melbourne, Australia. President of MDA National, Australia.

Peter Selvaratnam PhD(Anatomy), BAppSc (Physio), GradDipManipTherapy, DipAcupuncture, FACP
Specialist Musculoskeletal Physiotherapist, Anatomist. Director, Headache Centre of Victoria; Clinical Associate Professor, Faculty of Medicine, Dentistry and Health Sciences, The University of Melbourne; Adjunct Senior Lecturer, Department of Anatomy, Faculty of Medicine, Monash University, Australia.

Janaka Seneviratne MBBS, FRACP
Consultant Neurologist and Neurophysiologist. Monash Medical Centre, Australia.

Grant Shevlin BAppSc(Chiro)
Chiropractor. Director, St Kilda Road Chiropractic Clinic, Australia.

Cathy Sloan MBBS, Dip RANZCOG
General Practitioner. Clinician, Brighton Family and Women's Clinic; Surgical Assistant in Ophthalmology, Australia.

Iggy Soosay MBBS, FACNEM, FACoHM
Medical Practitioner, Doctor of Nutritional Medicine. Principal, Camberwell Medical Centre, Australia.

Diana Svendsen BAppSc(Physio), GradDipPhysio, Certified Feldenkrais Practitioner
Feldenkrais Physiotherapist, Australia.

Philip Tehan DipOsteo, DipPhysio, MHSc
Osteopath and Physiotherapist. Adjunct Associate Professor, School of Biomedical and Health sciences, Victoria University, Australia. Director, Spinal Manipulation Education Group, Australia. Adjunct Associate Professor, Department of Rehabilitation Sciences, College of Allied Health, Oklahoma University Health Science Center, USA. Clinical Instructor, Division of Biokinesiology and Physical Therapy, University of Southern California, USA.

Norman MR Thie BSc, MSc, DDS, MSc
Specialist Dental Practitioner. Director, TMD/Orofacial Pain Clinic; Clinical Associate Professor, Faculty of Medicine and Dentistry, University of Alberta, Canada.

Prabaker Rajan Thomas MBBS, DPM (India), DPM (Ireland), MRC Psych (UK), FRANZCP
Psychiatrist. Senior Consultant in Psychiatry, Delmont Private Hospital; Hon. Senior Lecturer, Faculty of Medicine, Monash University, Australia.

John Waterston MBBS, MD, FRACP
Neurologist. Consultant Neurologist, Alfred Hospital; Department of Medicine, Monash University, Australia.

Guy Zito DClinPhysio, MPhysio, Grad Dip (AdvManipTher), DipPhysio
Musculoskeletal Physiotherapist. Senior Lecturer, School of Physiotherapy, The University of Melbourne, Australia.

Maria Zuluaga BAppSc (Physio), Grad Dip (ManipTher), MWomen'sHlth
Musculoskeletal Physiotherapist. Clinician, Headache Centre of Victoria, Australia.

Foreword

Headache is one of the most complex and demanding areas of clinical practice. The challenge is to understand the pathophysiology, achieve an accurate diagnosis, and offer useful remedies. Secondary headache may be the key symptom of a major nervous system disorder which requires urgent diagnosis and treatment in itself. In an ill patient, who has other symptoms and signs of a major neuropathological problem, diagnosis may be straightforward, but that is not always the case – for example, in distinguishing a sentinel bleed due to a cerebral berry aneurysm from a migraine event.

Primary headache syndromes are common but there is some disagreement between experts both within and across fields as to the major pathogenic mechanisms. Most clinicians would now accept the view, long prevalent in neurology, that migraine is a discrete entity; it can be identified on the basis of established criteria and divided into migraine with or without aura (known previously as common and classical migraine respectively). The delineation of migraine leads the clinician and patient down a particular diagnostic and therapeutic pathway looking for identifiable triggers, establishing treatments that work for acute episodes, and developing a regimen for prophylaxis which is individualised for a particular patient.

The majority of patients with persistent headaches do not have secondary headaches, at least in terms of underlying major neuropathological disorders, and do not have migraine or vascular headache syndromes. This is perhaps the most contentious and difficult field in terms of understanding pathophysiology. Tension-type headache, the predominant headache type in this group, can be thought of either as being related predominantly to anxiety or emotional tension, or to muscle tension or myofascial pain. When I started neurological practice many years ago, a majority of patients in this category were probably thought to be suffering from stress or depression.

Undoubtedly that continues to be a factor in some patients but is the primary or major initiating factor in only a subset. Any patient with chronic headache may develop secondary anxiety or depressive features compounding the presentation. Over the last 30 years, a great deal of work has gone to identify factors which trigger myofascial headache. These include the whole field of temporomandibular disorders, bruxism, and the area of cervicogenic headache which are now recognised as major underlying pathophysiological factors.

Today the pathophysiological factors which underlie chronic primary headache are better understood. Healthcare workers have also become increasingly aware of the potential range of presentations of secondary headache that require urgent investigation and potential treatment. The plethora of factors which underlie chronic myofascial headache is also becoming an increasingly well understood pathophysiological domain.

As a result of these advances the treatment of primary headache in particular has become more and more a multidisciplinary task. Most patients with primary and secondary headache present to the family doctor and it is crucial that the doctor has a good understanding of the types of headache which require more urgent or specific investigation. Having excluded other pathologies as appropriate in particular presentations, the family doctor needs to know the presentations and diagnostic features of migraine and, increasingly, the range of factors which may trigger and prolong primary myofascial headache syndromes. This is an increasingly complex area which may require involvement of specialists from a number of domains to achieve the best result for individual patients. Chronic headaches are all too commonly a disabling problem that cause great personal discomfort and cause loss of a great deal of time from work as well as consuming resources in the healthcare system. Every effort should be made in patients with chronic headache to achieve an accurate diagnosis and institute an appropriate and often multidisciplinary treatment regimen.

This book is one of the best that I have seen in drawing together the various clinical issues paramount in the optimum management of headache not only for the family doctor but also for specialists active in headache management. There are chapters covering acute presentations of major neuropathology and the factors the family doctor and other primary health workers need to look for are well set out in early chapters. There is a good discussion of migraine and its unique aspects which opens specific therapeutic possibilities. Most importantly in the context of the book there is an excellent discussion of the various factors which underpin myofascial headache notably in the areas of psychology and psychiatry, temporomandibular disorders and bruxism and cervical spine problems which act as headache triggers and sustain chronic headache syndromes.

Clinicians who read this book from cover to cover will have a good grounding of modern diagnostic and management concepts in headache. They will recognise that it is often appropriate to involve a range of specialists in further investigation and management. The individual sections are self standing and the family doctor or therapist wanting to find more about any of the diagnostic areas and specific therapeutic approaches discussed in this book would find the information easily. I commend this book as an excellent multidisciplinary contribution to the management of headache syndromes at the beginning of the 21st century. It brings together a range of distinguished contributors from Australia and around the world, notable by having great clinical experience in the field of headache across all relevant disciplines. The section dealing with diagnosis is excellent and the chapters dealing with approaches in the area of chronic daily headache are particularly useful. Some knowledge of this area is essential for any clinician seeing large numbers of patients with headache and taken together the book provides an excellent overview of pathophysiology, diagnostic considerations and the range of approaches that have emerged. The editors of this excellent multi-author volume, Peter Selvaratnam, Ken Niere, and Maria Zuluaga, are to be congratulated for producing this timely contribution to the management of headache, orofacial pain and bruxism.

Ed Byrne
Dean of Medicine
University College London
London, February 2009

Preface

The impetus for this book comes from our clinical practice. Patients often present with headaches that clearly do not arise from a simple musculoskeletal source. It is our experience that the more complicated the patient's presentation, the more we have needed to involve other health practitioners in their management.

The overlap of symptoms in patients presenting with headache, orofacial pain and bruxism provides challenges in disentangling symptoms, identifying sources and contributing factors, and arriving at an accurate diagnosis. Because there are so many structures associated with this region it is often beyond the expertise of a single practitioner to address the problem without the assistance of colleagues from a variety of specialties.

This book has been written by clinicians for clinicians. It contains the collective knowledge of hundreds of years of clinical experience. Authors have described evidence-informed clinical practice derived from anatomical, physiological, and biomechanical concepts. Anecdotal evidence, based on clinical experience, is presented because it provides clinical instruction and the inspiration for more rigorous research to validate and refine practice. Some treatments have substantial evidence to support their use. Other treatments seem to work clinically but are yet to be validated by detailed research. Where it is available, empirical evidence for the management of headache, orofacial pain and bruxism has been provided by the authors.

The book aims to provide clinicians with the theoretical and clinical information to improve the management of patients with headache and orofacial pain and to appreciate the role of the different disciplines involved in the management of symptoms in these regions. Once this is achieved, patient care can be optimised through appropriate referral and an interdisciplinary team approach.

A substantial proportion of the book is devoted to the identification of contributing factors to aid accurate diagnosis of headache, orofacial pain, and bruxism. The process of diagnosis and appropriate management begins with the general practitioner and other primary contact practitioners. The recognition of conditions that require immediate and urgent medical treatment is introduced in Chapter 1 and explored more fully in Chapter 2. Migraine is singled out for special treatment because it is such a debilitating and often misdiagnosed condition. Headache in childhood and adolescence is also considered separately because of the concern that is always associated with severe headache in the young. The regions involved in and the underlying basis of the production of headache and orofacial pain are then discussed. Chapters 5 to 12 provide an account of the anatomy and physiology of the regions involved in the production of headache and orofacial pain. To justify any intervention we must be able to measure its effect on the patient and their lifestyle, thus issues involved in the measurement of pain and headache are discussed in Chapter 13. Chapters 14 to 22 present approaches from a range of disciplines: physiotherapy, chiropractic, osteopathy, integrative medicine, dentistry, psychology, and psychiatry. Where appropriate, specific treatment modalities are discussed in those chapters. Chapters 23 to 27 focus on specific interventions.

Those who read this book from cover to cover will find that some information is repeated across chapters. This illustrates a degree of commonality across disciplines. We have tried to ensure that each chapter can be read in isolation and thus some overlap is necessary. While there is no separate chapter on diagnostic imaging, even though it is vital to the differential diagnosis of certain conditions, we believe that is has been addressed appropriately in relevant chapters; as always, clinicians are urged to reconcile clinical presentations with clinical imaging. Although primary headaches such as tension-type headache and cluster headache have been mentioned in some chapters, we believe that a detailed account of the management of these and less common primary headaches is beyond the scope of this text.

Most texts have been discipline-specific in the management of headache and orofacial pain. This book draws on the knowledge and clinical expertise of a range of practitioners all of whom are frequently involved in the management of headache. It encompasses and acknowledges their role in working with patients who suffer from these often debilitating symptoms.

Our aim is for this book to inspire clinicians to use a multidisciplinary approach and to communicate with other health professionals in the management of headache and orofacial pain. Our hope is that our readers will remain open to new ideas and paradigms as they continue to strive for optimal patient management.

Peter Selvaratnam, Ken Niere
and Maria Zuluaga
Melbourne 2009

Acknowledgements

There are many people who have contributed to this book.

We are indebted to the authors who have so willingly given their time, knowledge and experience in the preparation, review, and final presentation of their chapters. We are confident that their contributions will be of assistance to clinicians in the management of headache, orofacial pain, and bruxism.

We particularly want to express our deepest thanks to Judy Waters. As style editor Judy initially liaised with Elsevier on the concept of this book and then spent innumerable hours reviewing and preparing each chapter for publication. Her unrelenting enthusiasm, encouragement, and support have been most stimulating and motivating. Judy has been a tower of strength throughout and her wise advice has been pivotal in the completion of this project.

We are also greatly indebted to Pamela Oddy for her guidance in preparing the submission to Elsevier, administrative expertise, and liaising with authors. Her input throughout this project was encouraging and reassuring.

We wish to express our gratitude to Dr Cathy Sloan and Dr Stephen Friedman, the Content Editors. Cathy's forthright editorial review of the medical chapters assisted in depicting current clinical practice and cutting edge medicine. We are grateful for Stephen's insight into the relationship between the orofacial and cervical regions, and for sharing his knowledge.

We are especially grateful to Dr Jonathon Tversky and Assoc Prof Ramesh Balasubramaniam, oral medicine specialists, for generously sharing their vast experience of the functional anatomy of the temporomandibular region and associated conditions, reviewing the dental chapters, and clarifying concepts and terminology in oral medicine. A special thanks to Dr Robin Hooper for his assistance.

Our sincere thanks to Professor Meg Morris, Head of Physiotherapy at the Faculty of Medicine, Dentistry and Health Sciences, The University of Melbourne, for providing access to the University photographer.

Many professional colleagues have been helpful during the course of this project in discussing and reviewing chapters. Their detailed peer review assisted in preparing the final content of this book and is much appreciated. We are most grateful for input from Dr Zita Marks, Katrina Schlager, and Dean Watson, and for the reviews by: Dr Naresh Arulampalam, Prof. David Barkla, Prof. Nik Bogduk, Tibor Boka, Kerrie Bolton, Prof. Peter Brukner, Dr Colin Clarey, Dr Kristian Coomar, Dr Mithran Coomaraswamy, Jodie Coster, Dr Megan Davidson, Dr Robert Delcanho, Dr Dhayanthi Devasayagam, Margaret Duncan, Dr Lorraine Elsass, Dr Phillip Feren, Dr Louise Field, Dr Burkhard Franz, Phillip Gabel, Dr Pathmini Gnanaharan, Dr Adrian Good, Lynne Haysman, Prof. Rob Helme, Prof. Keith Hill, Lindy Holbrook, David Kelly, Dr Peter Kent, Emma Kirk, Dr Henryk Kranz, Prof. Chelvarayan Barr Kumarakulasinghe, Dr Liisa Laakso, Prof. Gilles Lavigne, Prof. Frank Lobbezoo, Germarja Lomas, Janet Loundes, Dr Karen Lucas, Dr Mary Magarey, Dr Greg Malham, Prof. Tom Matyas, Leigh McCutcheon, Anne McGann, Diedrie McGhee, Dr Prithiva Moorthy, Max Neufeld, Dr Stewart Newland, Dr Louie Puentedura, Peter Roberts, Dr John Rogers, Dr Jal Sardana, Dr Janaka Seneviratne, Prof. Richard Stark, Dr Russell Vickers, Dr John Waterston, Dr Victor Wilk, Dr Thomas Wilkinson and Dr Guy Zito.

We wish to express our thanks to Ms Lee McRae of Media Services at The University of Melbourne, Australia, and Mr Paul Kubben from Holland for their excellent photographic work, and the models who posed patiently.

Our sincere thanks to the team at Elsevier: Sarena Wolfaard, Publisher; Claire Wilson, Commissioning Editor; Claire Bonnet, Associate Acquisitions Editor, and Nancy Arnott, Project Manager for their patience and encouragement during the project. We are also most grateful to Dr Lulu Stader for her valuable comments assisting us in the completion of the book.

Finally, we thank our families and friends who have generously provided the support necessary to complete this work. Their patience and forbearance during the many hours we were at the computer and in numerous editorial meetings are acknowledged gratefully. Jeya Selvaratnam catered generously and creatively for editorial meetings, and her hospitality is greatly appreciated. We also wish to thank Peter's children for sharing their home over so many weekends, providing unstinting IT back up, and for their patience during our meetings.

Section **One**

Diagnosis

Chapter One

Headache in general practice

Ian Devlin

Headache management and treatment is complex and patients often present to a general practitioner seeking help for a headache. In this chapter the author, a medical practitioner, introduces a rational basis for identifying when a headache patient needs to be referred to another health care professional.

Headache is a major public health burden. Studies show that the prevalence of tension-type headache in the population is around 40% (Headache Disorders and Public Health, Education and Management Implications 2000) and the prevalence of migraine is around 10% (Lipton et al 2001a). A majority of these migraine sufferers experience reductions in social activity and work capacity. A major US study published in 2001 demonstrated that migraine is grossly under-diagnosed in the community (Lipton et al 2001b). The researchers concluded: 'Diagnosis of migraine had increased over the decade but about half of migraineurs remain undiagnosed, and the increased rate of diagnosis of migraine has been accompanied by only a modest increase in the proportion using prescription medicines. Migraine continues to cause significant disability whether or not there has been a physician's diagnosis. Given the availability of effective treatments, public health initiatives to improve patterns of care are warranted.'

Headache is a frequent reason for presentation to general practitioners (GPs). In the Australian BEACH study of general practice activity, headache was given by patients as a reason for the encounter for around 2% of all encounters with Australian GPs (Charles et al 2005). In this study GPs were asked to record the problems they defined for management at each encounter. Analysis of these figures shows that the doctor defined a management problem as 'undefined headache' in 18.9% of these encounters. Migraine was defined as a problem for management in 14% of encounters, sinusitis in 12%, and tension headache in 9%. This evidence reinforces the likelihood that migraine is being under-diagnosed in the headache encounters with GPs.

Of concern is that the rate of nomination of sinusitis as a problem for headache encounters in the BEACH study at 12% (Lipton et al 2001b) is almost as high as the figure for migraine at 14%. In the author's experience sinus headache is not a very common presentation in general practice using the International Headache Society definition (International Headache Society 2004), while migraine is common.

The health system is not meeting the challenge of headache diagnosis and management.

This is further reinforced by evidence that large numbers of migraine sufferers self-medicate, and in one study only 1% had used specific migraine medication or narcotic analgesics (Heywood et al 1998). In the same study only 2% had used preventive medication for their migraines in the previous year.

Role of the general practitioner

The tasks for the GP when faced with a patient with headaches are to:

1. Exclude serious or life threatening causes of headache.

2. Establish a brief overview of the psychological context of the presentation and the individual's motivation and social supports.

3. Establish a working diagnosis.

4. Inform the patient about their headache and the expectations in management.

5. Work with the patient towards alleviating or attempting to resolve the problem.

It is useful to consider the needs of the patient. Von Korff (1999) demonstrated that people in pain are keen to: know exactly what their problem is, be reassured that it is not serious, be relieved of their pain, and receive information. Patients seek advice on how to manage their pain and return to normal activity. A management plan should be developed through two-way dialogue with the patient (Australian Acute Musculoskeletal pain Guidelines Group 2004). Trust and rapport needs to be established early to enable cognitive strategies to be used in pain management.

The challenge for the GP is considerable, and a failsafe framework is essential for success. The first priority is to identify any 'red flags' in the history or clinical signs indicating

Box 1.1

'Red flags' in the diagnosis of headache.
- Instantaneous headache
- Sub-acute headache in patients over 55
- Presence of neurological signs
- Fever
- Neck stiffness
- Headache worse on waking
- Recent head trauma

serious underlying pathology (see Box 1.1). The practitioner needs to take an adequate history and perform a brief neurological examination in the limited time available, sufficient to exclude any obvious underlying disorder. The blood pressure should be checked. It is important to gain an impression of the patient's demeanor, looking for features that may indicate depression.

Special tests need to be ordered if the results are likely to contribute to the patient's management. A plain CT brain scan without contrast may be required in cases of headache of recent onset to rule out underlying pathology and reassure the patient.

'Red flags'

The following examination findings should be regarded as 'red flags' that may require investigation or referral: history of severe headache or subacute onset; temporal headache in patients over 55; presence of neurological signs; fever and/or neck stiffness; headache on waking; history of recent head trauma.

1. History of severe headache of acute or subacute onset

A history of severe headache with no prior history could be indicative of possible intracranial hemorrhage or carotid or vertebral artery dissection. In the author's clinical practice, a young man presented with the following history: 'At 10 minutes to 11.00 this morning, I developed the worst headache I have ever had in my life'. This patient was referred to an emergency department where subsequent imaging revealed a subarachnoid hemorrhage (SAH). An algorithm for the assessment of instantaneous severe headache is given in Figure 1.1 and its management is given in Figure 1.2.

When patients present within a week of a suspected SAH, they should be referred to an emergency facility since a positive CT scan will require an urgent neurosurgical referral. A negative CT scan may necessitate lumbar puncture to exclude an SAH. In rural and remote areas, GPs may need to perform their own lumbar puncture if the CT is negative. If more than a week has elapsed since the onset of headache, CT angiography or magnetic resonance angiography (MRA) are appropriate investigations. This is because in SAH after about a week the blood may be reabsorbed and therefore the characteristic appearance of blood in the subarachnoid space will no longer be seen on CT. At this stage angiography will be required to identify the aneurism causing the bleed. Exertional or orgasmic headache can also cause SAH and would demand

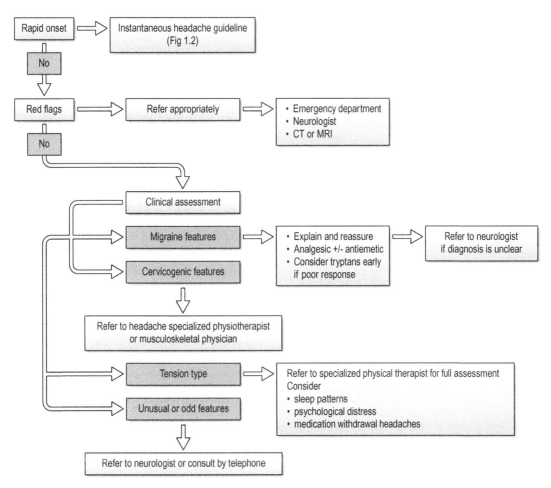

Figure 1.1 • Assessment of instantaneous severe headache.

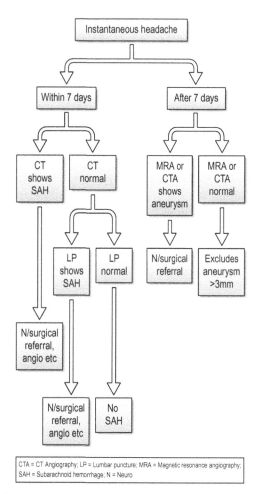

CTA = CT Angiography; LP = Lumbar puncture; MRA = Magnetic resonance angiography; SAH = Subarachnoid hemorrhage; N = Neuro

Figure 1.2 • Management of instantaneous severe headache.

similar investigation. The management of instantaneous severe headache is illustrated in Figure 1.2.

2. Temporal headache in patients over 55

Temporal arteritis should be excluded in patients over 55 years with subacute headache and is described in Chapter 2. Erythrocyte sedimentation rate and C reactive protein are helpful indicators in establishing the diagnosis. When temporal arteritis is suspected, temporal artery biopsy should be performed. Treatment

with steroids should not be delayed if the diagnosis is suspected, as permanent visual loss is a possible complication.

3. Presence of neurological signs

The presence of neurological signs such as altered consciousness and intellectual function, memory changes, delusions, hallucinations, emotional state, and speech changes need to be established. Similarly, papilledema, vomiting at night or early morning when the headache is severe, muscle weakness, involuntary movement, gait dysfunction, altered sensation, changes in urinary or bowel function, decreased male libido and potency, and unexplained amenorrhea in females need to be evaluated.

4. Fever and/or neck stiffness

The presence of fever or neck stiffness could indicate cerebral infection. If the patient is unwell, with a purpuric rash or septic shock, treatment should be commenced immediately with appropriate antibiotics or antiviral medications. In many cases the fever may simply be due to a benign viral infection.

5. Headache on waking

Headaches on waking in the mornings may suggest raised intracranial pressure. This pattern might also indicate sleep apnea or bruxism which is discussed later.

6. History of recent head trauma

A fall can cause headaches due to head trauma and is illustrated in the following case presentation. A 31-year-old man presented 1 week after he sustained a fall onto his occiput while snowboarding. There was a brief loss of consciousness, followed by an intense headache an hour later. The headache was severe and reminiscent of migraines he had suffered 12 years earlier. There had been episodes of mild vague paraesthesia in his left upper and lower limbs and torso lasting for fifteen

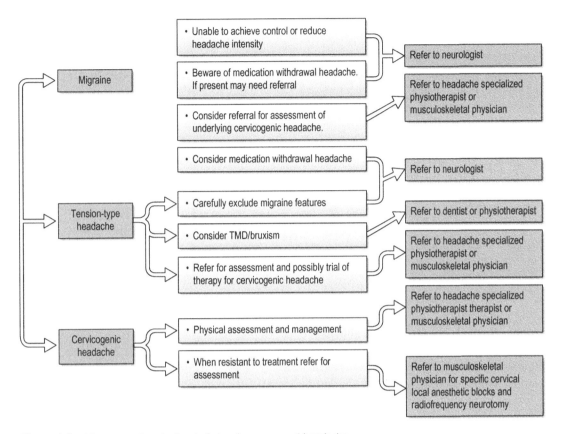

Figure 1.3 • Management and referral of chronic or recurrent headache.

minutes with a persistent generalized dull headache since the accident. A CT scan of the brain showed an SAH overlying the right parietal and occipital regions. He was referred to a neurosurgeon and required immediate decompression surgery. In this uncommon but serious trauma, the persistence of headache and neurological symptoms following trauma with loss of consciousness were 'red flags' demanding investigation.

Headache types

The International Headache Society (IHS) diagnostic criteria (see Ch. 2) are useful for communication with colleagues and when evaluating patients for therapeutic options. The role of the general practitioner is to diagnose and where necessary refer appropriately (Fig. 1.3.). The IHS classification is a large document but it is possible to condense from it criteria for the common headache types. The consistent use of the IHS criteria should lead to fewer errors in diagnosing headache types and may increase the number of patients correctly defined as migraineurs.

Migraine

Migraine headache is intense and associated symptoms are common. It is more likely to be unilateral, pounding, associated with nausea, photophobia, and phonophobia. Migraineurs tend to be helped by sleep, if they are able to achieve it. Migraines occur in episodes lasting 4–72 hours (International Headache Society 2004).

The use of a validated 3 question screening tool The ID Migraine ™ questionnaire can increase the frequency of migraine diagnosis in general practice. The questions posed are whether the headache causes nausea, disability, or photophobia. Patients who answer "yes" to 2 out of three questions are highly likely to have migraine, with a sensitivity of 81% and a positive predictive value of 93%.

The aim of management is to gain a good understanding of the patient, their symptoms, and the effect the migraine has on their work and lifestyle. Taking a detailed history can be time consuming and it may be necessary to set aside a longer appointment at the next consultation. Working with a practice nurse to conduct this assessment can be a very time efficient and effective approach. The interview needs to establish the pattern of the pain, location, time of onset, presence of visual aura, or focal neurological symptoms or signs. In order to establish differential management strategies it is important to ascertain whether the headache wakes them at night or is triggered during the day. Management with oral medication is less effective when a migraine wakes a patient as it is already quite severe at its onset, and nausea and vomiting will often preclude the use of medication.

Those who are woken by their migraine may be fortunate to have some warning symptoms the previous day. Migraineurs usually describe having excessive tiredness, déjà vu, or a feeling of excessive wellbeing prior to these attacks. An appropriate way of managing these attacks would be: a dose of ergotamine on the night prior to an expected attack: intranasal or injectable triptans may be required in those for whom this approach fails.

It is also important to involve the patient in a therapeutic partnership approach. The aim of therapy, which is primarily to reduce the intensity and either shorten or abort attacks of migraine, should be discussed. It is necessary to look at what has been prescribed previously,

and recommend simple analgesics with or without anti-emetic medications as a first line. This cocktail of medications should be prescribed as early as possible in the attack. It should be made clear that complete resolution may not be achievable, and that some trial and error with medication may be required.

At some point the chronic migraine sufferer should be offered a triptan as a trial. Even if the expense of these medications precludes their regular use, they may be kept on hand for use in particular circumstances. Referral is needed in cases of migraine when simple interventions have not improved the patient's quality of life to a level which can be tolerated. In this instance, a neurologist, preferably with an interest in headache management, would be the appropriate choice.

The role of physiotherapy in migraine treatment

In the author's experience the cervical spine has a very significant role in headache causation. Furthermore, some migraine sufferers report dramatic improvements in their migraine frequency and severity with competent management of their cervical spine dysfunction. In clinical practice, patients report that treatment of cervical spine dysfunction by physiotherapists can reduce the frequency of migraine episodes. This is supported by preliminary evidence (Bronfort et al 2005), and further research is needed.

Cervicogenic headache

The importance and prevalence of cervicogenic headache is under-recognized (Bronfort et al 2005). The primary care practitioner may recognize a very large group of patients presenting with headaches with a particular character, which is of an entirely different nature to migraines. Certain key features in the history will reveal the diagnosis.

These patients describe symptoms which will last for days to weeks, rather than the 4–72 hour range of migraine episodes. Sleep often does not help the headache. Although the intensity of the pain can be severe, it is usually described by patients as being in the pain intensity range of 5–7 out of 10 compared with migraine pain which is characteristically 7–10 out of 10. There may be associated features of mild dizziness or lightheadedness, and nausea may be present, but generally not at the same intensity of migraine headache, and vomiting is uncharacteristic. The pain is usually localized or predominantly localized to one side of the face, and is often described as a constant pain in a periorbital distribution, or less commonly in the maxillary or mandibular regions. An important feature of these headaches is that they are 'side locked' (the pain will consistently be on the same side), whereas in migraine it is characteristic for the side to change. Sinus headache may be confused with cervicogenic headache and is discussed later in this chapter.

A systematic examination of the neck should confirm if the cervical region is contributing to or causing the headache, particularly if manual examination provokes or eases the headache (see Chapter 9). Practitioners skilled in manual diagnosis are ideally placed to make this assessment (see Fig. 1.3). The clinical signs of cervicogenic headache may be subtle and require skill to elicit. Where a clear cause is not evident it is my practice to refer all patients with unilateral headache to physiotherapists with a special interest in headaches.

Treatment for cervicogenic headaches involves the use of physical therapy techniques outlined elsewhere in this book. Evidence exists for their use (Jensen 2005, Jull et al 2002). Another management option for refractory cervical headaches is specifically-targeted local anesthetic injection of certain cervical structures and nerves as described in Chapter 5.

Treatment with radiofrequency neurotomy has positive evidence based outcomes in patients with cervicogenic headaches (Lord et al 1996).

Tension-type headache

Tension-type headache is common and is a significant cause of distress and disruption to life. The typical pattern is a dull pressure or band-like pain that radiates from the forehead to the occiput and often radiates to the neck muscles. While tension-type headache has been defined in the International Headache Society classification of headache disorders, its pathogenesis remains elusive (Charles et al 2005). The IHS classification recognizes that it is certainly not simply a psychologically-mediated disorder, and that further research is needed. As with migraine, medication withdrawal or rebound headache needs to be considered. The GP's management role is often supportive but, importantly, a thorough assessment should be made to exclude the common and more readily treatable alternative diagnoses of migraine and cervicogenic headache. Patients may require referral to a physiotherapist or musculoskeletal physician or physiatrist for assessment. Management may also involve the use of pain modulators such as tricyclic antidepressants, relaxation training, and behavioral techniques.

TMD-related headache

Headache on waking in the morning may indicate TMD and bruxism. Where it is suspected, referral for assessment by a dentist (Chapter 7) or physiotherapist (Chapter 19) with an interest in this area is indicated.

Headaches which are present in the morning or on waking through the night may also suggest sleep apnea, especially when associated with snoring. Referral for a sleep study would be indicated.

Chronic daily and rebound headache

Migraine may change its pattern into one of chronic daily headache due to rebound or medication withdrawal. This may occur where migraines are frequent with little recovery between attacks. This phenomenon may also occur with tension-type headache. Even simple analgesics may be involved in a cycle of medication dependency where a headache occurs every time the patient stops the medication for a short time. It may be necessary to admit the patient to hospital, under specialist care, to achieve a complete and abrupt withdrawal of the medication, substituting an alternative medication for the control of the headaches.

Headache secondary to medication

Headache may commonly be associated with prescribed medication, as well as with over-the-counter medication and illicit drugs. Some common medications which are possible causes are tetracyclines, nifedipine, omeprazole, contraceptives, selective serotonin reuptake inhibitors, pseudoephedrine and vitamin A.

Sinus headache

As mentioned earlier, this disorder may be prone to over-diagnosis. Diagnosis errors can be avoided by strict adherence to the IHS guidelines which include clinical or imaging evidence of sinusitis being present simultaneously with the headache or facial pain. Consideration should be given to CT scanning of the sinuses and/or referral to an otolaryngologist before a patient is given this diagnosis. The diagnosis is particularly relevant since the pain distribution is often very similar to cervicogenic headache.

Other headaches

There are a multitude of less common headache types including cluster headache, and headache induced by various medications or chemicals. Many of these have such distinctive presenting symptoms that careful history taking will alert the GP to the nature of the headache. It should be remembered in these cases that specialist neurologists are always available for consultation by telephone (see Fig. 1.3).

Conclusion

GPs have the training to identify serious headaches requiring emergency management and if there is doubt about the diagnosis, or if red flags are present, referral to a neurologist or Emergency Department is warranted to determine a diagnosis and management plan. There is evidence that migraine and cervicogenic headache are under-diagnosed. Where there is suspicion about the cervical region as a possible cause of the patient's headaches, they will benefit from appropriate referral to a physiotherapist with an interest in headache management, or a musculoskeletal physician or physiatrist. Patients seek to have information about their condition, reassurance, and a positive approach emphasizing a quick return to normal function. GPs are also familiar with their particular patients' lifestyles and are used to providing an individualized management plan which may involve multiple modalities. As in most conditions encountered in general practice, management aims to be evidence-based, and often includes a mixture of empirical management based on a consensus of opinion amongst the profession and the practitioner's previous experience. The challenge is to apply evidence-based principles in clinical practice.

References

Australian Acute Musculoskeletal pain Guidelines Group 2004 Evidence-based Management of Acute Musculoskeletal Pain: A Guide for Clinicians. Australian Academic Press, Brisbane.

Bronfort G, Nilsson N, Haas M et al 2005 Non-invasive physical treatments for chronic/recurrent headache. The Cochrane Database of Systematic Reviews Issue 4.

Charles J, Ng A, Britt H 2005 Presentations of headache in Australian General Practice presenting figures from the BEACH program. Australian Family Physician 34:610-704.

Headache Disorders and Public Health, Education and Management Implications 2000 World Health Organisation, Geneva, WHO/MSD/MBD/00.9, Sept 2000.

Heywood T, Colgan C, Coffey J 1998 Prevalence of headache and migraine in an Australian city. Journal of Clinical Neuroscience 5:485.

International Headache Society 2004 The International Classification of Headache Disorders, 2nd edn. Cephalalgia 24 (Supplement 1).

Jensen S 2005 Neck related causes of Headache. Australian Family Physician 34:610-704.

Jull G, Trott P, Potter H et al 2002 A randomized controlled trial of exercise and manipulative therapy for cervicogenic headache. Spine 27:1835-1843.

Lipton R B, Dodick D, Sadovsky R et al 2003 A self-administered screener for migraine in primary care. Neurology 61:375-382.

Lipton R B, Stewart W F, Diamond S et al 2001a Prevalence and burden of migraine in the United States: Data from the American Migraine Study II. Headache 41:646-657.

Lipton R B, Stewart W F, Diamond S et al 2001b Migraine diagnosis and treatment: results from the American Migraine Study II. Headache 41: 638-645.

Lord SM, Barnsley L, Wallis BJ et al 1996 Percutaneous radio frequency neurotomy for chronic cervical zygapophysial joint pain. New Engl J Med 335:1721-1726.

Von Korff M 1999 Pain management in primary care: an individualised stepped/care approach. In: Gatchel DJ, Turk DC (eds), Psychological factors in pain. Guilford Press, New York.

Chapter Two

Catastrophic and sinister headache

Mark Faragher

Catastrophic headache is usually associated with conditions that if not diagnosed immediately may lead to permanent disability or death. Sinister headache, while associated with serious underlying pathology, may or may not cause great distress and interfere with quality of life. In this chapter the author, a neurologist, examines possible diagnoses and management options.

There was a time when many headaches were felt to be of a trivial nature, not worthy of rigorous scientific study. Fortunately, William Speed III (1918–2005), a physician and researcher at Johns Hopkins Hospital, helped establish migraine and other severe headache syndromes as legitimate medical disorders and developed medicines to treat them. Speed found his vocation in the diagnosis and treatment of headache; while an undergraduate he suffered from migraine and was struck by the dismissive reception of this condition by the medical establishment in the 1930s. At that time, many headaches were often considered to be psychosomatic in origin and usually without a physiological basis. Speed and others studied headache as clinicians and gradually began to document their view that head pain was frequently caused by vascular abnormalities or tumors, or were brought on by whiplash and other neck injuries. In the 1960s he formulated a new therapy involving the compound ergotamine, which constricts blood vessels and prevents the release of a protein that irritates nerve endings and causes headache. Speed's work has enabled medical practitioners to take a more scientific and structured approach to the diagnosis and management of headache.

Diagnosis

The classification of headache has been formalized by the International Headache Society (IHS) (Olesen et al 2004) as the International Classification of Headache Disorders. It lists over 100 different types of headache. The classification covers 14 main categories (Box 2.1). Categories 1 to 4 cover the primary headache disorders. For many of these diagnoses there are no specific tests and a high index of clinical suspicion of the primary headache is required as well as familiarity with the diagnostic criteria. Categories 5 to 12 cover secondary headaches. Secondary headache may come from extracranial pathology such as sinusitis, dental disease/temporomandibular disorders, cervical spine disorder, systemic infection, ophthalmological causes, or intracranial pathology such as mass lesion (including brain tumors), cerebral hemorrhage, and meningitis.

First level of the International Classification of Headache Disorders (Oleson et al 2004).

Part One: The primary headaches
Migraine
Tension-type headache
Cluster headache and other trigeminal autonomic cephalgias
Other primary headaches

Part Two: The secondary headaches
Headache attributed to head and/or neck trauma
Headache attributed to cranial or cervical vascular disorder
Headache attributed to non-vascular intracranial disorder
Headache attributed to a substance or its withdrawal
Headache attributed to infection
Headache attributed to disorder of homeostasis
Headache or facial pain attributed to disorder of cranium, neck, eyes, ears, nose, sinuses, teeth, mouth, or other facial or cranial structures
Headache attributed to psychiatric disorder
Cranial neuralgias and central causes of facial pain
Other headache, cranial neuralgia, central or primary facial pain

According to lifetime prevalence studies of headache mechanism (Steiner 2005), tension-type headache (primary and secondary) is the most common (69%), while headache from systemic infection is second in frequency (63%). Migraine is next (16%), followed by headache after head injury (4%), idiopathic stabbing headache (2%), exertional headache (1%), vascular disorders (1%), subarachnoid hemorrhage (< 1%) and brain tumors (0.1%). These data also illustrate that an individual may well experience multiple headache types throughout their lifetime.

Identification of sinister or potentially catastrophic headaches depends on a comprehensive history from the patient and/or other informant, and a thorough neurological and general clinical examination.

In the various headache syndromes the importance of the history cannot be over-emphasized. It is vital to gain a thorough understanding of the various aspects of the patient's particular headache. There is no substitute for obtaining fine detail regarding the exact circumstances of onset, and of provoking and relieving factors. On some occasions an accurate eyewitness account from family or friends may add a great deal. It is important to note that at any one time a patient may have more than one diagnosable headache syndrome, and throughout a patient's life they may swap diagnostic categories or conversely what appears to be superficially different headache syndromes at different times of a patient's life may be manifestations of the one underlying unifying diagnosis, e.g. migraine. The diagnostic process is fraught with traps for the unwary as sinister as well as relatively benign headaches may present in an identical fashion (Goadsby 2003). Thus a life-threatening process may mimic a benign one and vice versa. Headache pain of benign origin may be severe. Headache pain of sinister origin may be mild.

One clinical approach is to answer the following questions:

1. On a clinical basis, are there any suggestions of a secondary cause of headache? If so, what kind? (Box 2.2)

2. What is the appropriate ongoing investigation and management?

3. If secondary causes are thought unlikely, which primary headache syndrome could be responsible for the clinical scenario?

This process should lead to a clinical diagnosis or a list of possible differential diagnoses which are then tested by the appropriate use of investigations to confirm or refute the possible diagnoses. It should be reiterated that investigations are no substitute for a clinical diagnosis. A patient with a

Box 2.2

Differential diagnosis of the acute, severe new-onset headache ('First or Worst' headache).

Crash migraine
Cluster
Miscellaneous
    Benign exertional headache
    Benign orgasmic cephalgia
Post-traumatic
Associated with vascular disorders
    Acute ischemic cerebrovascular disease
    Subdural and extradural hematomas
    Parenchymal hemorrhage
    Unruptured saccular aneursym
    Sub arachnoid hemorrhage
    Systemic lupus erythematous
    Temporal arteritis
    Internal carotid and vertebral artery
      dissection
    Cerebral venous thrombosis
    Acute hypertension
    Pressor response
    Pheochromocytoma
    Pre-eclampsia
Associated with nonvascular intracranial disorders
    Intermittent hydrocephalus
    Benign intracranial hypertension
Post-lumbar puncture headache
    Related to intrathecal injections
    Intracranial neoplasm
    Pituitary apoplexy
Acute intoxications
Associated with non cephalic infections
    Acute febrile illness
    Acute pyelonephritis
Cephalic infection
Meningoencephalitis
Acute sinusitis
Acute mountain sickness
Disorders of the eyes
Acute optic neuritis
Acute glaucoma
Cervicogenic
Greater occipital neuralgia
Cervical myositis
Trigeminal neuralgia

Box 2.3

Entities causing catastrophic and sinister headache that may produce a 'normal' nondiagnostic CT brain scan.

Entities

Migraine
Cluster headache
Some tumors eg posterior fossa
Chronic meningitis
Trigeminal neuralgia
Temporal arteritis
Cervicomedullary lesions
Leptomeningeal disease
Venous sinus thrombosis

Suggested further Investigation

ESR
Temporal artery biopsy
CSF examination
MRI/A/V
CT venogram
Cerebral angiogram

normal CT brain scan may be harboring any of a number of serious conditions (Box 2.3).

The physician should be especially concerned if the patient has any of the following (Olesen et al 2004):

- New onset headache in a patient over the age of 50
- Sudden onset headache
- Headache that is subacute in onset and gets progressively worse over days or weeks
- Headache associated with focal neurologic symptoms or signs, such as papilledema, changes in consciousness or cognition (such as difficulty in reading, writing or thinking), or a stiff neck
- No obvious identifiable headache etiology.

Based on the rate of onset and duration, the clinical presentation of headaches can be broken down into: hyperacute/thunderclap, escalating, recurrent/episodic, or chronic/ongoing.

Hyperacute/thunderclap

When a patient presents with a hyperacute or thunderclap type headache the immediate concern is whether this represents a catastrophic cause such as subarachnoid hemorrhage.

Subarachnoid hemorrhage

Sudden, instantaneous or abrupt onset of severe headache with or without alteration in conscious state is a medical emergency. The diagnosis of exclusion is subarachnoid hemorrhage (SAH). Differential diagnoses are listed in Box 2.4. If SAH is a concern the investigations must be pursued until it can be confidently excluded. It is important to be aware of the diverse presentations of SAH. Classically, patients with SAH present with a very severe, rapid and even instantaneous onset headache. However there are other ways that SAH may present. Ten percent of patients have no headache at onset, and 8% describe a mild, gradually increasing headache. A stiff neck is absent in 36% of patients. SAH may present with a sentinel headache – a warning headache that is not crippling, which then resolves and is followed some hours or days later by a more typical catastrophic headache. SAH may occur spontaneously, or during physical exertion, or sex. Clinical examination may reveal altered conscious state, meningismus, subhyaloid hemorrhages, and even mild fever. However these findings may be absent and the clinical history is paramount. The wide variation in clinical presentations may be appreciated by reviewing the Hunt and Hess grading scale (Box 2.5). A patient might present anywhere along the spectrum from Grade 1 to Grade V. It is important to be aware of the diverse presentations of SAH and to initiate appropriate investigations if a patient presents with their worst ever headache or in a patient with previous headache syndrome who has a different type of an acute headache.

The initial investigation is an urgent CT brain scan, which may demonstrate subarachnoid blood. However the CT scan may be normal

---

Box 2.4

The causes of subarachnoid hemorrhage.

80% intracranial saccular aneurysm
5% intracranial arteriovenous malformation
15% negative angiogram
    50% benign mesencephalic hemorrhage
    50% other causes
Occult aneurysm
Mycotic aneurysm
Vertebral or carotid artery dissection
Dural arteriovenous malformation
Spinal arteriovenous malformation
Sickle cell anemia
Coagulation disorders
Drug abuse (cocaine and methamphetamine)
Primary or metastatic intracranial tumors
    (e.g. pituitary, melanoma)
Primary or metastatic cervical tumors
Central nervous system infection (e.g. herpes
    encephalitis)
Central nervous system vasculitis

Box 2.5

Hunt and Hess scale for grading subarachnoid hemorrhage (Hunt & Hess 1968).

Grade	Neurological status
I	Asymptomatic; or minimal headache and slight nuchal rigidity
II	Moderate to severe headache; nuchal rigidity; no neurologic deficit except cranial nerve palsy
III	Drowsy; minimal neurological deficit
IV	Stuporous; moderate to severe hemiparesis; possibly early decerebrate rigidity and vegetative disturbances
V	Deep coma; decerebrate rigidity; moribund appearance

especially if performed more than 24 hours after the onset of the headache. In such cases, examination of the cerebrospinal fluid for hemorrhage and xanthochromia may be appropriate. The opening pressure is checked and may be elevated in SAH. The CSF is examined in the laboratory for protein, glucose, and cytology, and most importantly the cell count should be checked for red cells and white cells, and the fluid examined for xanthochromia. Spectrophotometry should be used to diagnose xanthochromia since it is more accurate compared to visual examination (UK National External Quality Assessment Scheme for Immunochemistry Working Group 2003, van Gijn & Rinkel 2001).

The yield of CSF examination is highest when performed 12 hours following the onset; the down side to this is the highest risk of a re-rupture of an aneursym is within the first 6 hours. Therefore if the history is strongly suggestive of a SAH, and if CT scanning and CSF evaluation is not conclusive, further investigation with formal cerebral angiography or magnetic resonance angiography (MRA) and a neurosurgical consultation may be required in selective patients (van Gijn & Rinkel 2001).

The most common cause of SAH is ruptured cerebral aneurysm. Other underlying lesions that may cause SAH include cerebral arteriovenous malformation (AVM) and less often spinal AVM and metastatic melanoma (Box 2.4). In 'brainstem' SAH, hemorrhage in the vicinity of the brainstem/quadrigeminal cistern region, often no aneurysm is found and in this case conservative management would be appropriate.

Alternative diagnoses

Once the clinician is satisfied that SAH has been ruled out, alternative diagnoses will be entertained. Other possible causes of hyperacute/thunderclap headache are cervical artery dissection, retroclival hematoma, pituitary apoplexy, third ventricle colloid cyst, and intracranial infection. Crash migraine (migrainous vasospasm) and benign headache syndromes such as benign sex headache (orgasmic cephalgia) and exploding head syndrome are also possibilities (Schwedt et al 2006). MRI/MRA of the brain may help to clarify some of these diagnoses. It is possible that the patient might have more than one headache type and treatment must be directed at each entity to achieve resolution of pain.

Escalating headache

Causes of escalating headache include giant cell arteritis (temporal arteritis), subdural hematoma, cerebral venous sinus thrombosis, and benign intracranial hypertension.

Giant cell arteritis

Giant cell arteritis (GCA) is rare before 50 years of age and the incidence increases with age. There is no clear gender predilection. Stroke, transient ischemic attack, and dementia caused by GCA are usually preceded by other more common manifestations of GCA. Clinically the headache may be focal in the region of the temporal arteries, with the presence of temporal artery tenderness. Jaw claudication and neck stiffness may occur. There may be symptoms to suggest co-existing polymyalgia rheumatica such as generalized aches and pain, tiredness and lassitude, weight loss, and fatigue. Visual symptoms such as flashes, blurring, or transient scotomas may or may not precede visual loss. Visual loss is a feared component of GCA. Once visual loss has occurred, recovery is uncommon. Thus, funduscopic investigation is required to evaluate for ischemic optic neuropathy in GCA.

In GCA the ESR is typically increased. However the test has significant limitations: the ESR is not invariably elevated in association with GCA, and an elevated ESR is not specific for GCA and may mimic other forms of vasculitis.

Combining the results of ESR and C-reactive protein will increase the sensitivity and specificity of detecting GCA (Salvarni & Hunder 2001). Temporal artery biopsy remains the gold standard for diagnosis. Prompt administration of corticosteroids, even prior to biopsy, is appropriate treatment.

Subdural hematoma

Subdural hematoma may present in many ways and should be suspected in the elderly with new onset as well as escalating headache. Other presentations would include fluctuating confusion and decreased conscious state. There may be a history of trauma and often a fall. However, the actual incident is frequently forgotten or thought too trivial to rate a mention. The treating clinician must maintain a high index of suspicion especially in patients taking anticoagulants. Patients may experience a stable compensated honeymoon period before a rapid deterioration in conscious state that may lead to major disability and death. Thus it is important to make the diagnosis as early as possible so that definitive treatment can be instituted.

Cerebral venous sinus thrombosis

Patients may present with the combination of escalating headache and papilledema. Once optic disc swelling is confirmed the possibility of cerebral venous sinus thrombosis is explored with magnetic resonance scanning, in particular magnetic resonance venography. If venous sinus thrombosis is confirmed this may lead to further management such as anticoagulation or if the patient is clinically deteriorating another possibility is interventional radiology and thrombolysis. Some patients with cerebral venous sinus thrombosis may present without optic disc changes. 'Red flags' would include pregnancy, history of dehydration, underlying thrombotic disorder, or malignancy.

Benign intracranial hypertension

In the absence of signs of venous sinus thrombosis the patient may have benign intracranial hypertension (also know as pseudotumor cerebri and idiopathic intracranial hypertension) (see Chapter 11). In such cases, the next step is a lumbar puncture for cerebrospinal fluid pressure measurement and analysis of the fluid in the laboratory. If the pressure is elevated and the fluid is bland then draining 20–30 ml may normalize the cerebrospinal fluid pressure. Further management may involve repeated lumbar punctures and/or acetazolamide. If the cerebrospinal fluid pressure cannot be controlled in this way then optic nerve sheath fenestration and lumbo-peritoneal shunting remain options.

Recurrent/episodic headache

The primary headaches in this category may be divided according to frequency, i.e., by the number of headaches or headache days per month:

- low to moderate frequency (< 15 headache days per month) – episodic headaches
- high frequency (> 15 headache days per month) – chronic daily headaches.

The primary episodic headache disorders can then be further subdivided according to duration of attack. Four hours' duration can be used as the rough dividing line. Longer than four hours may suggest migraine, less than four hours may indicate cluster headache and related disorders.

Cluster headache

The pain in cluster headache tends to be excruciating, unilateral, located behind one eye, boring in character, and not affected adversely or beneficially by exercise or position. It occurs more in men than women and rarely shifts from one side to the other, but is usually 'side-locked'. Cluster headache is the archetype autonomic cephalalgia as it is associated with autonomic features in a sympathetic distribution such as ptosis, meiosis, chemosis, and nasal discharge. The cluster sufferer, in contrast to the typical migraineur, cannot sleep or lie quietly, and gets up and walks in an agitated or non-purposeful fashion. There may be bizarre elements such as head banging, contortions, or adopting unusual body positions. Some sufferers may run to ease the pain. In cluster headache, the onset is typically abrupt, with the pain reaching a crescendo in about five minutes, plateauing for about 30 minutes, and then a gradual decrement of about 20 minutes.

Alternative diagnoses

Other primary episodic headaches are:
- Episodic and chronic paroxysmal hemicrania
- Episodic and chronic cluster headache
- Short lasting, unilateral, neuralgiform headache attacks with conjunctival injection and tearing (SUNCT syndrome).
- Hypnic headache occurs primarily in the elderly, is relatively short lived and wakes patients' from sleep, often in the early morning hours. It is usually bilateral, and lacks the severity of cluster headache. There are no autonomic features.

Hemicrania continua is a rare, strictly unilateral headaches sometimes evolving from an intermittent pattern, and sometimes arising de novo, that has the features of cluster headache. The pain is usually moderately severe, but there can be severe pain during exacerbations. The autonomic features are not as pronounced as in cluster headache. It is dramatically responsive to indomethacin. Bilateral features and side shift are rarely documented.

Terms such as 'cluster-migraine' or 'migraine-cluster' often lead to confusion. They are best avoided or perhaps used sparingly, and only by those who are well versed in the nuances of the IHS classification system.

Miscellaneous primary headache disorders such as jabs and jolts or icepick pains, or benign orgasmic cephalalgia, may be brief or prolonged and have a clear precipitant.

Migraine

The World Health Organization ranks migraine among the top 20 causes in the world of years of healthy life lost to disability (http://www.who.int/mediacentre/factsheets/fs277/en/print.htm). Migraine ranks equally highly in other measures of quality of life such as days lost from school and work, and harm done to family and social relationships (Steiner 2005). As the derivation of the word suggests, the typical head pain of migraine is unilateral, moderate to severe throbbing headache – often frontal in location – but rather diffuse compared to the severe piercing nature of cluster pain.

In typical migraine attacks, the patient often lies down in a darkened room (photophobia), chooses silence (phonophobia), tries to sleep and finds sleep relieves the headache, and does not want to be disturbed. This may be mimicked by patients with SAH, encephalitis, and meningitis.

The IHS diagnostic criteria for migraine are (Olesen et al 2004):

1. The attack should be episodic with at least five attacks for migraine without aura and two attacks for migraine with aura.

2. The duration of the attack should not be shorter than four hours and not longer than 72 hours (pediatric migraines may be shorter, and occasionally migraines may be more prolonged).

3. The headache itself should be characterized by at least two of the following:

   (i) unilateral location

   (ii) throbbing quality of pain

(iii) aggravated by movement

(iv) moderate to severe intensity

One or both of the following characteristics should be present:

(i) nausea/vomiting

(ii) photophobia and phonophobia.

Many migraineurs will have prior warning of an attack in the form of a prodrome that occurs 24–48 hours before the aura or headache commences. It is rare for migraine patients to have an abrupt onset to their attacks. Occasionally episodes may be triggered by minor trauma. One example of this is footballer's migraine from heading the ball.

Migraines which are untreated, or treated unsuccessfully, last 4–72 hours. Cluster headaches are shorter, having a duration of 15–180 minutes. Episodic tension-type headache has a duration of 30 minutes to 7 days.

Chronic/ongoing headache

The examples of chronic/ongoing headache are: analgesic overuse, rebound, and chronic daily headache, chronic migraine, and low pressure headaches which occur spontaneously or post lumbar puncture.

Analgesics are commonly taken for headaches. Some patients enter an escalating spiral of taking increasing quantities of over-the-counter and/or prescription analgesics. The headache cycle may, in fact, be perpetuated by the increasing medication use. The drugs involved may include ergotamine, triptans, opioids, minor analgesics and combination medications, especially in those patients taking caffeine. There are significant regional variations: in Europe with triptans, in Australia drugs are often a combination of varying strengths of analgesics such as paracetamol and codeine; in North America, various combinations and permutations of aspirin, caffeine, butalbital (a barbiturate), paracetamol and codeine as

double, triple and quadruple combination analgesics may play a role in the evolution of rebound headache.

Analgesic rebound headache, or medication overuse headache, is increasingly recognized and is a relatively common cause of chronic headache. It is responsible for many of the cases of recurrent daily headache and the majority of referrals to headache specialists and specialist headache clinics. It may cause severe disruption to the patient's life and come to dominate it. Withdrawal of the inciting medications is the only effective treatment (Williams 2005). This may be performed gradually on an outpatient basis or as an inpatient with a short course of intravenous lignocaine or dihydroergotamine (DHE).

Triptans, ergot and nonopioid medications may be ceased abruptly. Nonsteroidal anti-inflammatory drugs may be used for withdrawal headache (e.g. naproxen 500 mg twice daily). Prophylactic drugs in migraine may be commenced prior to triptan or ergot withdrawal (e.g. propranolol 10–40 mg twice a day). Tricyclic antidepressants can be a useful 'prophylactic' drug to cover withdrawal of treatment for tension-type headaches (e.g. amitryptiline 10–25 mg at night).

It is important to recognize the high incidence of comorbid psychopathology and to apply a multidisciplinary approach to inpatient management when it is required in selected patients. In selected patients inpatient management may be of assistance. If self-weaning is not successful, then other options, remaining mindful of possible side effects, are a brief course of prednisolone (Krymchantowski & Barbosa 2000), naproxen, or intravenous lignocaine (Williams & Stark 2003).

As an alternative, behavioral strategies may help in overall management. Examples include relaxation therapy, stress management, meditation, and regular aerobic exercise. Specific recommendations need to consider patient interests and abilities as well as local availability.

Prevention of relapse is important. Once the overused medication(s) have been withdrawn migraine prophylaxis may be appropriate. Assessment of precipitants, counseling, a headache management plan, and clear limits on the use of analgesia may all be required in order to diminish the chances of relapse. In any case relapse may occur in up to 40% of patients in the first 12 months following withdrawal. Those who overuse combination analgesics are particularly prone to relapse and consideration should be given to complete avoidance of narcotic containing analgesics.

The pathophysiology of medication overuse headache is now partially understood. Triptans are agonists at serotonin 5HT 1b and 5HT 1d receptors. These receptors are rapidly down-regulated over 24–96 hours following drug exposure. Aspirin and nonsteroidal anti-inflammatory medications act on the enzymes cyclo-oxygenase 1 and 2. These enzymes are also down-regulated following drug exposure but much more slowly. Triptan use therefore results in in tachyphylaxis (less effect for the same dosage) more quickly, at lower frequency of use, and at lower dosage than other non-narcotic analgesics.

Receptor and enzyme down-regulation in structures responsible for the transmission and reception of nociceptive input creates increased sensitivity to such input, resulting in a lowered threshold for pain perception.

Daily headaches with underlying cause

Low pressure headache may follow lumbar puncture or may be spontaneous. Headaches following lumbar puncture may develop in 5–10% of patients. It is very characteristic in that it is postural: in the recumbent position the patient may be quite comfortable but sitting up, or more particularly standing with gradual rising crescendo, the patient will develop a severe generalized headache which may be relieved quite quickly on lying down again. Occasionally there may be no obvious precipitant and in these patients the low pressure state may have commenced following an occult event such as an otherwise asymptomatic dural tear.

Recognition is the key to further management as, in the cases following lumbar puncture, conservative measures may be attempted first. These may include prolonged bed rest, in a variety of positions, and vigorous hydration either orally or intravenously. Caffeine is an option. If these are ineffective, epidural blood patch may be spectacularly successful with rapid resolution of the symptoms. Sometimes the epidural blood patch needs to be performed more than once.

In spontaneous cases the diagnosis may be made clinically, changes may be seen on the brain MRI to suggest a low pressure state. Nuclear medicine studies may be undertaken to localize the site of CSF leakage. Management is similar, employing an epidural blood patch. As a last resort, dural repair is sometimes performed.

Conclusion

Catastrophic and sinister headaches may be linked to life-threatening conditions that, if left undiagnosed and thus untreated, will lead to death or severe disability. Prime examples are subarachnoid hemorrhage leading to death, and temporal arteritis leading to blindness. The neurologist's approach to catastrophic and sinister headaches relies upon a systematic approach to the history, a detailed physical and neurological examination, followed by judicious use of investigations. It should be remembered that in some cases physical findings and investigation results may not be pertinent to headache diagnosis. The challenge is to identify and assimilate the relevant clinical information to reach an accurate diagnosis.

References

Goadsby PJ 2003 Migraine: diagnosis and management. Intern Med J 33:436-442.

Hunt WE, Hess RM 1968 Surgical risk as related to time of intervention in the repair of intracranial aneurysms. J Neurosurg 28:14-20.

Krymchantowski AV, Barbosa JS 2000 Prednisone as initial treatment of analgesic-induced daily headache. Cephalalgia 20:107-113.

Olesen J, Bousser MG, Diener HC et al 2004 The international classification of headache disorders 2nd edn. Cephalalgia 24 (Suppl 1):1-160.

Salvarni C, Hunder GG 2001 Giant cell arteritis with low erythrocyte sedimentation rate: frequency of occurrence in a population based study. Arthritis Rheum 45:140-145.

Schwedt TJ, Matharu, MS, Dodick DW 2006 Thunderclap headache. Lancet: Neurology 5:621-631.

Steiner TJ 2005 Lifting the burden: the global campaign to reduce the burden of headache worldwide. J Headache Pain 6:373-377.

UK National External Quality Assessment Scheme for Immunochemistry Working Group 2003 National guidelines for analysis of cerebrospinal fluid for bilirubin in suspected subarachnoid haemorrhage. Ann Clin Biochem 40:481-488.

van Gijn J, Rinkel GJ 2001 Subarachnoid haemorrhage: diagnosis, causes and management. Brain 124:249-278.

Williams D 2005 Medication overuse headache. Aust Prescr 28:143-145.

Williams DR, Stark RJ 2003 Intravenous lignocaine (lidocaine) infusion for the treatment of chronic daily headache with substantial medication overuse. Cephalalgia 23:963-971.

Chapter Three

3

Migraine

Janaka Seneviratne

Migraine is a common headache that has a significant impact on quality of life and drives patients to seek treatment. The author, a neurologist, discusses the diagnosis of migraine and the pharmacological management of this debilitating condition.

A clear understanding of the definitions of migraine and its subtypes, underlying pathophysiology, and treatment, will optimize care for migraine sufferers. Migraine is a common cause of headache that is frequently misdiagnosed. When migraine is over-diagnosed, patients are often treated unnecessarily with medications that may be accompanied by adverse effects. There is also the risk that the underlying etiology will be overlooked. When migraine is under-diagnosed, patients may suffer debilitating symptoms that lead to underperformance at school and work, and to psychosocial difficulties.

Definition

Migraine is divided into two main types, migraine without aura (common migraine) and migraine with aura (classical migraine). The International Headache Society (IHS) revised criteria for migraine are summarized in Boxes 3.1 and 3.2 (International Headache Society 2004).

Epidemiology

Migraine occurs more frequently in females (15–17%) than in males (4–6%). Prevalence also varies according to ethnicity with migraine being most common in Caucasian, then African, then Asian people (Stewart et al 1996).

Breslau et al (1994) found that the incidence of migraine in subjects aged 21–30 years was 5 per 1000 person-years in men and 22 per 1000 person-years in women. This study provided the first body of evidence that the previously observed cross-sectional association between migraine and major depression can result from bi-directional influences, with each disorder increasing the risk for first onset of the other.

Lyngberg et al (2005) showed that in Denmark, the incidence of migraine was 8.1 per 1000 person-years (male:female ratio 1:6), and the incidence of frequent tension-type headache was 14.2 per 1000 person-years (male:female ratio 1:3). Both rates decreased with age.

Migraine with aura is considered an independent risk factor for stroke in young women (Etminan et al 2005, Kurth et al 2006). In a large prospective study of 27 840 women 45 years of age or older, Kurth and his colleagues concluded, 'In this cohort, active (i.e., experienced migraine

Box 3.1

Revised IHS criteria for migraine without aura (International Headache Society 2004).

A. Headache descriptions (at least two)

- Unilateral
- Pulsatile quality
- Moderate to severe (moderate generally defined as inhibiting daily activities, severe as prohibiting daily activities) pain intensity
- Aggravation by or causing avoidance of routine physical activity

Associated symptoms (one or both)

- Nausea and/or vomiting
- Photophobia and phonophobia

B. The headaches last 4–72 hours (untreated or treated unsuccessfully)

C. Must have 5 attacks fulfilling the above criteria and not attributed to another disorder.

Box 3.2

Revised IHS criteria for migraine with typical aura (International Headache Society 2004).

At least two attacks fulfilling criteria A–C.

A. Aura consisting of at least one of the following, but no motor weakness:

- fully reversible visual symptoms including positive features (e.g. flickering lights, spots or lines) and/or negative features (i.e. loss of vision)
- fully reversible sensory symptoms including positive features (i.e. pins and needles) and/or negative features (i.e. numbness)
- fully reversible dysphasic speech disturbance

B. At least two of the following:

- Homonymous visual symptoms and/or unilateral sensory symptoms
- At least one aura symptom develops gradually over $\geq$ 5 minutes and/or different aura symptoms occur in succession over $\geq$ 5 minutes
- Each symptom lasts $\geq$ 5 and $\leq$ 60 minutes

C. Headache fulfilling criteria A & B for migraine without aura begins during the aura or follows aura within 60 minutes

D. Not attributed to another disorder.

attacks in the previous year) migraine with aura was associated with increased risk of major CVD, myocardial infarction, ischemic stroke, and death due to ischemic CVD, as well as with coronary revascularization and angina. Active migraine without aura was not associated with increased risk of any CVD event.' When compared with women with no migraine history, the women who reported active migraine with aura were 1.91 times as likely to experience ischemic stroke. The study also found that after adjustment for traditional cardiovascular risk factors, migraine with aura was not associated with any of the elevated biomarkers. Therefore, the elevated biomarkers are an unlikely explanation of why women with migraine with aura are at increased risk for cardiovascular disease in this particular cohort.

Pathophysiology

In the last 30 years many theories have been put forward in an attempt to describe the pathophysiology of migraine, but the exact etiology is still unclear. The following is a brief overview of some of the proposed mechanisms and pathophysiology of migraine.

1. Vascular theory. It was once thought that the aura phase was due to cerebral vasoconstriction and the headache coincided with vasodilatation. But researchers have now discovered that the headache phase occurs while the cerebral arterioles are still constricted, and this theory has been largely refuted (Lance & Goadsby 2005, Olsen et al 1990).

2. Cortical spreading depression (CSD) theory. A wave of cerebral excitation and depression spreading forwards from the occipital cortex is thought to explain the aura phase of the migraine, and has been supported by functional brain imaging (Lance & Goadsby 2005). This theory does not provide an explanation for patients who suffer headache without an aura and patients who have an aura that does not lead to a headache. Current thinking is that many other neural pathways and stimuli contribute to the headache, rather than CSD alone.

3. Trigeminovascular theory. A plexus of large unmyelinated fibers arise from the ophthalmic division of the trigeminal ganglion and from upper cervical dorsal roots, surround the large cerebral vessels, large venous sinuses, pial vessels and the dura mater. Trigeminal fibers innervating cerebral vessels arise from neurons in the trigeminal ganglion that contain substance P (SP) and calcitonin gene-related peptide (CGRP), both of which can be released when the trigeminal ganglion is stimulated. It appears that CSD stimulates the trigeminal ganglion, which in turn releases SP and CGRP, which may cause the headache component of migraine (Lance & Goadsby 2005).

4. Cutaneous alloying and neuronal sensitization. Cranial allodynia, (perception of pain with a normally nonpainful stimulus), may occur during and sometimes after migraine attacks. Burstein and colleagues (2000) have described the presence of cranial allodynia, and allodynia in the upper limbs ipsilateral and contralateral to the headache. This finding is consistent with at least third-order neuronal sensitization, such as sensitization of thalamic neurons, and raises the possibility of the pathophysiology being within the central nervous system.

5. The trigeminocervical complex. The group of neurons from the superficial laminae of trigeminal nucleus caudal and C1 and C2 dorsal horns are functionally regarded as the trigeminocervical complex. Stimulation of branches of C1–C2 roots is thought to sensitize the distribution of the trigeminal nerve and vice versa. Experimental data suggest that a significant proportion of the trigeminal vascular nociceptive information comes through the most caudal cells. This may explain the referred pain to the back of the head during a migraine episode. Some of the anti migrainous agents, including the triptans and ergots, appear to act on these second order neurons, and this may explain their effectiveness in symptom control (Lance & Goadsby 2005). Extracranial structures can give rise to migraines through muscle contraction or trigger mechanisms involving the cervical region. Trigeminal and cervical distribution seems to overlap beyond their anatomical innervation. Trigeminal nucleus may extend beyond the traditional nucleus caudalis to the dorsal horn of the high cervical ganglion in a functional continuum (Lance & Goadsby 2005).

6. Serotonin depletion. Serotonin is a key neurotransmitter involved in CNS pain inhibition. Dysregulation of central serotonergic function is likely to be a key factor in the onset of migraine (see Ch. 9). The discharge of platelet serotonin at the onset of migraine is thought to reflect depletion of serotonin at central synapses (Anthony et al 1969).

7. Dopaminergic transmission. It has been proposed that dopaminergic activation may be an important factor in some types of migraine. Signs of dopaminergic activation such as hunger, yawning, thirst, irritability and depression can sometimes precede the headache.

Associated or predisposing factors

Twin studies and population-based epidemiological surveys strongly suggest that migraine without aura is a multifactorial disorder, caused by a combination of genetic and environmental factors. Some of the likely etiological factors are outlined below.

1. Genetic background. A positive family history is frequently seen in patients with migraine. The estimated risk of a child developing migraine is 70% if both parents suffer from migraine, 45% when one parent is affected, and 30% when a close relative has migraine. The genetic association is supported by studies on twins and first degree relatives. Familial hemiplegic migraine has been localized to chromosome 19 (May et al 1995).

2. Migraine, anxiety and depression may share common links. In one study migraine sufferers were found to be four times more likely to develop depression and 12 times more likely to experience anxiety attacks than those with no history of migraine (Breslau & Davis 1992).

3. Some migraine sufferers can identify certain food types and beverages that precipitate attacks. There is no convincing evidence to suggest that certain food types are directly linked to onset of migraine. However, these patients should be advised to avoid these food types.

4. Catamenial migraine (related to the menstrual cycle) is a well described phenomenon. The exact mechanism of this is unknown, but withdrawal of estrogen in the premenstrual period is a likely explanation. Migraine appears to be relieved by pregnancy in about 60% of women, and there is often no significant improvement after menopause.

5. Other precipitants for migraines may include stress, allergy and trauma. In clinical practice, if a patient describes a consistent association with a predisposing factor, avoidance of that precipitant should be encouraged.

Differential diagnosis

When the clinical history is consistent with migraine and the neurological examination is unremarkable, diagnosis is straight forward. When there is an atypical story or unusual clinical findings, other causes for headaches should be excluded. These include subarachnoid hemorrhage, cerebral tumor, cerebral abscess, encephalitis or meningitis, cerebral venous thrombosis, giant cell arteritis, and cervical artery dissection.

Migraine can progress to stroke in rare instances (Etminan et al 2005, Kurth et al 2006, Minan et al 2005). In a patient with a past history of migraines, an important question to ask is 'Is the current headache different to your usual migraines in any way?'

When the onset of the headache is sudden, and intensity is maximal, subarachnoid hemorrhage needs to be excluded. In this group of patients, the risk of a re-bleed is maximal within the first six hours. Therefore, if clinically suspected, a CT brain scan should be performed urgently. If the scan is negative for blood, further investigations including a lumbar puncture and an angiogram need to be considered.

Encephalitic illness or meningitis should be considered in every headache patient with a fever. This will be further supported if the patient is confused, photophobic or has evidence of meningism. Again, a CT brain scan followed by a spinal tap (if there is no potential intracranial mass lesion) should be done. Rarely, migraine patients can present with fevers or even CSF pleocytosis (HaNDL: headache with neurological deficits and CSF lymphocytosis) but this should be a diagnosis of exclusion.

Cerebral space occupying lesions usually present with gradual onset of dull headache with associated nausea or abnormal neurological examination. The headache is usually worse in the mornings and increases with coughing. It is vital to perform a funduscopic examination looking for evidence of papilledema. A brain MRI, or CT scan if MRI is not available, will usually reveal the lesion. It is important to remember that sometimes, a cerebral abscess can present without a systemic illness or rarely, can be sudden in onset.

The pregnant patient with first time migraine or 'different' or atypical migraine warrants an urgent neurological opinion.

Headache in a postpartum patient or a patient presenting with confusion and seizures could be secondary to cerebral venous thrombosis. If suspected, MR venography should be performed. In older patients, the differential diagnosis includes giant cell arteritis especially if there are associated visual symptoms, raised ESR or systemic symptoms. This is treatable with high dose steroids but, if treatment is delayed, complications including blindness and stroke may occur. Cervical artery dissection is usually associated with neck pain and other neurological deficits and, rarely, headache. This condition will need to be considered if the patient has a recent history of neck manipulation, trauma or neurological findings consistent with a dissection. An MR angiogram of the cervical region and MR brain scan will usually give positive results.

The other conditions that need to be considered in the differential diagnosis are tension headaches, cluster headaches (shorter duration, multiple times a day, headaches occur in clusters), trigeminal neuralgia (usually unilateral sharp facial pain lasting seconds), benign intracranial hypertension (bilateral papilledema, enlarged blind spot, body habitus and other risk factors), sinusitis and spontaneous intracranial hypotension.

In summary, if the history and clinical examination is atypical of migraine, or if there is a recent change in the character of the headaches in a patient with known headache, the clinician should proceed with further investigations.

Treatment

Effective treatment is imperative, given the social, emotional and financial impact of migraine in the community. Treatment options for migraine are conservative measures and pharmacological. The first option should be explored whenever possible, considering the adverse effects and possible high cost of some anti-migraine agents.

Conservative treatment

The cornerstone of conservative treatment is avoidance of trigger factors for the particular patient. Although not evidence-based, common sense approaches are useful, including healthy life style, good diet, and relaxation measures to combat stress.

Pharmacological treatment

There are multiple anti-migraine agents available. Most of the newer agents, although costly, are very effective. The choice of agent is decided by the tolerance and side effect profile of the patient (Table 3.1).

Treatment of acute attacks

1. Simple analgesics and nonsteroidal anti-inflammatory drugs (NSAIDs). NSAIDs are very useful anti-migrainous agents, and together with aspirin should be tried as first line agents if not limited by side effects and recurrence of headaches. The

Table 3.1 Migraine treatment and prophylaxis.

Acute treatment	Adult dose	Adverse effects (AE) Contraindications (CI)	Comments
NSAIDs Aspirin	Indomethacin: 50 g bid/tid Ibuprofen: 400 mg tid	AE: Gastrointestinal effects CI: Bleeding tendency	Effective for non-frequent, responding headaches Consider GI prophylaxis
Triptans (5 HT1 agonists)	Sumatriptan: Oral: 50 mg, maximum single oral dose is 100 mg, maximum daily dose 200 mg/day. Nasal spray: 20 mg spray. 1 spray, may repeat in 2 hr, max 40 mg/day. Injection: 6 mg subcutaneous, may repeat in 1 hr, maximum 12 mg/day Zolmitriptan: Start with 2.5 mg, may repeat in 2 hr, maximum 10 mg/day. 5 mg nasal spray Rizatriptan: 5, 10 mg tabs Almotriptan: 6.25, 12.5 mg tabs Naratriptan: 2.5 mg tabs	CI: Ischemic heart disease (IHD), uncontrolled hypertension, impaired hepatic function, MAOI use within 2 weeks, pregnancy and lactation Caution required in basilar artery or hemiplegic migraine	Avoid within 24 hr of receiving DHE If patient has vomiting consider zolmitriptan nasal spray or subcutaneous sumatriptan Decreased chest tightness with almotriptan Naratriptan has longer half life and is not contraindicated with MAOI If tablets are required to be taken without water: zolmitriptan and rizatryptan tablets are convenient, and melt in the mouth Patients respond differently to different triptans No clear evidence for continued use if first dose is ineffective
DHE (dihydroxy-ergotamine)	1 mg sc/IV tid slowly Can be used as a continuous infusion Maximum dose 6 mg/day or 10 mg per wk	CI: IHD, hypertension, peripheral vascular disease, pregnancy and lactation	Should be performed in a hospital setting Treat usually for 72 hr for intractable headaches Compatible with normal saline: refer to DHE infusion protocols in the hospital
Chlorpromazine	IV/IM 12.5–25 mg dilute with 0.9% NaCl (slow infusion: 1 mg/min) tid Oral: 25 mg tid	AE: sedation nausea hypotension	Subcutaneous not recommended Effective treatment in the emergency room for acute attacks

Table 3.1 Migraine treatment and prophylaxis—Cont'd

Acute treatment	Adult dose	Adverse effects (AE) Contraindications (CI)	Comments
Prophylaxis	**Adult dose**	**Adverse effects**	**Comments**
Tricyclic antidepressants	Amitriptyline: 10–25 mg nocte, can be increased up to 100 mg nocte Nortriptyline: 25–100 mg/day	Dry mouth, constipation, postural hypotension, urinary retention, drowsiness, cardiac arrhythmias Caution in the elderly Less sedating, anticholinergic effect	Very effective and low cost Caution in liver disease, glaucoma
Beta blockers	Propranalol: 60–240 mg/day Atenolol: 50–150 mg/day Metoprolol: 50–150 mg/day	Fatigue, bradycardia, impotence, sleep disturbance, depression	Avoid if possible in young, active patients Contraindicated in asthma, severe cardiac failure and heart block
Calcium channel blockers	Verapamil: 240–320 mg/day	Postural hypotension, constipation, peripheral edema	Effectiveness of this class not proven in large trials, but very effective in some patients
Antiepileptics	Valproic acid: 500–1500 mg/day Topiramate: 100–200 mg/day	Drowsiness, weight gain, tremors, alopecia, abnormal liver enzymes, paresthesia, cognitive disturbance, weight loss, renal calculi	Useful in patients with a seizure disorder plus migraine Consider when weight loss also useful Expensive
Other	Methysergide: 4–8 mg/day Pizotifen: 0.5–1 mg/day	Retroperitoneal, pulmonary and cardiac fibrosis, muscle cramps, nausea, diarrhea Weight gain, drowsiness, and anticholinergic effects	Proven effectiveness in controlled trials Should not be given for more than 6 months 1 month interruption prior to re-starting Taper dose over 1 week to avoid rebound headache

outcome is improved when combined with metoclopramide, probably due to the better absorption of aspirin and relief of nausea.

2. Triptans have revolutionized the treatment of migraines. Since the introduction of sumatriptan, many different triptans are available in the market today. Oral sumatriptan, particularly at a 100 mg dose has been shown to be significantly more effective than placebo at relieving migraine within 2 hours. In a meta-analysis comparing different triptans, Ferrari et al found that triptans at marketed doses were well tolerated and effective and that differences between them were relatively small. The authors concluded that rizatriptan 10 mg, eletriptan 80 mg, and almotriptan 12.5 mg provided the highest

likelihood of consistent success. Triptans can be given subcutaneously or intranasally. Intranasal treatment is especially good for patients who wake with migraine, as gastric absorption is altered in migraine and oral agents may not be absorbed once migraine has started.

3. Dihydroergotamine (DHE) preceded by an anti-emetic such as metoclopramide, given 1 mg IM or IV every 8 hr or by continuous IV infusion is a useful treatment for refractory migraine or status migrainosus. Typically, patients should be admitted to hospital and treated for a period of 2–3 days or more. Pregnancy, ischemic heart disease and untreated hypertension are contraindications.

4. Chlorpromazine (Largactil) given at a dose of 12.5–25 mg slow IV, with a normal saline bolus, is effective treatment for acute attacks. This can be followed by the oral form (25 mg bid). Major side effects are drowsiness, nausea and hypotension. In a trial comparing treatment of acute migraine with chlorpromazine 12.5 mg IV with DHE 1 mg IV and lignocaine 50 mg IV (Bell et al 1990) the chlorpromazine-treated group was found to do significantly better than the other two groups.

Prophylactic agents

Prophylactic treatment should be considered for migraine sufferers who experience frequent attacks, debilitating symptoms including neurological deficits or symptoms that interfere with lifestyle or daily activities (see Table 3.1).

Tricyclic antidepressants (TCA) and beta blockers are often effective as prophylactic agents. A systematic review of 26 randomized, placebo controlled trials showed that the beta blocker propanolol was clearly more effective than placebo in the short term prevention of migraine. In the elderly, TCA use is limited by postural hypotension, dry mouth, urinary retention and confusion. Amitriptyline is commonly used and is given as a night time dose to avoid side effects such as day time confusion.

Antiepileptic drugs including sodium valproate, and topiramate are also commonly used, though cost is a limiting factor with topiramate. The use of antiepileptic medication is supported by Level 1 evidence. A Cochrane review found that anticonvulsants are effective in reducing the frequency of migraine by 1–2 attacks per month. This review also found that patients taking anticonvulsants were more than twice as likely to reduce their migraine attacks by at least 50% when compared to patients who took an inactive placebo.

Oral ergotamine is not helpful, but magnesium, riboflavin, other vitamins and coenzyme Q10 are used by many patients with good results; these require further studies to confirm their effectiveness.

Conclusion

Migraine is a disorder associated with significant psychosocial impact. The diagnosis of migraine requires a good clinical history, and exclusion of other causes of headache. However, further investigations are needed when the findings from the history and clinical examination are atypical of migraine, or if there is a recent change in the character of the patient's headaches. Current pharmaceutical anti-migraine treatments have revolutionized migraine management. Optimal treatment needs to be individualized, taking into consideration side effects of medications, duration and severity of symptoms, and outcome of previous treatments.

References

Anthony M, Hinterberger H, Lance JW 1969 The possible relationship of serotonin to the migraine syndrome. Research and Clinical Studies in Headache 2:29-59.

Bell R, Montoya D, Shuaib A, Lee MA 1990 A comparative trial of three agents in the treatment of acute migraine headache. Ann Emerg Med 19:1079-1082.

Breslau N, Davis GC 1992 Migraine, major depression and panic disorder: a prospective epidemiologic study of young adults. Cephalalgia 12:85-90.

Breslau N, Davis GC, Schultz LR et al 1994 Joint 1994 Wolff Award Presentation. Migraine and major depression: a longitudinal study. Headache 34:387-393.

Burstein R, Cutrer M, Yarnitsky D 2000 The development of cutaneous allodynia during a migraine attack. Clinical evidence for the sequential recruitment of spinal and supraspinal nociceptive neurons in migraine. Brain 123:1703-1709.

Etminan M, Takkouche B, Isorna FC, Samii A 2005 Risk of ischaemic stroke in people with migraine: systemic review and meta-analysis of observational studies. BMJ 330:63-66.

International Headache Society 2004 The International Classification of Headache Disorders, 2nd edn. Cephalalgia 24 (suppl 1):1-160.

Kurth T, Gaziano JM, Cook NR et al 2006 Migraine and risk of cardiovascular disease in women. JAMA 296:283-291.

Lance J, Goadsby P 2005 Mechanism and management of headache, 7th edn. Elsevier, Philadelphia.

Lyngberg AC, Rasmussen BC, Jørgensen T, Jensen R 2005 Incidence of primary headache: A Danish epidemiologic follow-up study. Am J Epidemiol 161:1066-1073.

May A, Ophoff RA, Terwindt GM et al 1995 Familial hemiplegic migraine locus on 19p13 is involved in the common forms of migraine with and without aura. Hum Genet 96:604-608.

Minan M, Takkouche B, Isorna FC, Samii A 2005 Risk of ischaemic stroke in people with migraine: systematic review and meta-analysis of observational studies. BMJ 330:63-65.

Olsen J, Friberg L, Skyhoj-Olsen T et al 1990 Timing and topography of cerebral blood flow, aura headache during migraine. Ann Neurol 28: 791-798.

Stewart WF, Lipton RB, Liberman J 1996 Variation in migraine prevalence by race. Neurology 47:52-59.

4

Headache in childhood and adolescence

Andrew Kornberg and George Chalkiadis

Headache in children always requires careful evaluation, since a small number of headaches arise from life-threatening conditions. In this chapter the authors, a neurologist and a pain management consultant, address the factors that could lead to headaches in young people and propose management strategies.

The major concern for parents and for the treating physician when a child presents with headache, is the possibility that it is caused by a tumor. A detailed history and examination will be able to alleviate this anxiety in the majority of cases and provide the child and family with a specific diagnosis and appropriate therapy. Headache is the most common somatic pain complaint in children and adolescents (Perquin et al 2000). Studies of childhood headache have shown that the prevalence of recurrent headache in childhood may be as high as 29% (Zwart et al 2004). The prevalence increases with age and is more common in females (Dooley et al 2005, Laurell et al 2004, Zwart et al 2004). Other studies have demonstrated that headache prevalence ranges from 57% to 82% in 7–15 year-olds. However the prevalence of severe or recurrent headache occurring daily or almost daily is in the order of 2% (Larsson & Sund 2005). Migraine in childhood has been well studied and may have prevalence rates as high as 11% in some studies (Laurell et al 2004). Of the different types of headache encountered in childhood, chronic daily headache (tension-type headache) and migraine are the most common. Diagnostic criteria (International Classification of Headache Disorders [ICHD-2] and Silberstein-Lipton) exist for migraine and other types of headaches that occur in childhood (Bigal et al 2005, Lipton et al 2004).

Headaches are caused by the involvement of the pain-sensitive structures that include vascular and meningeal structures, cranial nerves (particularly those with sensory fibers – V, IX, X) and other neuromuscular structures surrounding the skull.

Children and adolescents who experience frequent headaches may also experience other somatization pain complaints such as abdominal pain, limb pain and backache (Fichtel & Larsson 2002, Ghandour et al 2004). In the US, over half of adolescent females who experience headache more than once each week also report abdominal pain more than once per week.

In the evaluation of a child with headache it is important to make a specific diagnosis as this is the key to providing the most appropriate therapy. The history and examination is the most important part of the evaluation of children presenting with headache. 'Routine' laboratory and imaging studies have no place, because these investigations should be used in a focused manner, depending on the differential diagnosis obtained from history and examination. The following details the important aspects of the history and examination that should be considered.

History

As the most important diagnostic attributes of headache are the chronological pattern and severity, a detailed and thorough account of the headache and associated problem(s) prompting the patient and/or parents to seek medical attention is essential. In addition, a full developmental and medical history should be obtained.

The headache history should elucidate chronologically the onset of headache, its chronicity, the setting in which it has developed, its manifestations and consequences and any previous treatment received.

The principal symptom or complaint (headache) should be well-characterized with descriptions of the following attributes:

- Location
- Quality
- Severity
- Timing which includes the onset, duration and frequency
- The setting in which the symptom(s) occur
- Factors that may have aggravated or relieved the symptom(s)
- Associated manifestations including the impact on normal functioning.

All of these attributes are invaluable for understanding the patient's symptom(s). Previous medications for headache and other disorders should be detailed with particular attention to caffeine

intake (including caffeine contained in soft drinks) and any illicit drug and alcohol use. Taking the past medical, family, and personal and social history is a very important component of history taking. The parents and patients should be asked about anxiety and depressive symptoms. A careful family history of headache or psychiatric illnesses should be obtained. These questions (see Box 4.1) may allow the clinician to make a diagnosis based on the headache type and to plan further management. Finally, a thorough systematic review is performed, concentrating on questions related to symptoms of raised intracranial pressure (ICP) or progressive neurological disease, such as ataxia, lethargy, seizures, visual disturbances, focal signs, personality change or intellectual change. Symptoms suggestive of a likely underlying serious cause include:

Box 4.1

Headache history questions.

How long ago did the headaches start?
Are the headaches the same, better or worse overall?
How often are the headaches occurring?
Do the headaches occur at any special time, or under any special circumstance?
Are the headaches related to any triggers you are aware of?
Are there any warning symptoms?
Where is the pain located?
What is the quality of the pain?
Are there any associated symptoms?
How long does it take from the onset of the headache to the peak of the headache?
How long does the headache last?
What do you do during the headache?
What makes the headache better?
What makes the headache worse?
In between headaches are you well?
Are you on any other medications?
Have you ever been treated for headaches before?
What do you think could be causing your headaches?
Is there a family history of headaches?

• Increased severity of headaches
• Waking from sleep
• Change in headache pattern.

Examination

A general physical examination should include blood pressure measurement, and examination of the skin for neurocutaneous stigmata of neurofibromatosis. Signs of trauma should be looked for. The head circumference should be measured, plotted and compared to previous measurements. A careful neurological examination is performed looking for focal neurologic findings. Eye movements and the optic fundi should be carefully examined. The sinuses should be palpated for tenderness and the neck and skull should be auscultated for bruits. Any abnormality in the neurologic examination requires further evaluation as this is normal in between attacks in individuals with migraine.

Pattern of headache

In the evaluation of a child with headache it is useful to classify headache clinically using a temporal pattern. Based on this, a number of patterns can be identified and used in the delineation of the most likely diagnosis. Patterns which are commonly encountered included:

• Acute
• Acute recurrent
• Chronic progressive
• Chronic non-progressive
• Mixed pattern.

The various patterns are shown in Figure 4.1.

Acute headaches are single events without a previous history of headache. Acute headaches in children are commonly associated with systemic illnesses such as viral or febrile illnesses often related to an upper respiratory tract infection. In teenagers, the concern is for an aneurysmal, arachnoid, or hemorrhagic cause. If an acute headache is associated with focal neurological findings or raised intracranial pressure one may need to consider an acute intracranial hemorrhage. Other causes of acute headache are listed in Box 4.2.

Acute recurrent headaches are usually migrainous and are described in more detail below.

Chronic progressive headaches worsen in frequency and severity over time. They are usually associated with symptoms of raised intracranial pressure such as early morning headache, vomiting and signs of papilledema or focal neurological

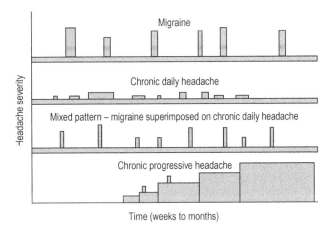

Figure 4.1 • Headache patterns.

Box 4.2

Causes of acute headache.

Infections including meningitis
Sinusitis
Postictal
Acute hypertension
Hypoglycemia
Trauma
Hemorrhage
Exertion
Dehydration

findings. The main differential diagnosis of this pattern of headaches includes brain tumors, hydrocephalus, subdural hemorrhage, and benign intracranial hypertension (BIH).

Chronic non-progressive headaches are often called tension-type headaches. They are not associated with symptoms of raised intracranial pressure or progressive neurological findings.

Mixed pattern headaches are a combination of migraine on chronic, non-progressive headaches.

Investigations

Headaches are frequently over-investigated. As discussed earlier, investigations should only be performed after a careful history and examination. Most children with headache will not require investigation. Laboratory tests yield little and are rarely necessary. Skull X-rays have little or no place in the investigation of headache. Imaging studies such as computed tomography (CT) of the brain or MRI have revolutionized the investigation of CNS disorders. Both modalities can be used to diagnose many congenital malformations, neoplasms, hydrocephalus, hemorrhage, vascular malformations or sinus pathology. However, MRI is more sensitive, particularly in the posterior fossa and in the area of the cranio-cervical junction. Lumbar puncture for CSF pressure measurement is necessary for the diagnosis of BIH.

Acute recurrent headache

Migraine

Migraine is an acute recurrent headache characterized by episodic, periodic, and paroxysmal attacks of pain, separated by pain-free periods. Migraine is often triggered by stress, anxiety, fatigue, lack of sleep, certain foods, exercise, and sunlight. A family history of migraine is common.

Prior to the onset of the headache there may be an aura which may consist of visual symptoms such as bright flashing lights, fortification spectra or an alteration of perception, the so called 'Alice in Wonderland' syndrome. Neurologic symptoms such as dysphasia, paresthesia, and hemiparesis may also begin at this stage. The headache then begins, usually frontal, lateralized, throbbing in quality, and gradually spreading. The child is often very pale and may be nauseous and begin to vomit. The child is usually photophobic and needs to go to sleep in a dark room. After sleep the child improves. In between headaches, the child is normal as is the neurological examination. Obviously, there are less severe headaches, and many children do not have an aura.

It is important to obtain from the history and examination the following aspects as these features essentially form the basis of the diagnostic criteria for migraine:

- Aura
- Lateralized
- Throbbing
- Nausea/vomiting
- Photophobia
- Normal intra-attack history and examination with no evidence of organic disease.

Migraine is common in childhood and has similar manifestations in childhood as it does in adults. The various complicated migraine syndromes described in adults such as hemiplegic migraine occur in childhood but other migraine syndromes appear to be seen exclusively in childhood. These include: benign paroxysmal vertigo, cyclic vomiting, and paroxysmal torticollis.

Management of migraine in childhood includes:

- identifying triggers and removing them
- aborting attacks by taking analgesia as early as possible into the attack (and at the onset of any aura)
- using non-pharmacological relaxation techniques
- taking prophylactic agents to prevent frequent disabling events.

As the remission rate of migraine is high, prophylaxis should not be used for long periods.

Chronic progressive headache

Chronic progressive headaches suggest that there is an ongoing pathologic process. It is usually associated with raised ICP. With this in mind, symptoms and signs are progressive over time. The symptoms (headache) typically worsen by becoming more frequent, more severe, associated with early morning wakening, a change in character, or associated with other neurologic symptoms. The headaches may worsen with coughing, bending over, or sneezing. Other symptoms will suggest an ongoing neurologic process. Symptoms may include a change in personality, focal weakness, ataxia, diplopia, visual loss, seizures, or lethargy. In between headaches the child will have ongoing symptoms. The general or neurologic examination will usually be abnormal or if normal, will show signs of raised ICP with evidence of cranial nerve palsies or papilledema.

Brain tumors are the second most common childhood malignancy after leukemia and are a common cause of this pattern of headache. Other causes include hydrocephalus from congenital anomalies.

In this scenario, imaging is mandatory and diagnostic. Lumbar puncture is contraindicated if a mass lesion is considered.

Benign intracranial hypertension

This condition is relatively common and presents with symptoms suggestive of raised ICP. It is termed 'benign' because the clinical features mimic a cerebral tumor.

An imaging study is required to exclude a tumor or hydrocephalus, and by definition no evidence for hydrocephalus or tumor is found on imaging. However, this disorder is not necessarily 'benign', as it is potentially associated with permanent and disabling visual loss. The pathogenesis has not been clearly elucidated. The next step to confirm the diagnosis is a CSF pressure measurement which will demonstrate a grossly elevated CSF pressure.

The disorder is associated with a number of risk factors including:

- adolescence
- female sex
- obesity
- recurrent otitis media
- medications: steroid withdrawal, oral contraceptives, tetracyclines, vitamin A, growth hormone treatment.

Management involves close monitoring of vision, withdrawal of risk factors (drugs), lowering of ICP by lumbar puncture and CSF drainage, and the use of drugs to decrease CSF production (acetazolamide). If vision is deteriorating despite active management, neurosurgical procedures such as lumboperitoneal shunting and optic nerve fenestration are necessary. **The protection of vision is the mainstay of therapy.** The prognosis for this disorder is generally good.

Chronic non-progressive headache

Tension-type headache

Tension-type headache (TTH) is classified as infrequent, frequent episodic, or chronic TTH. Primary chronic daily headache (CDH) is characterized by headaches not attributable to a secondary disorder, which last more than 4 hours per day and occur 15 or more days per month. CDH in turn is classified as chronic (transformed) migraine, chronic TTH, new daily persistent headache (NDPH) or infrequently in children, hemicrania continua. Chronic migraine and chronic TTH may co-exist. It is important to exclude analgesic induced headache that has been most frequently described in association with transformed migraine and NDPH in the adolescent population (Bigal et al 2005, Lipton et al 2004). NDPH also occurs after Epstein–Barr virus infection and minor head injury (with normal examination and neuroimaging) (Mack 2004).

The clinical features of these headaches have not been well defined. The headaches are most commonly described as being bi-frontal and pressure-like, or band-like. Unlike migraine headaches, they are not associated with a throbbing quality (although the mixed pattern headache has features of both types). There is no preceding aura, the headache may be present on a daily basis and be present throughout the day. Many adolescents will continue their activities, although evidence of functional disability (school absenteeism, social withdrawal, sleep disruption and physical inactivity) may be evident. School absenteeism may be more likely in adolescents with lower academic performance and higher scores on the Childhood Depression Inventory (although not meeting the criteria for clinical depression) (Breuner et al 2004). There

may be myriad other symptoms such as fatigue, dizziness, phonophobia and blurred vision. There may be some evidence of stressors, depressive symptoms and other psychosocial issues in the individual's life. A biopsychosocial approach is critical to identify and address contributing and maintaining factors for headache and its resultant consequences (Fig. 4.2).

Neurological examination and investigation is normal. Treatment can be difficult and is best managed in a multidisciplinary manner. There is good evidence that psychological treatments, principally relaxation and cognitive behavioral therapy, are effective in reducing the frequency of CDH in children and adolescents, although it remains unclear if these treatments are effective for other outcomes such as disability, school, and family functioning (Eccleston et al 2004). There is evidence that relaxation treatment for TTH administered by trained school nurses is effective although this is less likely when functional disability exists (Fichtel & Larsson 2004, Larsson et al 2005). Addressing parental response to pain behavior and their personal belief systems may be beneficial.

Other therapeutic techniques such as biofeedback, hypnotherapy and acupuncture have been described. Medication such as amitriptyline is sometimes effective (Hershey et al 2000) as are occipital nerve blocks where occipital neuralgia can be identified. Addressing impaired visual acuity and poor posture may help in some cases.

Labeling CDH functional or psychosomatic is often unhelpful, contributing to frustration with the medical system and encouraging families to seek alternative therapies to attenuate the symptom rather than focusing on the factors maintaining pain.

Without specific treatment, one-third of adolescents reported frequent headache one year later. Female sex, frequent headaches at initial assessment, reduced leisure time activity, and

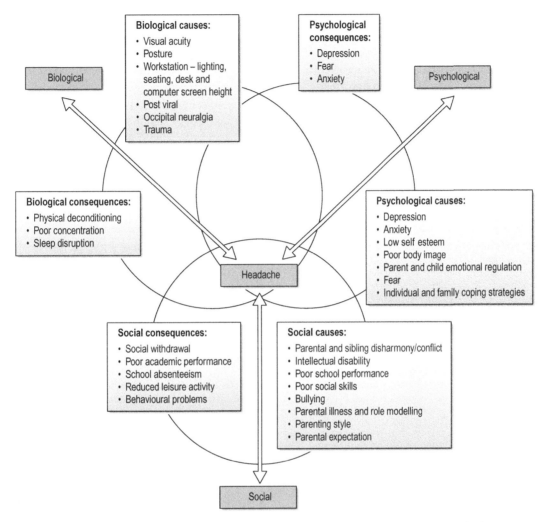

Biological causes:
- Visual acuity
- Posture
- Workstation – lighting, seating, desk and computer screen height
- Post viral
- Occipital neuralgia
- Trauma

Psychological consequences:
- Depression
- Fear
- Anxiety

Biological

Psychological

Biological consequences:
- Physical deconditioning
- Poor concentration
- Sleep disruption

Psychological causes:
- Depression
- Anxiety
- Low self esteem
- Poor body image
- Parent and child emotional regulation
- Fear
- Individual and family coping strategies

Headache

Social consequences:
- Social withdrawal
- Poor academic performance
- School absenteeism
- Reduced leisure activity
- Behavioural problems

Social causes:
- Parental and sibling disharmony/conflict
- Intellectual disability
- Poor school performance
- Poor social skills
- Bullying
- Parental illness and role modelling
- Parenting style
- Parental expectation

Social

Figure 4.2 • Biopsychosocial model showing the complex and bi-directional nature of factors contributing to and maintaining chronic daily headache and its consequences. These factors guide assessment and direct treatment.

higher reporting of depressive symptoms were associated with increased likelihood for headache persistence (Larsson & Sund 2005).

Other headaches

Headache can be seen as part of a variety of other conditions including:
- Connective tissue disease, e.g. systemic lupus erythematosus
- Systemic hypertension
- Hypoglycemia
- Sleep and obstructive apnea. A history of snoring with or without apnea, unrefreshed sleep and daytime somnolence in conjunction with morning headache are suggestive. A sleep study will quantify the problem, and adenotonsillectomy or nocturnal bipap ventilation may be indicated

- Post-dural puncture headache, characterized by frontal headache when sitting or standing with relief on assuming the supine position. More likely with large gauge spinal needles (< 25-gauge), less likely with Sprotte or Whitacre type needles. Simple analgesia, generous fluid intake, and caffeine may be helpful. If symptoms persist, epidural blood patch may be necessary
- Sinus infection
- Occipital neuralgia, characterized by pain at the base of the skull, which may be unilateral or bilateral, and associated with radiation or sudden shock-like paresthesias in the distribution of the greater and/or lesser occipital nerves. We have observed this in adolescents with dystonic cerebral palsy who communicate through head activated computer programs. Greater and lesser occipital nerve blocks with a local anesthetic and soluble steroid solution are diagnostic and therapeutic in the short-term (weeks). Longer lasting analgesia may be attained with scalp injection of botulinum toxin A
- Dental disease and malocclusion
- Bruxism (see Ch. 20).

These should be considered in an individual where they have the above risk factors or alternatively no other cause is found.

Case study 1

Helen is a 15-year-old girl who had developed daily headaches over a 6-month period. These were present on waking and on occasions were associated with vomiting without nausea. Recently, she had complained of intermittent double vision and transient episodes of loss of vision lasting seconds only.

On examination she was moderately obese; she was afebrile, and had no abnormal neurocutaneous stigmata. She had a moderate amount of acne over her face. Her blood pressure was 105/65. There were no bruits heard. Her general physical and neurological examinations were normal and there were no focal neurological findings. Her extraocular movements showed a partial left V1 nerve palsy and she had gross papilledema.

Questions

1. What is the differential diagnosis?
2. What investigations are required?
3. What other questions should be asked?
4. What is the management?

Discussion

The headache pattern is consistent with chronic progressive and the history is very suggestive of raised intracranial pressure (ICP). The child has focal neurological findings in that she has partial 6th nerve palsy. In addition, the papilledema confirms the historic suspicion of raised ICP. Based on this synthesis, the differential diagnosis is between a mass such as a tumor, hydrocephalus and its causes, or benign intracranial hypertension (BIH) or pseudotumor cerebri. The obesity and the adolescent onset are risk factors for BIH, as are some therapies for acne (see below).

An imaging study is required immediately. MRI scan is the investigation of choice, but if this cannot be obtained within a day or two, an urgent CT scan is indicated. Although a CT scan will be able to demonstrate a mass or hydrocephalus if present, an MRI may be required to more clearly define an abnormality in the posterior fossa. CT scanning through the posterior fossa can be associated with significant artifact whereas MRI provides wonderful anatomical detail. If the MRI scan is normal, then the diagnosis is most likely to be BIH and a lumbar puncture with confirmatory CSF pressure measurement is necessary.

BIH can be associated with a number of risk factors including being female, adolescence, obesity, recurrent otitis media, steroid withdrawal, oral contraceptives, tetracycline use, Vitamin A overuse and growth hormone treatment. Tetracyclines are used for acne. The major questions to be asked in this case are to ascertain whether any of the medications listed are being used as withdrawal may be helpful in management.

Even though this disorder is named 'benign', it is potentially serious with the potential for permanent visual loss. Management involves close monitoring of vision, withdrawal of risk factors (drugs), lowering of ICP by lumbar puncture, and the use of drugs to decrease CSF production (acetazolamide). If vision is deteriorating despite active management neurosurgical procedures such as lumboperitoneal shunting and optic nerve fenestration is necessary.

This patient had a normal MRI scan of the brain. Lumbar puncture confirmed a diagnosis of benign intracranial hypertension

Case study 2

Tara is a 12-year-old girl who presented with a 3-year history of headache, recurrent abdominal pain, and bilateral knee pain. The pains commenced just after the separation of her parents and she received counseling at the time. Her headaches became less frequent, but she continued to experience headaches every 3 weeks associated with vomiting and photophobia. On these occasions she would retire to bed and the headaches would have subsided by the time she woke the following morning. When younger, she would often experience headaches associated with vomiting when she had problems with her peers. Over the last 6 months, bi-frontal headaches have been present on a daily basis.

Of her various aches and pains, Tara found her headache the most troublesome in that she had difficulty concentrating at school and found the noise in the classroom intolerable at times. She had missed 15 days of school last term because of her headache and was experiencing headaches every 2 weeks in the afternoons associated with vomiting and photophobia. Tara had difficulty initiating sleep most nights and would often wake up unrefreshed. She had reduced her sporting activity at school because of knee pain, despite frequent physical therapy. She had been referred to a neurologist 12 months ago who diagnosed chronic daily headache with superimposed migraine.

Questions

1. Is further assessment necessary?
2. Are further investigations required?
3. What is the management?

Discussion

The chronic non-progressive history of headache is consistent with a mixed pattern of chronic TTH and migraine. No investigations for headache are required. The long history of symptoms which have not improved despite multiple visits to her local doctor and a neurologist, and which are causing functional disability, requires an interdisciplinary assessment of her pain complaints.

A team comprising a pain medicine specialist, a psychiatrist, a psychologist, a physiotherapist, and an occupational therapist assessed Tara. A number of issues relating to school were identified including that she had attended three different primary schools to date and was about to graduate to secondary school, that the current school rang her mother to pick her up from school whenever she complained of pain, and that she was being bullied at school. She had been attending her current school for 7 months. Tara received speech therapy when younger and was assigned an integration aide at a previous school. Psychometric tests had been performed 4 years ago that showed her intellectual functioning to be low normal. Although not clinically depressed, Tara had low self-esteem and would often ruminate at night about her peer relationships.

Tara visited her father on alternate weekends and was allowed to stay awake until midnight on these occasions when they often watched DVDs together. Her parents' relationship is not amicable.

Tara's diet consisted of mainly carbohydrates and fat, with little fresh fruit or vegetables. Bowel actions occurred once every 2 days, and suprapubic abdominal pain preceded opening of her bowels. Examination that included visual acuity was normal.

Contact was made with Tara's current school. They were not aware of any particular difficulties apart from pain issues. Psychometric tests were repeated, which confirmed her low normal functioning. Follow-up with the school was made to:

- provide strategies (for Tara, the school, and Tara's mother) to manage headaches at school
- address learning and social issues
- facilitate transition to secondary school the following year ensuring that the school is aware of her special needs

Tara was taught relaxation exercises to help facilitate sleep and manage her headaches. Tara's parents attended a Pain Education session that emphasized the nature of her social and learning problems, the impact of their unamicable relationship, the association of these with Tara's symptoms and what they could do to improve her sleep hygiene and diet. Taping of her knees whilst performing sport helped reduce her knee pain and the physiotherapist initiated vastus medialis strengthening exercises.

Improvements noted within 3 months included: headache free days, reduced frequency of headaches associated with photophobia and vomiting, less school absenteeism, less abdominal pain, and participation in sporting activities.

Conclusion

Headache is a common complaint in childhood and adolescence. It is imperative that secondary causes of headache are considered. Recent onset headache with increasing frequency and intensity, seizures, and focal neurological signs should alert the treating physician to investigate further. In the absence of secondary headache, one can proceed to diagnosing a primary headache, in which case a biopsychosocial approach to assessment and treatment is ideal.

References

Bigal ME, Rapoport AM, Tepper SJ et al 2005 The classification of chronic daily headache in adolescents – a comparison between the second edition of the International Classification of Headache Disorders and alternative diagnostic criteria. Headache 45:582-589.

Breuner CC, Smith MS, Womack WM 2004 Factors related to school absenteeism in adolescents with recurrent headache. Headache 44:217-222.

Dooley JM, Gordon KE, Wood EP 2005 Self-reported headache frequency in Canadian adolescents: validation and follow-up. Headache 45:127-131.

Eccleston C, Yorke L, Morley S et al 2005 Psychological therapies for the management of chronic and recurrent pain in children and adolescents. The Cochrane Database of Systematic Reviews Volume 4.

Fichtel Å, Larsson B 2002 Psychosocial impact of headache and co-morbidity with other pains in Swedish adolescents. Headache 42:766-775.

Fichtel Å, Larsson B 2004 Relaxation treatment administered by school nurses to adolescents with recurrent headaches. Headache 44:545-554.

Ghandour RM, Overpeck MD, Huang ZJ et al 2004 Headache, stomachache, backache, and morning fatigue among adolescent girls in the United States: associations with behavioral, sociodemographic, and environmental factors. Archives of Pediatrics & Adolescent Medicine 158:797-803.

Hershey AD, Powers SW, Bentti AL, deGrauw TJ 2000 Effectiveness of amitriptyline in the prophylactic management of childhood headaches. Headache 40:539-549.

Larsson B, Carlsson J, Fichtel Å, Melin L 2005. Relaxation treatment of adolescent headache sufferers: results from a school-based replication series. Headache 45:692-704.

Larsson B, Sund AM 2005 One-year incidence, course, and outcome predictors of frequent headaches among early adolescents. Headache 45:684-691.

Laurell K, Larsson B, Eeg-Olofsson O 2004 Prevalence of headache in Swedish schoolchildren, with a focus on tension-type headache. Cephalalgia 24:380-388.

Lipton RB, Bigal ME, Steiner TJ et al 2004 Classification of primary headaches. Neurology 63:427-435.

Mack KJ 2004 What incites new daily persistent headache? Pediatric Neurology 31:122-125.

Perquin CW, Hazebroek-Kampscheur AAJM, Hunfeld JAM et al 2000 Pain in children and adolescents: a common experience. Pain 87:51-58.

Zwart J-A, Dyb G, Holmen TL, Stovner LJ, Sand T 2004 The prevalence of migraine and tension-type headache; among adolescents in Norway. The Nord-Trøndelag Health Study (Head-HUNT-Youth). A large population-based epidemiological study. Cephalalgia 24:373-379.

5

Headache and the upper cervical zygapophyseal joints

Jayantilal Govind

In patients with refractory headaches injections are performed to the upper cervical zygapophyseal joints. Diagnostic blocks of these joints are considered the gold standard in the diagnosis of cervicogenic headache. In this chapter the author, a pain management consultant, describes the anatomy and neurophysiology related to these joints and management using joint blocks and radio frequency denervation.

Until June 2004 the diagnosis and management of headaches of cervical origin, or 'cervicogenic headaches', was polarized; within the medical profession there was major dissension between the European continent (Sjaastad et al 1998) and the rest of the world, in particular Australia and the United States (International Headache Society 1988). First mooted in 1983 (Sjaastad et al 1983), the concept and diagnosis of cervicogenic headache were conditional and contingent upon clinical features – variables that would not have survived the dictates of epidemiological scrutiny, including validity and reliability (Sackett et al 1991). Others argued that the lack of objective clinical signs and the absence of quantifiable tangibles such as imaging or electrophysiological studies implied a psychoneurotic causation (Edmeads 1978); but surprisingly, these same authors did not demand similar stringent criteria for the diagnosis of primary headaches such as migraine and its variants.

Definition

By definition, cervicogenic headache means pain that is perceived in the head but whose primary source lies in the cervical spine. Provided it is innervated, any structure of the cervical spine has the potential to be a source of headache. A number of studies have confirmed that the upper cervical synovial joints can be a potent source of neck pain and headaches, more so following trauma. Experimentally, the noxious stimulation of the atlanto-occipital, the lateral atlantoaxial (Dreyfuss et al 1994), and the C2–C3 zygapophyseal joints (Dwyer et al 1990) in normal human volunteers or patients, generated distinct patterns of replicable head pain (Fukui et al 1996). Conversely, relief of headache could be secured with the intra-articular injection of local anesthetic into the lateral atlantoaxial joint (Aprill et al 2002) or by third occipital nerve block for head pain emanating from the C2–C3 zygapophyseal joint (Lord & Bogduk 1996). Of all the potential sources of cervicogenic headaches, only the cervical zygapophyseal joint has survived scientific rigor.

Background

By 1940 occipital or 'neuralgic' headaches were attributed to gout, trauma, syphilis, malaria (Perelson 1947), fibrositis (Holmes 1913), fibrotic nodules (Cyriax 1938), and cervical arthritis (Hadden 1940). In a persuasive clinicoradiological observation, (Brain 1963) reported that headache was one of the commonest presenting symptoms of upper cervical apophyseal joint spondylosis; but, establishing an unambiguous biological correlation was elusive.

A year later, Trevor-Jones (1964) demonstrated the surgical correlation between occipital headaches, the C2–C3 zygapophyseal joint, and the third occipital nerve. Surgical exploration of patients presenting with occipital headaches, upper cervical tenderness, and radiological features of C2–C3 osteoarthrosis, revealed the third occipital nerve to be entrapped within an osteophytic mass. Complete relief of headache soon followed once the osteophytes were excised and the nerve freed. Some 50 years later, other investigators reported the complete relief of the headache following fusion of the osteoarthritic lateral atlanto-axial (C1–C2) joints (Ehni & Benner 1984, Ghanayem et al 1996, Schaeren & Jeanneret 2005, Star et al 1992).

Pre-surgical diagnostic accuracy was improved with the introduction of diagnostic nerve blocks. In an earlier uncontrolled study, headaches, that were refractory to trigeminal nerve blocks, were completely relieved by selectively anesthetizing the upper cervical spinal nerves (Pentecost & Adriani 1955). The advent of fluoroscopy permitted the precise deposition of minute aliquots of local anesthetic upon the targeted nerve. Bogduk and Marsland (1986) then first described the technique whereby headaches emanating from the C2–C3 zygapophyseal joint could be alleviated by blocking the third occipital nerve (TON), and the concept of 'Third Occipital Headache' thus evolved.

Validation came from a subsequent controlled study in which Lord et al (1994) investigated 100 consecutive patients presenting with headache after whiplash injury. In this cohort, the prevalence of headache was deemed to be 27%, and where headache was the dominant symptom, the prevalence was 53% (95% CI 37% to 68%). At least 50% of all headaches were mediated by the third occipital nerve, making the C2–C3 zygapophyseal joint the most common source of upper neck pain and headaches. These findings were replicated in a subsequent unrelated study (Govind et al 2005). Not only did the latter study reaffirm that the C2–C3 zygapophyseal joint was the most common known source of cervicogenic headaches, but also in 6% of patients, the lateral atlantoaxial (C1–C2) joint was implicated. The lower synovial joints contributed to a lesser extent. Additionally, these studies did not identify any specific clinical or X-ray feature pathognomonic for cervicogenic headache.

Anatomy

The juxtaposition of two consecutive cervical vertebrae creates three joints: the large central intervertebral joint and the two posterolateral synovial joints known as the zygapophyseal (facet) joints. These synovial joints bridge the vertebrae behind the intervertebral foramina, unlike the atlanto-occipital (C0–C1) and the lateral atlantoaxial (C1–C2) joints, which lie anterolateral to the vertebral foramen. Commencing at the level of the second cervical vertebrae, the facets of the inferior and superior articular processes of each consecutive vertebrae articulate to form the zygapophyseal joint, and because of their semi-vertical inclination, the opposing articular pillars create a 'chisel-upon-chisel' effect. A loosely applied capsule surrounds the articular margins of each synovial joint. Attached to the capsules are the intra-articular meniscoids which lubricate and protect the joint surfaces during its movements. The integrity of the ipsisegmental intervertebral disc and the posterior neck muscles ensure joint stability.

Neuroanatomy

Peripheral

The atlanto-occipital (C0–C1) and the lateral atlantoaxial (C1–C2) joints receive their innervation from the ventral rami of the C1 and C2 spinal nerves respectively (Bogduk 1982).

Unlike the joints distal to it, the C2–C3 zygapophyseal joint is innervated by a single nerve, the TON. Derived from the third spinal nerve, the TON is the superficial branch of the C3 dorsal ramus. It passes around the lateral and then the posterior aspect of the C2–C3 zygapophyseal joint, and supplies articular branches from its deep surface as it crosses the joint transversely. Additional articular branches may arise from a communicating loop between the third occipital nerve and the C2 dorsal ramus (Bogduk 1982).

Synovial joints distal to the C2–C3 zygapophyseal joint have a dual innervation. Articular branches originate from the deep medial branches of the cervical dorsal rami as they cross the posterolateral aspect of their respective articular pillars, sending ascending branches to the joint above, and descending branches to the joint below (Bogduk 1982).

The joint capsules and subsynovial loose areolar tissue are richly innervated by nociceptive and mechanoreceptive nerve endings (McLain 1994), thus establishing the neuronal circuitry for proprioception and the transmission of pain impulses.

Central connections

The trigeminocervical nucleus provides the neuronal conduit by which pain from the posterior cranial fossa and the upper cervical structures can be perceived as headache. The nucleus is represented by a continuous column of grey matter containing the pars caudalis of the spinal nucleus of the trigeminal nerve and the apical grey matter of the dorsal horns of the upper three segments of the cervical spinal cord (Bogduk 2001).

Afferents from the upper three cervical spinal nerves and from the spinal tract of the trigeminal nerve converge onto the trigeminocervical nucleus. The trigeminal afferents ramify principally within the upper three cervical cord segments, but may descend as far as C4 (Torvik 1956). Within the nucleus the central terminals of the upper three cervical nerves overlap extensively. In experimental animals, the C2 spinal nerve sends communicating branches to the C1 and C3 segments; the C3 spinal nerve has a similar distribution pattern whilst the C1 spinal nerve is restricted to its own segment (Escolar 1948). This extensive relay system facilitates convergence not only between the cervical afferents (cervicocervical) but also between the cervical and trigeminal (cervico-trigeminal) afferents: this means that pain may be referred between different cervical fields and between cervical and trigeminal fields.

Neurophysiology

Convergence provides the neurophysiological basis by which pain originating in the cervical spine can be perceived as headache. In neurological terms, headache is perceived to arise or occur in a region innervated by nerves other than those that innervate the actual source of pain (International Association for the Study of Pain 1994). In this regard headache is a sensory illusion (Bogduk 1984) and does not imply spinal nerve compression. Within the pars caudalis, the ophthalmic division of the trigeminal nerve extends most caudally and is most densely represented: hence, referred pain is most likely to be perceived as frontal headaches.

Physiological confirmation of convergence has been provided under experimental conditions. In laboratory animals, stimulation of the greater occipital nerve increased the metabolic activity in the ipsilateral caudal brain stem, upper cervical cord, and in the dorsal horn at the level of C1 and C2 (Goadsby et al 1997). This pattern of neural activation was contiguous with the pars caudalis and was in the same distribution when trigeminally innervated structures were stimulated (Goadsby & Hoskin 1997). In human volunteers, ipsilateral headache was produced in the parietal and frontal regions by stimulating the greater occipital nerve. Occasionally, these second order neurons also received input from the contralateral greater occipital nerve and this might explain why primary headaches may be experienced bilaterally (Bartsch & Goadsby 2005, Piovesan et al 2001). In normal volunteers, distending the C2–C3 joint capsule with contrast medium produced headache in the occipital region (Dwyer et al 1990). Because the ophthalmic nerve is most densely represented, referred pain is commonly perceived as frontal headaches; but pain may also be perceived as originating from cutaneous distribution of the maxillary and mandibular divisions of the trigeminal nerve (Bogduk 1984, Goadsby et al 1997, Kerr 1961). Either trigeminal or cervical stimulation can generate central sensitization of the trigeminocervical nucleus, and this may account for the shared clinical features between migraine and cervicogenic headaches (Bartsch & Goadsby 2005, Bogduk 1984, Goadsby et al 1997, Goadsby & Hoskins 1997, Kerr 1961, Piovesan et al 2001).

Clinical features

There are no distinguishing features either in the history, physical examination or imaging studies that are pathognomonic for cervicogenic headaches. The headache is described as having a deep, dull aching quality which may be unilateral or bilateral. Pain emanating from the upper cervical zygapophyseal joints, i.e. the C2–C3 or the C3–C4 joints, is most often felt in the occipital/suboccipital region and may radiate proximally to terminate as frontal headaches: with lateral atlantoaxial joint (C1–C2) pain, frontal or supraorbital headaches are more common (Fig. 5.1). Headaches are usually constant and the variable intensity may be activity dependent. Whilst there are no definitive physical findings diagnostic of cervicogenic headache, tenderness over a painful joint however increases the likelihood (Lord et al 1994).

Not dissimilar to arm pain associated with cardiac ischemia, cervicogenic headache is one

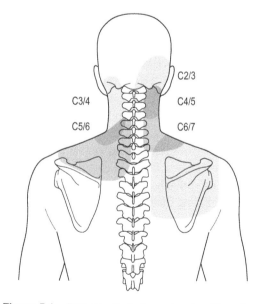

Figure 5.1 • Pain map illustrating pain referral from the cervical zygapophyseal joints.

form of somatic referred pain and does not imply a distinct neurological abnormality. Cervicogenic headache is not a neurological disorder; therefore, altered neurological signs, and electrophysiological or imaging abnormalities should not be expected.

Several studies report that cervicogenic headaches share many clinical features with other forms of primary headaches including drug-induced headaches (Antonaci et al 2001, Fishbain et al 2001, Leone et al 1998, Sanin et al 1994). In one study, not only did the symptoms overlap by as much as 75%, but also drug-induced headache was a common confounder (Sanin et al 1994). Complementary studies confirmed the substantial co-existence of different types of headaches in any one patient and at least 60% were post-traumatic in origin; of these, 84% also complained of neck pain (Fishbain et al 2001). Further, unremitting severe pain, misdiagnosis, and the side effects of medications collectively and severely disrupted the patients' social and vocational goals, accelerated physical deconditioning, and accentuated the levels of psychosocial distress (Fishbain et al 2001).

Radiological investigations are of limited value in the diagnosis of cervicogenic headaches. Morphological features (Fredriksen et al 1989) and range of motion (Zwart 1997) are generally non-specific and show no difference between headache patients and normal subjects (Pfaffenrath et al 1987).

Nevertheless, certain features may be predictive of cervicogenic headaches. These might include history of trauma, localized tenderness and diminished mobility. The pattern of pain referral, commonly of suboccipital origin and parietofrontal radiation may simulate and be similar to patterns generated under experimental conditions (Aprill et al 2002, Dreyfuss et al 1994, Dwyer et al 1990, Fukui et al 1996). Ultimately diagnostic blocks are the only means by which a firm and unambiguous diagnosis can be secured.

Diagnostic nerve blocks

Like the primary headaches, there are no specific biological markers, imaging, or electrophysiological tests for cervicogenic headaches. The diagnosis of cervicogenic headache is only made by isolating a cervical source of pain. Likely sources would be those structures innervated by the upper three cervical nerves, including contents of the posterior cranial fossa (Bogduk & Lord 1998).

Pertinent to cervicogenic headaches, nerve blocks are diagnostic and not therapeutic. The nerve block is a physiological test that determines whether the patient's pain is mediated by the targeted nerve, i.e. one or more of the medial branches of the dorsal rami that innervate the posterior elements of the cervical spine including the intervertebral discs, the zygapophyseal joints, and the posterior neck muscles. Such blocks are advocated once all conventional forms of investigations and treatment have been exhausted, red flags excluded, and the patient remains symptomatic. Because of their physiological mechanism, nerve blocks have biological *plausibility* and thus represent a rational and logical diagnostic utility.

In this regard diagnostic blocks have both face and construct validity. Face validity means that a block actually blocks what it is supposed to block and no other structure. Construct validity reaffirms that the relief of pain can be ascribed to the block and not to some other confounder such as a placebo response. Unlike imaging studies, a diagnostic block addresses the patient's experience of pain. By anesthetizing ('blocking') the actual source of pain or its nerve supply, with minute aliquots of precisely placed local anesthetic, index pain may be eliminated and the source of pain can be inferred.

Patient expectations and observer bias may generate a false positive response of at least 27% if single blocks are relied upon (Barnsley et al 1993a). False-positive blocks can be minimized by using double-blind controlled blocks whereby the patient and the investigator remain blind to the nature of the active agent. However, ethical and logistic considerations will severely limit the usefulness of a conventional 'placebo'/saline block. Additionally, injecting saline increases the likelihood of generating a false-negative response, particularly when investigating the C2–C3 zygapophyseal joint. The TON, which innervates the C2–C3 synovial joint, also has a constant cutaneous distribution over the occiput (Bogduk 1982). Anesthetizing the TON as it crosses the C3 superior articular process will generate a small patch of numbness over the occiput. Whilst headache and/or neck pain may or may not be relieved, occipital numbness should always follow. It is this latter feature that validates the technical efficiency of TON block. Saline does not have this capability: consequently, unblinding and possible false-negative responses will erode the diagnostic accuracy and genuine cases will be missed. It is for these reasons that comparative blocks are preferred.

With comparative blocks two different types of local anesthetics are administered on separate occasions (Barnsley et al 1993b). This utility minimizes both the false positive and false negative responses; the rationale being that the duration of pain relief would be commensurate with the known pharmacological duration of the injectate (Barnsley et al 1993b, Rubin & Lawson 1968, Watt et al 1968). Hence, the patient would obtain short-term relief when a short acting local anesthetic is used (e.g. lignocaine) and longer lasting relief with a long acting agent (e.g. bupivacaine). Comparative blocks may still generate a 12% false positive response (Lord et al 1995) but, conversely, the chance of a false-negative at 46% is also high (Lord et al 1995). Thus comparative blocks may fail to detect a proportion of patients who have the condition and who are not placebo responders.

Diagnostic medial branch nerve blocks have certain advantages over intra-articular blocks. They are easier and safer to perform than intra-articular injections. Unnecessary puncture of sterile joints increases the risk of infection, damages the articular cartilage and provides access for the injectate into the epidural space.

The side effects of nerve blocks are minimal. With third occipital nerve blocks there is loss of proprioception and this may cause slight disequilibrium but nearly all patients recover within 10–15 minutes. A slow injection of extremely small amounts of local anesthetic (0.3 to 0.4 ml) precisely onto the targeted nerve ensures confinement of the injectate to the target area and no other structure is anesthetized (Barnsley & Bogduk 1993).

Nerve blocks and intra-articular injections require special facilities and skills; they must be performed using aseptic technique and under fluoroscopic guidance. For a joint to be deemed symptomatic it should respond consistently to repeated blocks. Failure to do so indicates that the targeted joint may not be the primary source of pain. A block is accepted to be positive only if the patient reports complete pain relief for the entire pharmacological duration of the active agent used. To date, comparative diagnostic blocks are the only means by which a cervical source of pain, and hence headaches, can be identified. Accordingly, the International Headache Society (2004) stipulates controlled diagnostic blocks as an essential and integral pre-requisite for the diagnosis of cervicogenic headaches.

For suspected lateral atlantoaxial (C1–C2) joint pain, intra-articular blocks are performed. Unlike the TON, the technical finesse to selectively and accurately anesthetize the nerves innervating either the lateral or the medial atlantoaxial joints has not been devised. Greater occipital nerve blocks are inappropriate. Distal to the C1–C2 joint, the greater occipital nerve is not known to innervate any of cervical synovial joints. Injecting local anesthetic percutaneously without X-ray guidance may render the scalp numb, but has neither diagnostic nor therapeutic utility.

Of all the potential sources of cervical pain and headaches, only the zygapophyseal joints have been validated scientifically (Bogduk & Lord 1998). As a source of headache, the C2–C3 zygapophyseal joint predominates, with a prevalence ranging between 50% and 70%: the lateral atlantoaxial (C1–C2) joint contributing to a lesser extent (Aprill et al 2002, Govind et al 2005, Lord et al 1994).

Treatment

Contrary to the notion of biological plausibility, the management of headaches of cervical origin has been empirical, symptomatic, and often dissonant with the known neurobiology of somatic referred pain. In some instances headache may be the dominant feature and hence recognising its extracranial origin should alleviate the potential for misdiagnosis and inappropriate treatment.

Non-specific treatment

For headache *per se* there is no known specific medication and the commonly prescribed analgesics, including opioids, exert a modulatory effect at the primary source. Studies that report favorable outcomes with physical therapies are undermined by severe methodological limitations and no study has established any biological correlation between the presumed diagnosis and the mechanism of treatment (Astin & Ernst 2002) though the clinical study by Jull et al (2002) show that patients with chronic cervicogenic headache benefit from spinal mobilization and a specific craniocervical flexion program (see Ch. 15).

Equally, there is no published evidence to advocate the use of epidural steroids or local anesthetics. Although widely publicized, the usefulness of botulinum toxin remains unsubstantiated and its mode of action is dissonant with the known pathophysiology of cervicogenic headache (Evers et al 2002, Sycha et al 2004). The notion of 'muscle spasm' or the 'pain-spasm-pain' cycle in the genesis of headaches has no electrophysiological validation (Mense et al 2001).

In one study, subcutaneous injection of lignocaine and corticosteroid relieved the headaches for a mean duration of 23.5 (range 10–77) days (Anthony 2000). However, the subsequent disequilibrium experienced by some patients implied imprecise needle placement and anesthetization of upper cervical afferents other than just the occipital nerves, as intended. The neural mechanism by which relief was secured was not described.

Specific treatment

C2–C3 zygapophyseal joint headache

Intra-articular steroids. Technically, the intra-articular deposition of an active agent is target specific. In one small-uncontrolled trial, patients who suffered chronic daily headaches and whose headache was completely relieved with diagnostic blocks, had steroids injected into their C2–C3 synovial joints (Slipman et al 2001). Of these, 11% reported total relief of their index pain for as long as 19 months, and in a further 50% headache frequency was reduced to three per month with the latter responding to oral analgesics.

Thermal radiofrequency neurotomy. The one form of treatment that has been most efficacious is thermal or continuous radiofrequency neurotomy (RFN). When precisely executed in properly selected patients, RFN confers complete relief of pain for substantial periods (Fig. 5.2).

Unlike the destructive effects of conventional cautery, the relief of pain with RFN is secured by coagulating the nerve that transmits pain impulses from an identified source. This is achieved by placing the exposed tip of a teflon-covered electrode parallel and adjacent to the target nerve and permitting the passage of a high frequency, low energy current between the exposed tip and the ground plate attached to the patient (International Spine Intervention Society 2004). The current density is greatest around the exposed tip. The intense friction of the protein molecules due to the passage of an alternating current generates sufficient heat

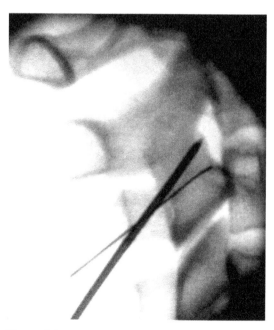

Figure 5.2 • Radiofrequency neurotomy. Electrode placement at the peak of the C3 articular process to coagulate the third occipital nerve at its highest projection.

to coagulate the surrounding tissue, which, in turn incorporates and coagulates the target nerve thereby creating a mechanical barrier to the transmission of pain impulses. Anatomical continuity is retained, neuromas are avoided, and the nerve is able to regenerate. Pain may return and the relief can be reinstated by repeating the procedure.

By controlling the rate of heating, RFN generates well-circumscribed, smooth and regular lesions that are confined to the target area and which ensure long-lasting beneficial effects with no major neurological complications, including Charcot's joints. The procedure is generally performed under local anesthetic.

The only indication for cervical medial branch RFN is the total abolition of the index pain following controlled diagnostic blocks of the target nerve. This caveat is absolute given the unreliability of clinical features (King et al 2007). In patients who are poorly selected, or in whom the procedure is inappropriately administered, RFN will fail (Stovner et al 2004).

One form of cervicogenic headache where RFN has been exceptionally effective is in the management of third occipital headache. It is the one form of cervicogenic headache that has been the most extensively investigated and validated. Third occipital headache or the *Headache of Bogduk* (Edmeads & Soyka 1997) is so named because the headache perceived is mediated by the third occipital nerve (TON), the only nerve that innervates the C2–C3 zygapophyseal joint. To date the latter remains the commonest known source of post-traumatic headache of cervical origin (Govind et al 2005, Lord & Bogduk 1996).

When RFN is executed meticulously and precisely in properly selected patients, some 88% of patients can expect complete relief of their headache for a median duration of 297 days (Govind et al 2003). At the time of publication of this study, some patients enjoyed continuing relief and in those in whom pain had returned, repeating the procedure successfully reinstated complete relief.

Lateral atlantoaxial joint headache

The diagnosis of lateral atlantoaxial (C1–C2) joint pain is secured by controlled intra-articular blocks. Articular branches innervating the lateral C1–C2 joints emanate from the C2 spinal nerve and close to the C2 ganglion (Bogduk 1982). There are no valid means by which a selective nerve block can be safely executed without harming the C2 ganglion. Consequently, intra-articular blocks offer a safer and more precise option.

The treatment for proven lateral atlantoaxial (C1–C2) joint pain is limited to surgical arthrodesis. Observational studies report the complete relief of index pain for as long as seven years (Ghanayem et al 1996, Schaeren & Jeanneret 2005).

Published data in support of any other treatment, including corticosteroids and physical modalities, are lacking. Articular branches that innervate the lateral C1–C2 joints are not accessible for coagulation, and there is no known technique by which thermal radiofrequency can be administered safely and effectively. By its very nature, radiofrequency will severely compromise the viability of the cervical cord, the vertebral artery, the C2 ganglion, and the C2 ventral ramus.

Conclusion

Cervicogenic headache is common and is a type of somatic referred pain, mediated via the trigeminocervical nucleus in the cervical cord. It is the one form of headache that is best understood anatomically and physiologically. A failure to recognize its relevance is often associated with significant pain and suffering. Diagnostic features are sparse and hence the condition is commonly either misdiagnosed or under-diagnosed. Because cervicogenic headache is a form of somatic referred pain, abnormal clinical, neurological, radiological, or electrophysiological findings are unlikely. Controlled diagnostic blocks are the only means by which the diagnosis can be confirmed. For third occipital headache, radiofrequency neurotomy meticulously executed confers total relief of pain for periods greater than three months. Thus diagnostically and therapeutically, the algorithm for the management of third occipital headache, the most common known form of cervicogenic headache, fully satisfies the criteria recently enunciated by the International Headache Society (2004).

References

Anthony M 2000 Cervicogenic headache: prevalence and response to local steroid therapy. Clin Exp Rheumatol 18(suppl 119):S59-S64.

Antonaci F, Ghirmai S, Bono G et al 2001 Cervicogenic headache: evaluation of the original diagnostic data. Cephalalgia 21:573-583.

Aprill C, Axinn MJ, Bogduk N 2002 Occipital headaches stemming from the lateral atlanto-axial (C1–2) joint. Cephalalgia 22:15-22.

Astin JA, Ernst E 2002 The effectiveness of spinal manipulation for the treatment of headache disorders: a systematic review of randomised clinical trials. Cephalalgia 22:617-523.

Barnsley L, Bogduk N 1993 Medial branch blocks are specific for the diagnosis of cervical zygapophyseal joint pain. Reg Anaesth. 18:343-350.

Barnsley L, Lord S, Wallis B et al 1993a False-positive rates of cervical zygapophyseal joint blocks. Clin J Pain 9:124-130.

Barnsley L, Lord S, Bogduk N 1993b Comparative local anaesthetic blocks in the diagnosis of cervical zygapop-hyscal joint pain. Pain 55: 99-106.

Bartsch T, Goadsby PJ 2005 Anatomy and physiology of pain referral patterns in primary and cervicogenic headache disorders. Headache Currents 2:42-48.

Bogduk N 1982 The clinical anatomy of the cervical dorsal rami. Spine 7:319-330.

Bogduk N 1984 The rationale for patterns of neck and back pain. Patient Management 13:17-28.

Bogduk N 2001 Cervicogenic headache: anatomic basis and pathophysiologic mechanisms. Curr Pain Headache Rep 5:382-386.

Bogduk N, Lord SM 1998 Cervical zygapophyseal joint pain. Neurosurg Quarterly 8:107-117.

Bogduk N, Marsland A 1986 On the concept of third occipital headache. J Neurol Neurosurg Psychiatry 49:775-780.

Brain L 1963 Some unsolved problems of cervical spondylosis. BMJ 1:771-777.

Cyriax J 1938 Rheumatic Headache. BMJ 2:1367-1368.

Dreyfuss P, Michaelsen M, Fletcher D 1994 Atlanto-occipital and lateral atlanto-axial joint pain patterns. Spine 19:1125-1131.

Dwyer A, Aprill C, Bogduk N 1990 Cervical zygapophyseal joint pain patterns I. a study in normal volunteers Spine 15:453-457.

Edmeads J 1978 Headaches and head pains associated with diseases of the cervical spine. Med Clin North Amer. 62:533-544.

Edmeads J, Soyka D 1997 Headache associated with disorders of the skull and cervical spine, In: Olesen J, Tfelt-Hansen P, Welch KMA. (eds) The Headaches, Raven Press, New York, pp 741-755.

Ehni G, Benner B 1984 Occipital neuralgia and the C1–2 arthrosis syndrome. J Neurosurg 61: 961-965.

Escolar J 1948 The afferent connections of the 1st, 2nd and 3rd cervical nerves in the cat: an analysis by the Marchi and Rasdolsky methods. J Comp Neurol 89:79-92.

Evers S, Rahmann A, Vollmer-Haase J et al 2002 Treatment of headache with botulinum toxin A: a review according to evidence-based criteria. Cephalalgia 22:699-710.

Fredriksen TA, Foughner R, Teengerund A et al 1989 Cervicogenic headache. Radiological investigations concerning head/neck Cephalalgia 9:139-146.

Fishbain DA, Cutler R, Cole B et al 2001 International Headache Society. Headache Diagnostic Patterns in pain facility patients. Clin J Pain 17: 78-93.

Fukui S, Ohseto H, Shiotani M 1996 Referred pain distribution of the cervical zygapophyseal joints and the cervical dorsal rami. Pain 68:78-73.

Ghanayem AJ, Leventhal M, Bohlman HH 1996 Osteoarthrosis of the atlanto-axial joints: long-term follow-up after treatment with arthrodesis. J Bone Joint Surg Am 78A: 1300-1307.

Goadsby PJ, Hoskin KL 1997 The distribution of trigemino-vascular afferents in the nonhuman primate brain Macaca nemestrina: a c-fos immuno-cytochemical study. J Anat 190:367-375.

Goadsby PJ, Knight YF, Hoskin KL 1997 Stimulation of the greater occipital nerve increases metabolic activity in the trigeminal nucleus caudalis and the central dorsal horn of the cat. Pain 73:23-28.

Govind J, King W, Bailey B, Bogduk N 2003 Radiofrequency neurotomy for the treatment of third occipital headache. J Neurol Neurosurg Psychiatry 74:88-93.

Govind J, King W, Giles P et al 2005 Headache and the cervical zygapophyseal joints (cervicogenic headache). (Orthopaedic Proceedings). J Bone Joint Surg 87B: (suppl III):399-440.

Hadden SB 1940 Neuralgic headache and facial pain. Arch Neurol Psychiatry 43:405-408.

Holmes G 1913 Headaches of organic origin. Practitioner 1:968-984.

International Association for the Study of Pain 1994 In: Mersky H, Bogduk N. (eds) Classification of Chronic Pain, 2nd edn. IASP Press, Seattle, pp 12-1.

International Headache Society 1988 Classification and diagnostic criteria for headache disorders, cranial neuralgias and facial pain Cephalalgia 8 (suppl 7):1-96.

International Headache Society 2004 The International Classification of Headache Disorders, 2nd edn. Cephalalgia 24 (suppl 1):115-116.

International Spinal Intervention Society 2004 Percutaneous radiofrequency cervical medial branch neurotomy. In: Bogduk N (ed) Practice guidelines for spinal diagnostic and treatment procedures. International Spinal Injection Society, San Francisco, pp 249-284.

Jull G, Trott P, Potter H et al 2002 A randomized controlled trial of exercise and manipulative therapy for cervicogenic headache. Spine 27:1835-1843.

Kerr FEL 1961 Structural relation of the trigeminal spinal tract to the upper cervical roots and the solitary nucleus in the cat. Exp. Neurol. 4:134-148.

King W, Lau P, Lees R, Bogduk N 2007 The validity of manual examination in assessing patients with neck pain. Spine Journal 7:22-26.

Leone M, D'Amico D, Grazzi L et al 1998 Cervicogenic Headache: a critical review of the current diagnostic criteria. Pain 78:1-5.

Lord SM, Bogduk N 1996 The cervical synovial joint as a source of post-traumatic headache. J Musculoskel Pain 4:81-94.

Lord SM, Barnsley L, Wallis BJ et al 1994 Third occipital headache: prevalence study. J Neurol Neurosurg Psychiatry 57:1187-1190.

Lord SM, Barnsley L, Bogduk N 1995 The utility of comparative local anaesthetic blocks versus placebo-controlled blocks for the diagnosis of cervical zygapophyseal joint pain. Clin J Pain 11:208-213.

McLain R 1994 Mechanoreceptor endings in human cervical facet joints. Spine 19:495-501.

Mense S, Simons DG, Russell IJ 2001 Muscle pain. Understanding its nature, diagnosis and treatment. Lippincott Williams and Wilkins, Philadelphia, pp 62-83.

Pentecost SP, Adriani J 1955 The use of cervical plexus block in the diagnosis and management of atypical cephalalgia of cervical origin. Anesthesiology 16:726-732.

Perelson HN 1947 Occipital nerve tenderness: a sign of headache. South Med J. 40:653-656.

Pfaffenrath V, Dandekar R, Pollman W 1987 Cervicogenic headache—the clinical picture, radiological findings and hypotheses on its pathophysiology. Headache 27:495-499.

Piovesan EJ, Kowacs PA, Tatsui CE et al 2001 Referred pain after painful stimulation of the greater occipital nerve in humans: evidence of convergence of cervical afferents on the trigeminal nuclei. Cephalalgia 21:107-109.

Rubin AP, Lawson DIF 1968 A controlled trial of bupivacaine. A comparison with lignocaine. Anaesthesia 23:327-330.

Sackett DL, Haynes RB, Guyatt GH et al 1991 Clinical epidemiology. A basic science for clinical medicine, 2nd edn. Little Brown and Company, Boston.

Sanin LC, Mathew NT, Bellmeyer LR et al 1994 The International Headache Society (IHS) Headache Classification as applied to a headache clinic population. Cephalalgia 14:443-444.

Schaeren S, Jeanneret B 2005 Atlantoaxial osteoarthritis: case series and review of the literature. Eur Spine J 14:501-506.

Sjaastad O, Saunte C, Hovdahl H et al 1983 'Cervicogenic' headache. A hypothesis. Cephalalgia 3:249-256.

Sjaastad O, Fredriksen TA, Pfaffenrath V 1998 Cervicogenic headache: diagnostic criteria. Headache 38: 442-445.

Slipman CW, Lipetz JS, Plastara C et al 2001 Therapeutic zygapophyseal joint injections for headache emanating from the C2–3 joint. Am J Phy Med Rehabil 80: 182-188.

Star MJ, Curd JG, Thorne P 1992 Atlantoaxial lateral mass osteoarthritis: a frequently overlooked cause of severe occipitocervical pain. Spine 17 (suppl 6) S71-S76.

Stovner LJ, Kolstad F, Helde G 2004 Radiofrequency denervation of the facet joints, C2–C6 in cervicogenic headache: a randomised double blind sham study. Cephalalgia 24:821-830.

Sycha T, Kranz G, Auff E. et al 2004 Botulinum toxin in the treatment of rare head and neck pain syndromes: a systematic review of the literature. J Neurol 251(suppl 1): 1/19-1/30.

Torvik A 1956 Afferent connections to the sensory trigeminal nuclei, the nucleus of the solitary tract and adjacent structures. J Comp Neurol. 106:51-141.

Trevor-Jones R 1964 Osteoarthritis of the paravertebral joints of the second and third cervical vertebrae as a cause of occipital headaches. S. Afr. Med J.38:392-394.

Watt MJ, Ross DM, Atkinson RS 1968 A double-blind trial of bupivacaine and lignocaine. Anaesthesia 23:331-337.

Zwart JA 1997 Neck mobility in different headache disorders. Headache 37:6-11.

Chapter Six

6

Sleep structure, bruxism and headache

Norman Thie, Pablo Kimos, Gilles Lavigne and Paul Major

Sleep bruxism may be associated with temporomandibular disorders and headache. In this chapter the authors, dental and orofacial pain researchers, critically evaluate the literature investigating the links between sleep bruxism, temporomandibular disorders and headache with emphasis on the role of altered sleep structure in precipitating or maintaining particular headache types.

Orofacial pain includes temporomandibular disorders (TMD), neuropathic pain, and some forms of headaches. Sleep bruxism (SB), an involuntary motor activity during sleep associated with tooth grinding, may be related to temporomandibular joint problems including joint sounds or movement limitation and myofascial pain of the jaw and neck muscles (Bader et al 1997, Dao et al 1994, Kampe et al 1997 a & b, Lobbezoo & Lavigne 1997, Magnusson et al 2000). Currently, in sleep medicine sleep bruxism is classified into the group of 'movement sleep-related disorders' (American Academy of Sleep Medicine 2005). It is common for patients with SB who present to a TMD/ Orofacial Pain Clinic to report headaches and it has been identified that up to 70% of patients in TMD clinics report headache-related complaints (Zarb et al 1994).

A recent attempt (Woda et al 2005) to revise the taxonomy of chronic orofacial pain in relation to sign and symptom commonalities, revealed three clusters:

1. Neuralgia: trigeminal and post-traumatic

2. Neurovascular and tension-type: tension-type headache, migraine and cluster headache

3. Persistent idiopathic orofacial pain: atypical facial pain or undifferentiated orofacial pain, arthromyalgia and stomatodynia.

Headache classification was recently revised and simplified, at least for headaches not associated with a traumatic event or medical condition, with primary headaches divided into four major categories: migraine, tension-type headaches, cluster and other autonomic cephalgias and other primary headaches (Headache Classification Subcommittee of The International Headache Society 2004). It is important to mention that headache may also be associated with respiratory sleep disorders such as a limitation of airflow (upper airway resistance syndrome, UARS) or cessation of breathing (sleep apnea) (Gold et al 2003).

To our knowledge, there is a paucity of prospective studies that address the cause-and-effect relationship between headaches and sleep bruxism (SB). Most of the information available comes from case reports, expert opinion, case-control studies or epidemiological surveys. Correlation analyses from these studies suggest that SB may be a risk factor in the initiation or maintenance of some forms of headache, but do not support a cause and effect relationship. Interestingly, there are some studies that suggest that sustained muscle activity, such as clenching, may trigger orofacial pain of muscular and joint origin (Arima et al 1999, Clark et al 1991, Glaros & Burton 2004, Svensson & Arendt-Nielsen 1996). It should be noted that most of these studies were done with normal subjects who clenched their teeth for a certain time during wakefulness but not during sleep. Furthermore, because SB is usually characterized by rhythmic jaw muscle contraction and not clenching, the extrapolation of these findings to a SB population may not be valid (Jensen & Olesen 1996, Lavigne et al 1996, Plesh et al 1998).

The aim of this chapter is to provide a critical review of the literature on sleep-related bruxism and headaches to aid clinicians in developing definitive diagnosis, management and referral strategies. The chapter is divided into five sections. The first provides a general background on sleep and bruxism. The second provides details on SB diagnosis. The third focuses on the literature that reports on headaches and SB. The fourth discusses sleep-related and morning headaches. The final section provides a summary and criteria for differential diagnosis, management and referral strategies.

Sleep structure and bruxism

Sleep structure

Sleep is a state of conscious disengagement from the environment that may include conditions such as sleep-walking, sleep-talking, and tooth grinding (SB) (Carskadon & Dement 2005). Sleep duration is between 6 and 9 hours in most healthy persons over a 24-hour circadian rhythm. Sleep architecture is divided into two major periods: non-rapid eye movement (nonREM) followed by rapid eye movement (REM) (Fig. 6.1). The nonREM and REM sleep

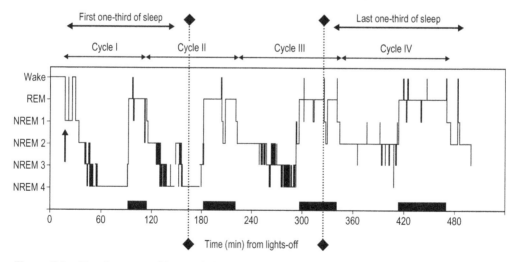

Figure 6.1 ● Sleep hypnogram (histogram) of a normal 23-year-old subject with 4 sleep cycles. Small vertical arrowhead indicates when sleep initiated after lights out. Note the dominance of stages 3 and 4 of nonREM in the first one-third of sleep compared to REM dominance (thick horizontal bars on time axis) in the last one-third of sleep. nonREM is usually 75–80% of sleep, REM sleep usually 20–25% and wakefulness usually less than 5% of sleep.

periods are repeated every 70–120 minutes and three to five times per sleep period; they are known as the ultradian sleep cycles. NonREM sleep is further subdivided into four stages. Stages 1 and 2 are considered to be light sleep stages, a period associated with most body movements and SB; while stages 3 and 4 are deep sleep stages associated with a 'sleep recovery effect' (Kato et al 2003a). REM sleep covers 20–25% of total sleep time and is characterized by fast low-voltage cortical electro-encephalographic (EEG) activity, phasic eye movements, rapid heart rate and profound muscle relaxation (Kato et al 2003a, Lavigne et al 2003). REM sleep can be sub-divided in phasic or tonic (less eye rolling) phases. While nonREM sleep stages 3 and 4 are characterized by a dominance of slow EEG activity (slow wave activity) most notable in the first third of the sleep period, REM sleep is characterized by fast EEG waves that predominate during the last third (early morning hours) of the total sleep cycle. Under the above described circadian (24-hour shift of wake and sleep) and ultradian (nonREM and REM repetition) sleep oscillations, sleep is characterized by cyclic reactivation, every 20–40 seconds, of the brain and autonomic (cardiorespiratory) systems. These last for 3–10 seconds and act to provide the sleeping individual an indication of the body's external surroundings to readjust body temperature, heart and respiratory rate. These rapid and transient reactivations are named sleep micro-arousals (differentiated from awakenings); they are part of the micro-structure of sleep architecture and are repeated at a rate ranging from 12–20 times per hour of sleep (Terzano et al 2002). A good way to remember their role is to see these microarousals as physiological 'sentinels' that prepare a 'sleeping' brain for transient physiological adjustments to preserve sleep continuity or to initiate an awake reaction if bodily threat is perceived. In

this way then, the brain filters the external milieu and makes instant adjustments of its internal functions during sleep; these oscillations are named the cyclic alternating pattern (CAP). When microarousals repeat too frequently, the CAP is in an active phase with a high probability of arousal from sleep; conversely, when the brain is more quiescent, EEG activity is reduced and heart and respiratory rates lower to preserve sleep continuity (Parrino et al 2006). In a sleep laboratory, most SB episodes are observed on sleep traces during the active phase of the CAP, specifically sleep stages 2 or 1 of nonREM (Lavigne et al 2005a).

Bruxism

The term 'bruxism' has been used to describe the gnashing and grinding of teeth for no apparent reason. Bruxism during wakefulness is usually a semi-voluntary mandibular activity, generally with no associated sounds (Bader & Lavigne 2000, Lavigne et al 2003) and needs to be distinguished from SB, which was formerly classified as a parasomnia – a disorder intruding or occurring during sleep (Thorpy 1997). As stated previously, this classification has recently changed and SB is now considered an oromotor movement disorder occurring during sleep (Thorpy 2005).

Sleep bruxism is present in approximately 8% of adults, tends to decrease with age, and does not appear to have a significant gender bias (Lavigne & Montplaisir 1994, Ohayon et al 2001). The pattern of inheritance of SB is unknown and the influence of familial and environmental factors requires study (Lavigne et al 2005a). In the absence of a medical cause, SB is considered to be primary or idiopathic, whereas SB associated with a medical condition may be considered secondary, as in medical and psychiatric conditions, or iatrogenic, as in drug withdrawal (Lavigne et al 2005a). In young adult SB subjects, more than 80% of SB episodes occur during sleep stages 1 and 2 of nonREM and approximately 5–10% in REM (Huynh et al 2006a, Lavigne et al 2005a). Interestingly, 74% of SB episodes are observed to occur in the supine position, a sleep position in which airway obstruction is frequently observed in patients with obstructive sleep apnea (OSA) (Lavigne et al 2005a).

The etiology of SB is not completely understood but is believed to be multifactorial and probably the product of biologic and psychosocial influences (Lavigne et al 2005a). Currently, three etiological explanations have been proposed: peripheral factors, central factors, and psychological influences – e.g. life stress and anxiety (Ohayon et al 2001, Lavigne et al 2005a). Current research tends to consider SB as a centrally-mediated process related to sleep micro-arousals (Kato et al 2001a, 2003b, Lobbezoo & Naeije 2001, Macaluso et al 1998) (Fig. 6.2). Neurotransmitters may be involved in the genesis of characteristic rhythmic jaw movements

and the modulation of muscle tone during sleep (Ellison & Stanziani 1993, Lavigne et al 2003, Lobbezoo & Naeije 2001, Lobbezoo et al 1997 a & b, 2001, Por et al 1996, Winocur et al 2003). Tooth contact in SB is the last in a sequence of physiological events that are likely to occur in the following order:

1. Increase in autonomic cardiac activity 4 to 8 minutes preceding tooth grinding or phasic jaw muscle contractions (this rise is prevented with clonidine pre-treatment).

2. Increase in cortical activity (alpha waves) 4 seconds before SB.

3. Increase in cardiac rhythm 1 second before SB.

4. Increase in suprahyoid muscle tone (probably involved in jaw opening or airway patency) 0.8 seconds before SB.

5. Onset of activity of jaw-closer muscle (phasic muscle contractions – termed rhythmic masticatory muscle activity) with possible tooth grinding (Lavigne et al 2005a, Huynh et al 2006a).

The association of SB with sleep microarousal is also supported by findings from other laboratories (Bader et al 1997, Macaluso et al 1998).

Clinical diagnosis

Initial recognition of SB may be reliably based on a sleep partner's complaints of tooth grinding or occasionally tooth tapping. To a lesser extent the patient may be aware of jaw clenching during sleep or upon awakening, tooth sensitivity to cold or warm stimuli (e.g. food, liquid, oral respiration), jaw pain or tenderness or temporal headache on awakening. In our laboratory definitive diagnosis of SB is made through polysomnographic studies. It can also be established in the home environment using ambulatory systems, preferably with audio-video signals to rule out other oromotor

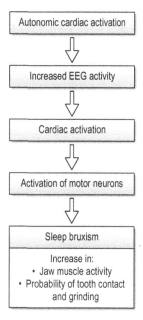

Figure 6.2 ● Physiological sequence of events in sleep bruxism genesis.

movements such as swallowing, smiling, chewing or orofacial myoclonia that can represent up to 30% of non specific oromandibular activities during sleep. Unfortunately, these studies are complex, not readily available, time-consuming, and expensive. Consequently, diagnosis generally relies on clinical observations and patient history. The clinical predictors and differential diagnoses for SB are outlined in Table 6.1 (Kato et al 2001b, Lavigne et al 1999, 2005a).

Headache and sleep bruxism

When an evidence-based approach is applied to the literature, we find that there are very few studies that have found a causal relationship between SB and headache and there are no randomized control trials (RCT) or cohort studies in this area (Table 6.2). A case-controlled study (Macfarlane et al 2001) represents the highest level of evidence in this area to date, however, the study did not specifically address headache but rather a relationship between SB and pain dysfunction syndrome (PDS). The authors did report frequent headaches as a part of PDS. Of the five case series published, three reported a relationship between headache and SB (Kampe et al 1997 a & b, Miller et al 2003); the other two did not (Magnusson et al 2000, Watanabe et al 2003). The survey of three expert opinions described SB as a common finding in patients with headaches but also as a cause of headaches (Bailey 1990, Biondi 2001, Rugh & Harlan 1988).

Sleep-related and morning headaches

The lifetime prevalence of headache in the general adult population is 85–95% (Biondi 2001). Headaches are classified as primary or secondary: primary headaches are those which are not a result of structural abnormalities or disease; secondary headaches are those resulting from an underlying pathologic process (Biondi 2001). As mentioned earlier, there is no RCT to support an association between SB and headache pain. A similar lack of RCT is evident within the literature pertaining to a cause and effect relationship between bruxism and headache during wakefulness (Kampe et al 1997a, Molina et al 1997). Molina et al (1997) have reported that approximately two-thirds of bruxism patients report headache pain, Hamada et al (1982) reported that approximately 90% of bruxism subjects have headaches and Yustin et al (1993) reported approximately 60% of bruxism subjects have headaches and neck pain. With a SB patient population spanning from 23 to 67 years of age, 65% reported morning headache (Bader et al 1997).

How sleep affects headache has been of interest to health care providers and researchers for years. For instance, in a clinical setting, patients may report that sleep terminates their headache attack (e.g. migraine headache), their headache may awaken them in the middle of the night (e.g. cluster headache), or they may awaken in the morning with headache (e.g. OSA, SB). According to the International Classification of Sleep Disorders, primary headaches that are sleep-related include: migraine and cluster headache, tension-type headache, chronic paroxysmal hemicrania (CPH), hypnic headaches (Thorpy 2005) and headache stemming from other medical conditions.

Migraine and cluster headache

Patients with migraine and cluster headache may report headache attacks occurring during sleep (Culebras 2005). The onset of nocturnal migraine has been associated with an abrupt decline of serotonin levels during REM sleep (Dexter & Weitzman 1970, Biondi 2001, Rasmussen 1993). Cluster headache has been linked to REM stage and sleeping in, and is characterized by severe

Table 6.1 Clinical predictors and differential diagnosis of SB.

Clinical predictors of SB	Clinical consideration and differential diagnosis
Grinding or tapping sounds reported by bed partner	Sleep bruxism Other sounds caused by other orofacial movements (e.g. temporomandibular joint clicking, throat grunting)
Dental wear facets	Sleep bruxism Coarse diet Acidic diet Past dental restorative work Tooth wear due to normal aging
Fractures in teeth and/or dental restorations	Sleep bruxism Coarse diet (e.g. popcorn kernels) Occlusal trauma
Tooth mobility	Sleep bruxism Periodontal disease or occlusal trauma independent of SB
Tooth discomfort or sensitivity upon waking	Sleep bruxism Dental or periodontal problems independent of SB
Masticatory muscle pain upon waking	Sleep bruxism Chronic masticatory myalgia or facial pain independent of SB Localized myofascial pain Fibromyalgia or widespread pains
Masseter hypertrophy	Sleep bruxism Inflammatory swellings Tumor Parotid-masseter syndrome (blockade of parotid ducts by sustained contraction of the masseter muscle – characterized by: episodic swelling, pain, inflammation, and abnormal mouth dryness
TMJ locking and clicking upon waking	Sleep bruxism TMJ disc adherences or displacement TMJ disc displacement, independent of SB
Waking headache	Sleep bruxism Sleep apnea and/or upper airway resistance syndrome (limitation or cessation of airflow with daytime sleepiness = medical hazard) Insomnia (greater than 20 minutes required to fall asleep or difficulty resuming sleep if waking during the night) Raised intracranial pressure
Tongue and/or cheek indentation	Sleep bruxism Tongue pushing

Table 6.2 Literature evaluating a possible relationship between SB and headaches.

Authors	Study design	EBM level*	Conclusion
Rugh & Harlan 1988	Expert opinion	5	Temporal tension headaches are an effect of SB due to excessive temporal muscle contraction.
Bailey 1990	Expert opinion	5	Headaches are a common finding in SB patients.
Kampe et al 1997a	Case series n = 29 Patient survey for reported symptoms and health history	4	A statistically significant correlation between headaches and SB was found.
Kampe et al 1997b	Case series n = 29 Personality inventory (Karolinska Scales of Personalities)	4	A statistically significant correlation between headaches and SB was found.
Magnusson et al 2000	Case series n = 135 Clinical examination and questionnaire	4	Weak and non-significant correlation was found between headaches and oral parafunction, including SB.
Biondi 2001	Expert opinion	5	SB can cause headaches, which are muscular in origin.
Macfarlane et al 2001	Case control n = 317 Questionnaire collecting socio-demographic, mechanical and psychological factors	3a	Frequent headaches are part of the pain dysfunction syndrome (PDS). Nocturnal teeth grinding was significantly associated with PDS.
Miller et al 2003	Case series n = 118 Children's Sleep Habits Questionnaire and standardized questionnaire for headache characteristics	4	The frequency of migraines is positively related to SB.
Watanabe et al 2003	Case series n = 12 Correlation between a telemetric system to monitor SB and patient's rating of symptoms	4	Headache pain or sleep disturbances were not found to be related to SB.

*Levels of evidence for etiology/harm (Oxford Centre for Evidence-based Medicine): 1a. Systematic review of randomized controlled studies (RCT); 1b. Individual RCT (with narrow confidence interval); 2a. Systematic review of cohort studies; 2b. Individual cohort studies (including low-quality RCT; e.g., < 80% follow up); 2c. 'Outcomes' research; ecologic studies; 3a. Systematic review of case control studies; 3b. Individual case control study; 4. Case series (and poor-quality cohort and case control studies); 5. Expert opinion without explicit critical appraisal, or based on physiology, bench research, or 'proof of principle study'.

unilateral temporal, malar and periorbital pain with associated features of forehead perspiration, nasal congestion, lacrimation and rhinorrhea (Culebras 2005). Interestingly, a recent report estimated that a diagnosis of sleep apnea is 8.8 times more likely in cluster headache patients when compared to controls and that a body mass index of over 25 kg/m^2 and an age greater than 40 years increase the risk of OSA by 24 and 13 times respectively (Nobre et al 2005). Hypoxemia has been postulated as a headache trigger in cluster headache patients when morning headache is reported, although there is debate on whether the duration of hypoxemia relates to headache complaints in sleep apnea patients (Chervin et al 2000, Greenough et al 2002).

Tension-type headache

Tension-type headaches related to sleep disorders tend to be present on morning waking (Bader et al 1997, Kampe et al 1997a). They may be episodic or chronic and characterized by pressing, aching, non-pulsating pain. Sleep disorders related to this type of headache are reported to include sleep apnea, SB, insomnias, parasomnias, UARS and periodic limb movement disorder (Biondi 2001, Guilleminault et al 2005, Kayed & Sjaastad 1985, Poceta 2003).

The sleep quality of patients with tension-type headaches is frequently reported to be poor during headache periods (Jennum & Jensen 2002). Interestingly, experimental studies in humans have shown that nitric oxide (NO) may play a critical role in initiating primary headaches and a recent study suggests that infusion of glyceryl trinitrate (a nitric oxide donor) may trigger the production of NO in patients with chronic tension-type headache (Ashina et al 2004). Further research is required to elucidate whether this molecule influences the sleep quality of patients with chronic headache complaints.

In a recent study, headache was reported by 48% and 49% of patients with a definitive diagnosis of insomnia and OSA respectively; and in OSA patients the headaches had a tension-type pattern (Alberti et al 2005). Morning headaches lasting < 2 hours occurred in 74% of the patients with OSA, compared to 40% of insomnia patients. Patients with morning headache also showed greater oxygen desaturation ($SaO_2 = 82.5\%$) than patients without headache ($SaO_2 = 86.1\%$), but interestingly REM sleep and total sleep time under desaturation ($SaO_2 < 90\%$) was similar in both groups (Greenough et al 2002, Alberti et al 2005). An additional study (Gold et al 2003) found headache symptoms in 15–25% of patients with mild to severe OSA and in slightly greater than 50% of patients with UARS. Moreover, the prevalence of SB

was also slightly greater than 50% in patients with UARS and the general prevalence of SB was greatest in UARS patients compared to those patients with mild to severe OSA (Gold et al 2003).

Chronic paroxysmal hemicrania and hypnic headache

Chronic paroxysmal hemicrania is considered a variant of cluster headache with attacks in close association with REM sleep (Culebras 2005) and responds quasi-specifically to the nonsteroidal anti-inflammatory drug indomethacin. Hypnic headache is an uncommon, benign headache that only occurs during sleep and affects an elderly population (Biondi 2001, Culebras 2005, Mahowald & Schenck 1996, Poceta 2003). Headache episodes can occur 15 times per month for at least one month and, unlike cluster headache and CPH, occurs as a diffuse headache pain in two-thirds of patients (Culebras 2005). There may be associated nausea and most patients do not have autonomic symptoms (e.g. lacrimation, rhinorrhea, nasal congestion).

Other medical conditions and headache

Sleep-related or morning headaches can commonly be secondary to insomnia, medication and/or alcohol abuse, mental stress, post-traumatic and respiratory disturbances (Jennum & Jensen 2002). A recent European study revealed that morning headaches were more frequent in patients with concomitant depression, using anxiolytic medications for insomnia, and those patients with circadian rhythm and sleep-related breathing disorders (Ohayon 2004). Inspiratory airflow limitations may play a key role in the development of somatic complaints in fibromyalgia patients such as widespread body pain and tenderness, sleep-maintenance and sleep onset insomnia and headaches (Gold et al 2004).

Other headaches that may occur during sleep and cause awakening, although rare, include hemicrania horologica, or 'exploding head syndrome' (once called 'snapping of the brain') intracranial tumor or abscess, cerebrospinal fluid obstruction, subarachnoid hemorrhage and cerebrovascular ischemia or stroke (Biondi 2001, Culebras 2005). It should be noted that neurologic conditions with brain damage from infectious or demyelinating encephalitides, multiple sclerosis and traumatic brain injuries may also alter sleep (Culebras 2005). There are also reported cases of referred headaches and facial pain originating from cardiovascular ischemia (Durso et al 2003, Lipton et al 1997) and there have been 32 reported cases of patients with lung tumors, of which nine had pain referral to the temporal skull areas and six cases with pain referral to the orbital area (Sarlani et al 2003).

Referral and management strategies

From the differential diagnoses provided in Table 6.3, headaches not secondary to SB require referral or collaboration with:

- A neurologist if the headaches are of cluster, CPH, hypnic, migraine types, or facial pain of a neurological origin (e.g. trigeminal neuralgia);
- A sleep clinic if a respiratory disorder is suspected. This may include: sleep partner report of cessation of breathing, daytime sleepiness, memory problems, physical examination revealing large neck and long palate with macroglossia, hypertension, patient reports of restless legs and limb movements during sleep, if sleep onset is delayed by more than

Table 6.3 Patient symptoms and differential diagnosis.

Patient reported symptoms	Differential diagnosis
Headache upon waking	Poor quality of sleep due to other sleep disorders (e.g. sleep apnea, insomnia, UARS Sleep bruxism Myofascial pain Chronic or recurrent tension-type headache independent from SB Fibromyalgia or widespread pains
Nocturnal headache and/or facial pain	Chronic or recurrent tension-type headaches independent from SB Sleep bruxism Migraine Cluster headache Chronic paroxysmal hemicrania Hypnic headache Myofascial pain independent from SB Fibromyalgia or widespread pains

30 minutes or if sleep cannot be resumed in the middle of a sleep period;

- A dentist for an occlusal splint if tooth grinding and headaches are not related to sleep respiratory disorders. Mandibular advancement devices (MAD) may be indicated for patients with snoring or mild to moderate OSA, who prefer them to continuous positive airway pressure (CPAP) therapy, who do not respond to or fail attempts with CPAP therapy, or are not appropriate candidates for CPAP therapy (Kushida et al 2006);
- A rheumatologist if widespread pains such as in fibromyalgia or systemic inflammatory disease are suspected to be contributing to symptoms;
- An allergist if breathing is affected by allergens;
- An ear, nose and throat specialist if nasal or sinus pathology is identified or suspected.

Immediate referral to a hospital emergency department is required if patients report headache pain that is unremitting, progressive and worsening, with symptoms including the first or worst-ever headache experienced, unremitting fever, nausea or vomiting, confusion, fatigue or neck stiffness (Culebras 2005).

Once other causes have been excluded, the management of sleep bruxism related headaches may involve a number of strategies.

1. Mild cases without sleep related breathing disorder. Home relaxation exercises (imagery, abdominal breathing), stress management, lifestyle changes, avoidance of large meals and alcohol in the evenings, improvement in sleep hygiene and sleep environment (proper temperature, low or no light, minimal noise etc.) may be utilized. However, there is a lack of controlled studies to support their efficacy. Medication can be used to reduce sleep-related anxiety causing insomnia, including anxiolytic medications (e.g. a small dose of clonazepam for short term periods) or hypnotic medications (e.g. zaleplon, zolpidem, zopiclone). These may be used for short periods of time if patients are informed that excessive daytime sleepiness may occur. The benefit of headache-related medication (e.g. topiramate, triptans) remains to be demonstrated in RCTs with objective sleep and respiratory measures (Brousseau et al 2003, Lampl et al 2006, Lavigne et al 2005a,b, 2006, Saletu et al 2005, Stepanski & Wyatt 2003).

2. Where limitation or cessation of airflow during sleep is present (Bondemark & Lindman 2000, Cistulli et al 2004, Ferguson & Lowe 2005, Gagnon et al 2004, Gotsopoulos et al 2004, Kushida et al 2006, Landry et al 2006, Lindberg et al 2006, Oksenberg & Arons 2002), a MAD may be prescribed for use in patients with primary snoring and mild to moderate OSA, in those patients that have not responded to CPAP therapy, prefer a MAD, or are not the appropriate candidates for CPAP therapy. As recommended by the American Academy of Dental Sleep Medicine and the sleep medicine guidelines developed by the American Academy of Sleep Medicine, the efficacy and safety of such devices need to be determined with polysomnography or a Type 3 sleep study in the months following treatment initiation. Furthermore, long-term follow-up with dental appliances is required to monitor patient adherence, appliance fit and integrity and patient signs and symptoms of worsening OSA.

Patients may expect a 50% reduction in headache symptoms, diastolic blood and SB when using a MAD. Although CPAP therapy is the gold standard treatment for sleep apnea in patients with morning headache, its use in patients with SB has only been reported in one severe apneic case. However, compliance may be a problem in SB patients since it has been observed in our sleep laboratory that most severe SB cases without headache remove the facial mask used for CPAP therapy during their sleep due to factors such as discomfort, mask pressure, air dryness, hoses that limit body movements. There are no firm data on long-term compliance for patients with severe SB who utilize a MAD. Where sleep apnea is present, caution is advised when using occlusal splint appliances as respiratory disturbance indices may be adversely affected.

3. There are also new avenues of treatment available (Huynh et al 2006b, Kast 2005, Pirelli et al 2004, Powell et al 2005, Saletu et al 2005). In patients with SB, clonidine (an alpha agonist), used to assess the mechanism of SB in a randomized polygraphic study (not a drug efficacy and safety study), was shown to reduce the muscle contractions during SB by 60%, although 20% of patients subsequently had severe hypotension lasting several hours after waking. Thus, the efficacy and safety of cardioactive medications in the clinical management of SB and related headache remains to be demonstrated. In a self report case series study, tiagabine (a gamma-aminobutyric acid uptake inhibitor) was reported to reduce bruxism associated with temporomandibular pain. The long-term efficacy/safety ratio using clonazepam, (a benzodiazepine with addiction potential) needs to be established before final recommendations can be made. A potential new avenue is orthognathic surgery (e.g. palatal expansions, mandibular advancement) that may be a more permanent alternative for patients with persistent morning headache related to sleep respiratory disturbances.

Conclusion

It is important to consider SB as a factor contributing to headache even though current literature displays a weak causal relationship. Nonetheless, signs and symptoms such as jaw clenching and facial tightness on waking, tooth wear or thermal sensitivity, headaches, and reports of tooth grinding are important indicators of SB. Sleep-related headaches include tension-type headache, migraine and cluster headache, but sleep time respiratory disturbances (e.g. sleep apnea) should not be overlooked. The influence of respiratory variables, such as sleep apnea, on SB and future treatment options await research and recommendations in this exciting and expanding field of health care.

References

Alberti A, Mazzotta G, Gallinella E et al 2005 Headache characteristics in obstructive sleep apnea syndrome and insomnia. Acta Neurologica Scandinavica 111:309-316

American Academy of Sleep Medicine 2005 The International classification of sleep disorders: Diagnostic and coding manual, 2nd edn. Westchester, Illinois

Arima T, Svensson P, Arendt-Nielsen L 1999 Experimental grinding in healthy subjects: a model for post exercise jaw muscle soreness? Journal of Orofacial Pain 13:104-114

Ashina M, Simonsen H, Bendtsen et al 2004 Glyceryl trinitrate may trigger endogenous nitric oxide production in patients with chronic tension-type headache. Cephalalgia 24:967-972

Bader G, Lavigne G 2000 Sleep bruxism; an overview of an oromandibular sleep movement disorder. Sleep Medicine Reviews 4:27-43

Bader G G, Kampe T, Tagdae T et al 1997 Descriptive physiological data on a sleep bruxism population. Sleep 20:982-990

Bailey D R 1990 Tension headache and bruxism in the sleep disordered patient. Cranio 8:174-182

Biondi D M 2001 Headaches and their relationship to sleep. Dental Clinics of North America 45: 685-700

Bondemark L, Lindman R 2000 Craniomandibular status and function in patients with habitual snoring and obstructive sleep apnoea after nocturnal treatment with a mandibular advancement splint: a 2-year follow-up. European Journal of Orthodontics 22:53-60

Brousseau M, Manzini C, Thie N M R et al 2003 Understanding and managing the interaction between sleep and pain: An update for the dentist. Journal of the Canadian Dental Association 69:437-442

Carskadon M A, Dement W C 2005 Normal human sleep: an overview. In: Kryger M H, Roth T, Dement W C (eds) Principles and practice of sleep medicine, 4th edn. Elsevier Saunders, Philadelphia, p 13-23

Chervin R D, Zallek S N, Lin X et al 2000 Sleep disordered breathing in patients with cluster headache. Neurology 54:2302-2306

Cistulli P A, Gotsopoulos H, Marklund M et al 2004 Treatment of snoring and obstructive sleep apnea with mandibular repositioning appliances. Sleep Medicine Reviews 8:443-457

Clark G T, Adler R C, Lee J J 1991 Jaw pain and tenderness levels during and after repeated sustained maximum voluntary protrusion. Pain 45:17-22

Culebras A 2005 Other neurological disorders. In: Kryger M H, Roth T, Dement W C (eds) Principles and practice of sleep medicine, 4th edn. Elsevier Saunders, Philadelphia, p 879-888

Dao T T, Lund J P, Lavigne G J 1994 Comparison of pain and quality of life in bruxers and patients with myofascial pain of the masticatory muscles. Journal of Orofacial Pain 8:350-366

Dexter J D, Weitzman E D 1970 The relationship of nocturnal headaches to sleep stage patterns. Neurology 20:513-518

Durso B C, Israel M S, Janini M E et al 2003 Orofacial pain of cardiac origin: a case report. Cranio 21:152-153

Ellison J M, Stanziani P 1993 SSRI-associated nocturnal bruxism in four patients. Journal of Clinical Psychiatry 54:432-434

Ferguson K A, Lowe A A 2005 Oral appliances for sleep disordered breathing. In: Kryger M H, Roth T, Dement W C (eds) Principles and practice of sleep medicine, 4th edn. Elsevier Saunders, Philadelphia, p 1098-1108

Gagnon Y, Mayer P, Morisson F et al 2004 Aggravation of respiratory disturbances by the use of an occlusal splint in apneic patients: A Pilot Study. International Journal of Prosthodontics 7:447-453

Glaros A G, Burton E 2004 Parafunctional clenching, pain, and effort in temporomandibular disorders. Journal of Behavioral Medicine 27:91-100

Gold A R, Dipalo F, Gold M S et al 2003 The symptoms and signs of upper airway resistance syndrome: A link to the functional somatic syndromes. Chest 123:87-95

Gold A R, Dipalo F, Gold M S et al 2004 Inspiratory airflow dynamics during sleep in women with fibromyalgia. Sleep 27:459-466

Gotsopoulos H, Kelly J J, Cistulli P A 2004 Oral appliance therapy reduces blood pressure in obstructive sleep apnea: a randomized, controlled trial. Sleep 27:934-941

Greenough G P, Nowell P D, Sateia M J 2002 Headache complaints in relation to nocturnal oxygen saturation among patients with sleep apnea syndrome. Sleep Medicine 3:361-364

Guilleminault C, Poyares D, Rosa A et al 2005 Heart rate variability, sympathetic and vagal balance and EEG arousals in upper airway resistance and mild obstructive sleep apnea syndromes. Sleep Medicine 6:451-457

Hamada T, Kotani H, Kawazoe Y et al 1982 Effect of occlusal splints on the EMG activity of masseter and temporal muscles in bruxism with clinical symptoms. Journal of Oral Rehabilitation 9:119-123

Headache classification subcommittee of the international headache society 2004 The international classification of headache disorders, 2nd edn. Cephalalgia 24 (supplement1): p 9-160

Huynh N, Kato T, Rompré P H et al 2006a Sleep bruxism is associated to micro-arousals and an increase in cardiac sympathetic activity. Journal of Sleep Research 15:339-346

Huynh N, Lavigne G J, Lanfranchi P A et al 2006b The effect of 2 sympatholytic medications–propranolol and clonidine–on sleep bruxism: experimental randomized controlled studies. Sleep 29:307-316

Jennum P, Jensen R 2002 Sleep and headache. Sleep Medicine Reviews 6:471-479

Jensen R, Olesen J 1996 Initiating mechanisms of experimentally induced tension-type headache. Cephalalgia 16:175-182

Kampe T, Tagdae T, Bader G et al 1997a Reported symptoms and clinical findings in a group of subjects with longstanding bruxing behaviour. Journal of Oral Rehabilitation 24:581-587

Kampe T, Edman G, Bader G et al 1997b Personality traits in a group of subjects with long-standing bruxing behaviour. Journal of Oral Rehabilitation 24:588-593

Kast R E 2005 Tiagabine may reduce bruxism and associated temporomandibular joint pain. Anesthesia Progress 52:102-104

Kato T, Rompre P, Montplaisir J Y et al 2001a Sleep bruxism: an oromotor activity secondary to micro-arousal. Journal of Dental Research 80:1940-1944

Kato T, Thie N M R, Montplaisir J Y et al 2001b Bruxism and orofacial movements during sleep. Dental Clinics of North America 45:657-684

Kato T, Thie N M R, Huynh N, et al 2003a Topical review: sleep bruxism and the role of peripheral sensory influences. Journal of Orofacial Pain 17:191-213

Kato T, Montplaisir J Y, Guitard F et al 2003b Evidence that experimentally induced sleep bruxism is a consequence of transient arousal. Journal of Dental Research 82:284-288

Kayed K, Sjaastad O 1985 Nocturnal and early morning headaches. Annals of Clinical Research 7:243-246

Kushida C A, Morgenthaler T I, Littner M R et al 2006 Practice parameters for the treatment of snoring and obstructive sleep apnea with oral appliances: An update for 2005: An American academy of sleep medicine report. Sleep 29:240-243

Lampl C, Marecek S, May A et al 2006 A prospective, open-label, long-term study of the efficacy and tolerability of topiramate in the prophylaxis of chronic tension-type headache. Cephalalgia 26:1203-1208

Landry M-L, Rompre PH, Manzini C et al 2006 Reduction of sleep bruxism using a mandibular advancement device: An experimental controlled study. International Journal of Prosthodontics 19:549-556

Lavigne G J, Montplaisir J Y 1994 Restless legs syndrome and sleep bruxism: prevalence and association among Canadians. Sleep 17:739-743

Lavigne G J, Rompre P H, Montplaisir J Y 1996 Sleep bruxism: validity of clinical research diagnostic criteria in a controlled polysomnographic study. Journal of Dental Research 75:546-552

Lavigne G J, Goulet J P, Zuconni M et al 1999 Sleep disorders and the dental patient: an overview. Oral Surgery, Oral Medicine, Oral Pathology, Oral Radiology, and Endodontics 88:257-272

Lavigne G J, Kato T, Kolta A et al 2003 Neurobiological mechanisms involved in sleep bruxism. Critical Reviews in Oral Biology and Medicine 14:30-46

Lavigne GJ, Manzini C, Kato T 2005a Sleep Bruxism. In: Kryger M H, Roth T, Dement W C (eds) Principles and practice of sleep medicine, 4th edn. Elsevier Saunders, Philadelphia p 946-959

Lavigne G J, McMillan D, Zucconi M 2005b Pain and Sleep. In: Kryger M H, Roth T, Dement W C (eds) Principles and practice of sleep medicine, 4th edn. Elsevier Saunders, Philadelphia p 1246-1255

Lavigne G J, Morisson F, Khoury S et al 2006 Sleep-related pain complaints: morning headaches and tooth grinding. Insom (7):4-11

Lindberg E, Berne C, Elmasry A et al 2006 CPAP treatment of a population-based sample-what are the benefits and the treatment compliance? Sleep Medicine 7:553-560

Lipton R B, Lowenkopf T, Bajwa Z H et al 1997 Cardiac cephalgia: a treatable form of exertional headache. Neurology 49:813-816

Lobbezoo F, Lavigne G J 1997 Do bruxism and temporomandibular disorders have a cause-and-effect relationship? Journal of Orofacial Pain 11:15-23

Lobbezoo F, Lavigne G J, Tanguay R et al 1997a The effect of catecholamine precursor L-dopa on sleep bruxism: a controlled clinical trial. Movement disorders 12:73-78

Lobbezoo F, Soucy J P, Hartman N G et al 1997b Effects of the D2 receptor agonist bromocriptine on sleep bruxism: report of two single-patient clinical trials. Journal of Dental Research 76:1610-1614

Lobbezoo F, Naeije M 2001 Bruxism is mainly regulated centrally, not peripherally. Journal of Oral Rehabilitation 28:1085-1091

Lobbezoo F, van Denderen R J, Verheij J G et al 2001 Reports of SSRI-associated bruxism in the family physician's office. Journal of Orofacial Pain 15:340-346

Macaluso G M, Guerra P, Di Giovanni G et al 1998 Sleep bruxism is a disorder related to periodic arousals during sleep. Journal of Dental Research 77:565-573

Macfarlane T V, Gray R J M, Kincey J et al 2001 Factors associated with the temporomandibular disorder, pain dysfunction syndrome (PDS): Manchester case-control study. Oral Diseases 7:321-330

Magnusson T, Egermark I, Carlsson G E 2000 A longitudinal epidemiologic study of signs and symptoms of temporomandibular disorders from 15 to 35 years of age. Journal of Orofacial Pain 14:310-319

Mahowald M W, Schenck C H 1996 NREM sleep parasomnias. Neurologic Clinics 14:675-696

Miller V A, Palermo T M, Powers S W et al 2003 Migraine headaches and sleep disturbances in children. Headache 43:362-368

Molina O F, dos Santos J Jr, Nelson S J et al 1997 Prevalence of modalities of headaches and bruxism among patients with craniomandibular disorder. Cranio15:314-325

Nobre ME, Leal AJ, Filho PMF 2005 Investigation into sleep disturbance of patients suffering from cluster headache. Cephalalgia 25:488-492

Ohayon M M 2004 Prevalence and risk factors of morning headaches in the general population. Archives of Internal Medicine 164:97-102

Ohayon M M, Li K K, Guilleminault C 2001 Risk factors for sleep bruxism in the general population. Chest 119:53-61

Oksenberg A, Arons E 2002 Sleep bruxism related to obstructive sleep apnea: the effect of continuous positive airway pressure. Sleep Medicine 3:513-515

Oxford centre for evidence-based medicine. Accessible at http://www.cebm.net/

Parrino L, Halasz P, Tassinari C A et al 2006 CAP, epilepsy and motor events during sleep: the unifying role of arousal. Sleep Medicine Reviews 10:267-285

Pirelli P, Saponara M, Guilleminault C 2004 Rapid maxillary expansion in children with obstructive sleep apnea syndrome. Sleep 27:761-766

Plesh O, Curtis D A, Hall L J et al 1998 Gender difference in jaw pain induced by clenching. Journal of Oral Rehabilitation 25:258-263

Poceta J S 2003 Sleep-related headache syndromes. Current Pain and Headache Reports 7:281-287

Por C H, Watson L, Doucette D et al 1996 Sertraline-associated bruxism. Canadian Journal of Clinical Pharmacology 3:123-135

Powell N B, Riley R W, Guilleminault C 2005 Surgical management of sleep-disordered breathing. In: Kryger M H, Roth T, Dement W C (eds)

Principles and practice of sleep medicine, 4th edn. Elsevier Saunders, Philadelphia p 1081-1097

Rasmussen B K 1993 Migraine and tension-type headache in a general population: precipitating factors, female hormones, sleep pattern and relation to lifestyle. Pain 53:65-72

Rugh J D, Harlan J 1988 Nocturnal bruxism and temporomandibular disorders. Advances in Neurology 49:329-341

Saletu A, Parapatics S, Saletu B et al 2005 On the pharmacotherapy of sleep bruxism: Placebo-controlled polysomnographic and psychometric studies with clonazepam. Neuropsychobiology 51:214-225

Sarlani E, Schwartz A H, Greenspan J D et al 2003 Facial pain as first manifestation of lung cancer: a case of lung cancer-related cluster headache and a review of the literature. Journal of Orofacial Pain 17:262-267

Stepanski E J, Wyatt J K 2003 Use of sleep hygiene in the treatment of insomnia. Sleep Medicine Reviews 7:215-225

Svensson P, Arendt-Nielsen L 1996 Effects of 5 days of repeated submaximal clenching on masticatory muscle pain and tenderness: an experimental study. Journal of Orofacial Pain 10:330-338

Terzano M G, Parrino L, Rosa A et al 2002 CAP and arousals in the structural development of sleep: an integrative perspective. Sleep Medicine 3:221-229

Thorpy M J 1997 American sleep disorders association; The international classification of sleep disorders. Allen Press, Rochester

Thorpy M J 2005 Classification of sleep disorders. In: Kryger M H, Roth T, Dement W C (eds) Principles and practice of sleep medicine, 4th edn. Elsevier Saunders, Philadelphia p 615-625

Watanabe T, Ichikawa K, Clark G T 2003 Bruxism levels and daily behaviors: 3 weeks of measurement and correlation. Journal of Orofacial Pain 17:65-73

Winocur E, Gavish A, Voikovitch M et al 2003 Drugs and bruxism: a critical review. Journal of Orofacial Pain 17:99-111

Woda A, Tubert-Jeannin S, Bouhassira D et al 2005 Towards a new taxonomy of idiopathic orofacial pain. Pain 116:396-406

Yustin D, Neff P, Rieger M R et al 1993 Characterization of 86 bruxing patients with long-term study of their management with occlusal devices and other forms of therapy. Journal of Orofacial Pain 7:54-60

Zarb G A, Carlsson G E, Sessle B J et al 1994 Temporomandibular joint and masticatory muscle disorders, 2nd edn. Munksgaard, Copenhagen

Temporomandibular disorders and related headache

Ramesh Balasubramaniam and Robert Delcanho

Painful dysfunction of the temporomandibular joint and associated muscles can cause headache. In this chapter the authors, both dental practitioners, describe the etiology of temporomandibular-related symptoms and management of temporomandibular disorders and related headache.

Pain involving the head and orofacial regions is very common and in one study affected 26% and 12% respectively of the general population in the previous six months (Von Korff et al 1988). One of the most common causes of oro-facial pain is a group of musculoskeletal conditions known as temporomandibular disorders (TMD). These conditions are primarily associated with pain and dysfunction involving the masticatory apparatus. It has long been presumed that there is an intimate relationship between bruxism and the development of TMD. It is the purpose of this chapter to review the common TMD, including etiological factors and also to discuss the relationship of TMD to the primary headaches.

Temporomandibular disorders

Temporomandibular disorder is defined by the American Academy of Orofacial Pain as 'a collective term that embraces a number of clinical problems that involve the masticatory muscles, the temporomandibular joint (TMJ), and the associated structures' (De Leeuw 2008) (Fig. 7.1). Pain is the most common symptom and may be associated with jaw dysfunction such as interference to or limitations in mouth opening, asymmetric jaw movements, and TMJ sounds (clicking or crepitation). Other associated signs and symptoms may include earache, tinnitus, headache, neck pain, altered bite and accelerated tooth wear. The prevalence of TMD in the general population is difficult to determine and the reported prevalence varies depending on the criteria used and the population studied. Similarly, signs and symptoms of TMD fluctuate over time (Magnusson et al 2005). Schiffman et al (1990) investigated the signs and symptoms of TMD in the general population based on established diagnostic criteria and reported the prevalence of joint disorders and masticatory muscle disorders to be 33% and 41% respectively. However, only 7% of the subjects had signs and symptoms of TMD that warranted treatment.

The etiology of TMD remains an enigma and is likely multifactorial. The masticatory apparatus usually functions normally until interrupted by an event. For example, a direct blow to the jaw may result in ligamentous strain to the TMJ

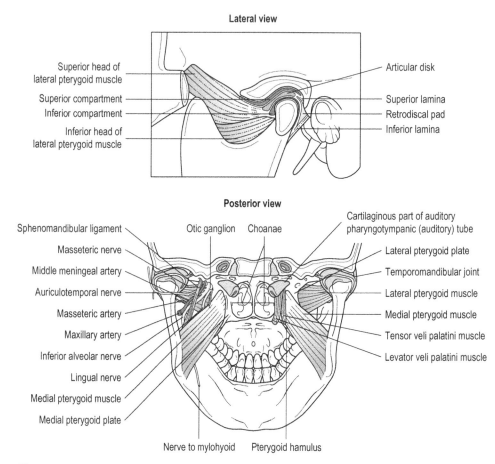

Lateral view

Superior head of lateral pterygoid muscle

Superior compartment

Inferior compartment

Inferior head of lateral pterygoid muscle

Articular disk

Superior lamina

Retrodiscal pad

Inferior lamina

Posterior view

Sphenomandibular ligament

Masseteric nerve

Middle meningeal artery

Auriculotemporal nerve

Masseteric artery

Maxillary artery

Inferior alveolar nerve

Lingual nerve

Medial pterygoid muscle

Medial pterygoid plate

Otic ganglion   Choanae

Cartilaginous part of auditory pharyngotympanic (auditory) tube

Lateral pterygoid plate

Temporomandibular joint

Lateral pterygoid muscle

Medial pterygoid muscle

Tensor veli palatini muscle

Levator veli palatini muscle

Nerve to mylohyoid   Pterygoid hamulus

Figure 7.1 • Overview and topographical anatomy of the temporomandibular joint (lateral and posterior view).

complex and associated masticatory muscles causing pain and dysfunction (Pullinger & Seligman 1991). Other local events include inadvertent placement of a 'high' dental restoration, toothache, dental surgical procedures, chewing on hard food for a prolonged period, yawning, and severe bruxism. Also, indirect traumatic events such as cervical whiplash injury due to a motor vehicle accident may be an etiological factor for TMD (Carroll et al 2007, Eriksson et al 2007). In a controlled prospective study, one in three whiplash trauma subjects had delayed symptoms of TMD (Salé & Isberg 2007). In fact, any source of deep pain input associated with the

orofacial region, regardless of whether it is directly or indirectly related to the temporomandibular and masticatory apparatus, may predispose these structures to pain and dysfunction. Systemic factors such as joint laxity and fibromyalgia are also considered risk factors for TMD (Balasubramaniam et al 2007, Kavuncu et al 2006). Of interest is the relationship between stress and TMD. Curran et al (1996) showed an increase in resting electromyographic activity of masticatory muscles in subjects exposed to experimental stressors. Likewise, the relationship between post-traumatic stress disorder and TMD has been reported to be partially related to genetic vulnerability (Afari et al 2008). A case-control study reported that tooth clenching, trauma and female gender were associated with chronic masticatory myalgia; irrespective of the subjects' psychological symptoms of anxiety and depression (Velly et al 2003). It remains unclear if TMD is influenced by psychosocial factors or vice versa. Table 7.1 summarizes possible associative factors for TMD.

Over the years there have been numerous classification systems for TMD compiled by various organizations; these lacked validity and contributed to confusion among clinicians and academics. In order to address this problem, the Research Diagnostic Criteria for Temporomandibular Disorders (RDC/TMD) was developed (Dworkin & LeResche 1992). The criteria are now widely accepted and are considered valid and reliable for use in TMD research (John et al 2005). However, in everyday clinical practice the RDC/TMD is limited in its use as its criteria are rigid and difficult to translate to patient care. The following discussion reviews the diagnosis of common TMD and is divided into muscle disorders and joint disorders.

Muscle disorders

TMD encompass numerous muscle disorders. For the purpose of this chapter, the discussion is limited to the common clinical presentation of muscle disorders in TMD, namely protective co-contraction, local myalgia, myofascial pain, myospasm, and centrally mediated myalgia.

Protective co-contraction

The initial response of the masticatory musculature to an event is protective co-contraction (muscle splinting/trismus) (Stohler & Ash 1986). It is the reaction of antagonist muscles in order to protect the injured muscles from further injury as explained by the pain-adaptation model (Lund et al 1991, Stohler et al 1988). When the jaw elevator muscles are involved, jaw opening is limited and pain is elicited when the jaw is stretched open. This condition is not strictly pathological and usually resolves within a few days if the affected muscles are rested and further stimulus is avoided.

Local myalgia

Local myalgia is a non-inflammatory muscle disorder caused by a noxious event and presents clinically as tender, painful muscles along with sensations of jaw fatigability, muscle stiffness, weakness, and limited mouth opening. Also known as 'post-exercise soreness or delayed onset muscle soreness' local myalgia is associated with excessive use of the masticatory muscles (Dao et al 1994a, Lieber & Friden 2002). Local masticatory myalgia may be viewed as a progression from unresolved protective co-contraction.

Table 7.1 Factors associated with temporomandibular disorders.

Factor	Example
Trauma	
Direct trauma	Blow to the face, yawning, iatrogenic prolonged mouth opening
Indirect trauma	Flexion-extension injury (whiplash)
Microtrauma	Forward head posture, pencil chewing, muscle hyperactivity
Occlusal factor	Large (> 6 mm) overjet Minimal overbite and anterior skeletal openbite Unilateral posterior crossbite Occlusal slides greater than 2 mm
Systemic factors	Generalized joint laxity Fibromylagia
Psychosocial factors	Emotional distress, anxiety, depression, somatization, post-traumatic stress disorder

Myofascial pain

Myofascial pain (MFP) is a regional muscle pain involving the skeletal muscles, tendons, and ligaments associated with myofascial trigger points (MTPs) within hypersensitive taut bands. The pain may involve the area of the MTP (source) which refers to a distant site which is the perceived source of pain (Gerwin 2001, Travell & Rinzler 1952). Also, central excitatory effects such as secondary hyperalgesia, co-contraction, and autonomic activation may be associated with MFP (Fricton 1990). For example, upon palpation, an active MTP involving the sternocleidomastoid muscle may refer pain to the TMJ, temple, and jaw mimicking TMD (Fig. 7.2). Likewise, MFP involving the temporalis muscle may refer to upper teeth mimicking dental pain (Fig. 7.3). The various possible mechanisms involved in MFP are often debated and the scientific validity of MFP is yet to be established. In spite of this, myofascial trigger point injections are frequently used in clinical settings to treat MFP. A discussion of MFP and MTPs may be found in Chapter 23.

Myospasm

Myospasm is an infrequent CNS mediated acute muscle disorder characterized by brief, involuntary tonic contraction. The etiology of myospasm is unknown but thought to be related to deep pain input, muscle fatigue,

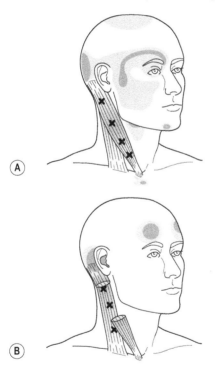

Figure 7.2 • Referred pain patterns (*solid* shows essential zones and *stippling* shows the spill over areas) with location of common myofascial trigger points (Xs) in the right sternocleidomastoid muscle. **A**, the sternal (more anterior and more superficial) division. **B**, the clavicular (more posterior and deeper) division.

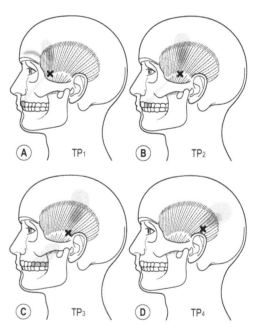

Figure 7.3 • Patterns of pain and tenderness referred from trigger points (Xs) in the left temporalis muscle (essential zone *solid*, spill over zone *stippled*). Three of the trigger points are attachment trigger points (AMTPs) which occur at musculotendinous junction. One is a central trigger point (CMTP) which occurs in the midfiber region of the muscle. **(A)** = anterior 'spokes' represent referred pain arising from AMTP1 in the anterior fibers of the muscle. **(B** and **C)** = middle 'spokes' represent referred pain and tenderness arising from AMTP2 and AMTP3. **(D)** = posterior supra-auricular 'spoke' referred from CMTP4.

and electrolyte imbalances. Clinically, myospasm is represented by firm, tight, and painful muscles that are aggravated during function often resulting in acute trismus and malocclusion. The inappropriate use of the term myospasm to describe various masticatory muscle pains remains common in spite of studies showing that increased electromyographic activity is a rare finding (Lund et al 1991, Curran et al 1996).

Centrally mediated myalgia

Centrally mediated myalgia (chronic myositis) is a centrally driven chronic, persistent muscle pain. It is thought to be the result of neurogenic inflammation due to a prolonged noxious stimulus that remains untreated (Sessle 1999). It may also be perpetuated by upregulation of the autonomic nervous system and unremitting emotional stress. Unlike other muscle diagnoses, centrally mediated myalgia is characterized by constant, long-term pain that worsens with function. The involved muscles are hyperalgesic to palpation and associated with dysfunctional masticatory apparatus (Okeson 2005).

Temporomandibular joint disorders

The TMJ disorders include congenital disorders, disc derangements, dislocation, ankylosis, inflammatory, and noninflammatory disorders. The discussion in this chapter is limited to the more common TMJ disorders.

Disc derangements

Disc derangements are characterized by abnormal condyle-disc relationships which are subdivided into disc displacement with reduction and disc displacement without reduction. Typically, the disc displaces anteromedially or anterolaterally due to elongation and tearing of the articular discal ligaments (Farrar & McCarty 1983, Isberg-Holm & Westesson 1982, Larheim 2005, Stegenga et al 1991). A disc displacement with reduction is associated with altered position of the disc in its relationship to the mandibular condyle in the closed mouth position that relocates with a clicking sound (< 35 mm) when the mouth is opened. This phenomenon may or may not be associated with pain. Occasionally, both an opening and closing click may be heard (reciprocal) with deviation of the jaw opening movement coinciding with the click. It is estimated that 33% of the general population have moderate and severe derangement which are asymptomatic and do not require treatment (Greene & Laskin 1988, Kircos et al 1987, Larheim et al 2001).

In contrast, disc displacement without reduction, also known as 'closed lock', is characterized by more severe malpositioning of the disc in the closed mouth position that does not improve with jaw opening. The mouth opening is often painful and limited with deflection of the jaw opening pathway towards the affected joint and limited excursive movement to the contralateral side (Stegenga et al 1989). Upon questioning, patients will most often report a history of joint clicking noise that progressed acutely into a closed locked situation. In chronic closed lock cases, the pain becomes less prominent, mouth opening improves, and ultimately osteoarthritic changes may develop which are usually associated with joint crepitation (Luder 1993, Minakuchi et al 2001, Stegenga et al 1993). To date, there is no scientific evidence to suggest that over time disc displacements can progress and lead to degenerative changes of the TMJ.

Dislocation

Temporomandibular joint dislocation (open lock) is characterized by wide mouth opening without the ability to close due to the anteriorly subluxed position of the condyle out of its fossa beyond the crest of the articular eminence. Dislocation is not the result of a pathologic condition. It is postulated that excessive pterygoid muscle activity maintains the condyle in this hyperextended position (De Leeuw 2008). This condition is a medical emergency if the patient is unable to self-reduce the joint and requires special jaw manipulation by a dentist or may result in an emergency room visit whereby the joint is reduced under intravenous or general anesthetic sedation.

Inflammatory disorders

Common inflammatory disorders of the TMJ include synovitis and capsulitis. Since it is not possible to differentiate the two conditions clinically, we will discuss them together. In synovitis and capsulitis there is inflammation of the TMJ synovial lining and capsular ligament respectively which may be the result of trauma, autoimmune disease, or infection (Schille 1986). Clinically, these conditions present with TMJ pain that worsens with function and joint loading. In cases with significant joint effusion, patients may report a slight ipsilateral posterior openbite.

There are a group of polyarthritides that include rheumatoid arthritis, juvenile rheumatoid arthritis, ankylosing spondylitis, psoriatic arthritis, infectious arthritis, Reiter syndrome and gout which can also involve the TMJ. Likewise, autoimmune and connective tissue diseases may have TMJ involvement. These conditions are beyond the scope of this chapter and further information may be found elsewhere (De Leeuw 2008, Klasser et al 2007, Laskin et al 2006).

Non-inflammatory disorders

Osteoarthritis of the TMJ is a degenerative condition of the joint that results in deterioration and remodeling of the articular cartilage and subchondral bone (De Bont et al 1985). It is classified as primary/idiopathic or secondary osteoarthritis. In secondary osteoarthritis, a known etiology such as direct trauma or infection is identified. Clinically, patients may be asymptomatic or may report pain and jaw dysfunction which correlates with the degree of inflammation superimposed on this condition. Over time, radiographic evidence of condylar erosion, osteophyte formation, subchondral sclerosis and joint space narrowing may be found. There is evidence to suggest that this is typically a non-progressive condition that rarely requires treatment (Boering 1966).

Bruxism

Bruxism is an involuntary activity of the jaw musculature typified by parafunctional activities such as jaw clenching, tooth gnashing, and grinding (Lavigne et al 2003). It is important to differentiate between awake bruxism (AB) and sleep bruxism (SB). AB involves jaw clenching and jaw bracing without tooth contact in awake individuals often related to a stress reaction. Its prevalence is between 5% and 25% of the general population and decreases with age (Allen et al 1990, Egermark-Eriksson et al 1981, Glaros 1981, Gross et al 1988). AB can occur with or without SB.

SB is a stereotypical movement disorder characterized by both tooth clenching and grinding that occurs during sleep (Medicine AAoS 2005). SB may be subdivided into primary (idiopathic) or secondary SB. Secondary SB may be related to an underlying neurological or psychiatric disorder such as Parkinsonism or schizophrenia, or as a side effect of medication or illicit drug use (Balasubramaniam & Ram 2008). The prevalence of SB declines with age; occurring in 14% of children and decreases to 8% and 3% in adults greater and less than 60 years respectively (Laberge et al 2000, Lavigne & Montplaisir 1994, Ohayon et al 2001, Reding et al 1966). It is likely that the prevalence of SB is greatly under-reported as many individuals may not be aware of nocturnal parafunctional habits and there is a large variability in frequency of SB over time (Lavigne et al 2001). In fact, 85–90% of individuals have reported periods of bruxism (Bader & Lavigne 2000, Okeson et al 1990, 1991, 1994).

The etiology of SB has in recent years undergone a paradigm shift. Previously, SB was thought to be related to occlusal factors and treatment of occlusal discrepancies was advocated (Ash & Ramfjord 1995, Guichet 1977, Ramfjord 1961). Likewise, the role of emotional stress as causative of SB was supported by its association to nocturnal muscle activity and pain with increased stress levels (Clark et al 1979, Rugh & Solberg 1975, Solberg et al 1975). More rigorous studies have disputed the role of occlusal factors and its treatment for SB (Clark et al 1999, Kardachi et al 1978, Rugh et al 1984, Tsukiyama et al 2001). Similarly, more recent studies have found that only a percentage of SB patients have an association between SB and stress (Dao et al 1994b, Pierce et al 1995, Watanabe et al 2003). Currently, the most accepted theory of SB is that it is a movement disorder involving a cascade of physiological events characterized by autonomic-cardiac activities as related to sleep arousal (Kato et al 2003, 2001, Macaluso et al 1998, Medicine AAoS 2005).

Clinically, 20% to 30% of SB patients have reported orofacial pain (Dao et al 1994a, Goulet et al 1993). The orofacial/dental consequence of SB includes TMJ and masticatory muscle pain, jaw locking, tooth wear and headaches (Bader & Lavigne 2000, Lavigne et al 2005). The odds ratio of TMD in the presence of clenching or grinding is between 4.2 and 8.4 (Huang et al 2002, Velly

et al 2003). Also, close to 65% of SB patients report headaches (Bader et al 1997, Camparis & Siqueira 2006). Dao et al (1994b) reported that myofascial pain was more intense among bruxers even if pain is not a primary complaint compared to myofascial pain patients without evidence of bruxism. Pain patients regardless of being bruxers or myofascial pain patients had reduced quality of life compared to bruxers who were pain-free. Also post-exercise related muscle soreness among bruxers was worse in the morning suggestive of nocturnal oral parafunction as the etiology for the pain.

The diagnosis of SB without a sleep study relies on the patient's partner or parent reporting observed episodes. Additionally, patients may report jaw muscle tightness, fatigue, and pain, typically upon awaking. Also, the clinician may observe accelerated tooth wear patterns as evidence of SB. The problems with relying on the above mentioned correlates of SB are numerous. Unscientific reporting of SB may include other jaw motor activities such as swallowing, sleep talking, or myoclonus. Also, observed wear facets may be the result of other causes such as food texture and acidity, previous history of bruxism, acid reflux disease or other oral parafunctional habits (Kato et al 1999, Lavigne et al 1996, 1999, 2005, Pergamalian et al 2003).

Occlusion

The subject of the dental occlusion (bite) and its relationship to TMD is perhaps the most controversial of all areas in dentistry. With advances in scientific methodology, there is a shift away from previously held beliefs that malocclusion or bite discrepancy is causative for TMD; however it continues to provoke passionate debate. Okeson (2008) summarized 57 epidemiological studies on the relationship between occlusion and TMD and found

35 studies suggesting a relationship compared to 22 studies that suggested no relationship. Although, there were more studies that were suggestive of a relationship between occlusion and TMD, these studies varied greatly with respect to the occlusal conditions implicated in causing TMD. It should be noted that the so called malocclusion cited in these studies is prevalent among many symptom free individuals. At this stage, no serious conclusion can be drawn from these studies.

McNamara et al (1995) reviewed the interaction of morphological and functional occlusal factors with respect to TMD and found a weak relationship between occlusal schemes and TMD. Specifically, occlusal features such as skeletal anterior open bite, overjets greater than 6–7 mm, intercuspal position slides greater than 2 mm, unilateral lingual crossbite, and five or more missing posterior teeth were found to be associated with subcategories of TMD (Pullinger et al 1993). The authors suggested a minor relationship between occlusion and TMD may exist. Koh and Robinson (2004) reviewed the literature pertaining to occlusal adjustments for treating and preventing TMD. The specific outcomes that were discussed included global measures of symptoms, pain, headache and limitation of movement. The authors reported that there was no evidence for the use of occlusal adjustment procedures for either the treatment or prevention of TMD.

A possible explanation for the failure of past studies in ascertaining a definitive relationship between occlusion and TMD is due to the focus on dental malocclusion (static tooth-tooth relationship) rather than functional disturbances. For example, placement of a high restoration and the resultant hyperocclusion can induce acute masticatory muscle pain secondary to an increased tonus of the elevator muscles (protective co-contraction) (Rugh et al 1984). On the other hand, a chronic occlusal interference is dealt by the individual's ability to adapt and alter muscle engrams (jaw movement patterns) to avoid potential nociception (high restoration). Failure to adapt may in certain individuals, result in continued elevator muscle pain (Okeson 2008).

Management of temporomandibular disorders

The treatment of TMD is aimed at resolving pain and jaw dysfunction. TMD is a cyclical, self-limiting and rarely progressive condition (Schiffman et al 1990, Von Korff et al 1988, Yatani et al 1997). With this in mind, non-invasive, conservative and reversible treatments have been shown to be beneficial (Randolph et al 1990, Skeppar & Nilner 1993). Current treatment standards advocate a biopsychosocial approach to chronic TMD; that is, a therapeutic approach to both Axis I (physical) and Axis II (psychological) diagnosis will lead to greater treatment success (Ohrbach & Dworkin 1998). Table 7.2 summarizes the various modalities commonly used for the treatment of TMD. For a more complete review of the management of TMD readers are encouraged to peruse recent texts on this subject (De Leeuw 2008, Laskin et al 2006, Okeson 2008, Balasubramaniam et al 2008).

Temporomandibular disorders and headache

Headache is one of the ten most common presenting symptoms to general medical practices, afflicting a large proportion of the population and frequently associated with disruption of daily activity and economic loss. Lipton et al (1993) surveyed 45 711 American households and found that 22% of the general population

Table 7.2 Treatment of temporomandibular disorders.

Approach	Example
Patient education and self management	Reassurance on the benign nature of TMD
Pain-free jaw function	Avoid aggravating factors and jaw function that results in pain
Behavioral modification	Avoid chewing on hard foods and gum, oral sex
Parafunctional modification	Awake clenching and bruxing, cheek biting, pencil chewing
Self-administered physiotherapy	Application of warm and cold compresses, soft tissue mobilization of muscles and passive jaw stretching within a pain free range
Cognitive and behavioral interventions	Habit reversal
	Counseling, and progressive muscle relaxation
	Hypnosis
	EMG biofeedback
Pharmacological therapy	
Analgesics	Aspirin, nonacetylated aspirin, choline magnesium trisalicylate, salsalate, opioids
Nonsteroidal anti-inflammatory drugs	
Corticosteroids	
Benzodiazepines	Diazepam
Muscle relaxants	Tizanidine, cyclobenzaprine
Low dose antidepressants	Amitriptyline
Physiotherapy	
Posture training	Orthostatic head, neck, shoulder and tongue posture
Exercises	Guided exercises within pain free range may include: gentle active stretching to mobilize the TMJs; isotonic and isometric exercises to stabilize TMJs; jaw postural and co-ordination exercise to reduce joint clicking
Progressive muscle relaxation therapy	
Myofascial trigger-point treatment	Injections, dry needling and acupuncture
Oral appliance therapy	Stabilization appliance
	Anterior positioning appliance
Surgery	Arthrocentesis
	Arthroscopy

over 18 years of age had experienced some orofacial pain in the prior six months. By far the most common are the primary headaches, and in particular tension-type and migraine. Tension-type headache affects about 30% of the population and are usually associated with pericranial and upper quarter regional muscle tenderness and pain. There is only a slight female preponderance (male:female ratio of 4:5) with average age of onset of 25–30 years (Rasmussen et al 1991). By contrast, migraine affects 18% of females and 6% of males. The age of onset is younger than for tension-type headache and in females is associated with menarche. Peak prevalence is in the reproductive years, between age 18 and 40 years.

Cross sectional studies of selected non-patient adult populations have found that 40–75% of subjects have at least one sign of TMD (e.g. interference with jaw movement, muscle tenderness) whilst 33% have at least one symptom (e.g. pain) (Dworkin et al 1990). Myogenous pain involving the temporal and pre-auricular regions are the most common type of TMD affecting about 10% of the population over 18 years, predominantly in young women of reproductive age. In a general population study of TMD patients, 41% had masticatory muscle disorders (Schiffman et al 1990).

Given the epidemiological data, it is not unreasonable to speculate that some patients suffering headaches may actually have TMD. Indeed, a significant percentage of headache patients may have undiagnosed TMD and vice versa. In one study, headaches in the general population were more frequent among subjects with TMD symptoms (27.4%) compared to those without TMD symptoms (15.2%) (Ciancaglini & Radaelli 2001). This has led to the assumption that TMD may be causative of headaches and treatment directed at jaw pain and dysfunction will likely lead to resolution. However, the mechanism of TMD-related headache is so far unknown.

The frontotemporal, periorbital and preauricular regions are often involved during a primary headache. This can be easily confused with TMD pain which often affects the same anatomical locations. Consideration must also be given to the possibility of referred pain arising from regional cervical structures. Adding to the dilemma it is presumed that etiologic factors often associated with the development of TMD such as stress, anxiety, sleep disturbance, tooth clenching and grinding and cervical dysfunction are commonly linked to tension type headache. Another clinical manifestation, palpation tenderness of the pericranial muscles,

is a predominant finding in tension-type headache, but is also notable during migraine attacks. Similarly, tenderness and pain involving the masticatory muscles are considered as primary clinical features of a muscle disorder in TMD. Although neurologists and primary care physicians seek to rule out organic causes of headache, it is fair to say that TMD is usually not considered. In the International Classification of Headache Disorders-II (ICHD) published in 2004, TMD are only mentioned in section 11.7 as 'Headache or facial pain attributable to temporomandibular joint disorders' (ICHD 2004).

Some studies have investigated the relationship between TMD and headache. De Rossi et al (2000) found significantly higher prevalence of TMD in patients presenting to a neurology clinic with headaches than a control population. In unpublished work utilizing the RDC/TMD, Ohrbach et al (1998) found 40% of 362 subjects with masticatory myalgia/TMD pain satisfied ICHD criteria for tension-type headache. Eighty-five percent of that group reported headache as a symptom. In 184 subjects diagnosed with temporalis myalgia, 49.5% satisfied the ICHD criteria of tension-type headache and 99.5% of that group reported headache. Jensen and Oleson (1996) found prolonged experimental tooth clenching induced significantly more headaches and tenderness in tension-type headache subjects than healthy controls, and that the tenderness preceded the headache.

Therapeutic intervention for TMD, tension-type headache, and to a lesser degree migraine have similarities in the response to analgesic, anti-inflammatory, antidepressant and anxiolytic medications, physical medicine modalities and cognitive-behavioral treatments for stress reduction. Occlusal splints have been used for many years to treat TMD and a number of studies have suggested that this treatment may also benefit headaches, although the mechanism remains unknown. Schokker et al (1990a & b) found that occlusal splint treatment of TMD resulted in a decrease in headache in some patients, sometimes better than conventional neurology treatment. The best results were seen where the TMD pain was bilateral and the clinical features were suggestive of myogenous rather than arthrogenous TMD.

Recently a type of occlusal splint called Nociception Trigeminal Inhibition Tension Suppression System (NTI-tss) has been marketed aggressively as being more effective in reducing the symptoms of tension-type headache and migraine, compared to conventional occlusal splint therapy (Shankland 2002). In fact, the quoted NTI-tss study was seriously flawed and definitive conclusions cannot be drawn from it. Subsequently, more scientifically rigorous studies investigating the NTI-tss have since reported that it is not superior to conventional occlusal splints (Al Quran & Kamal 2006, Jokstad et al 2005, Magnusson et al 2004). Additionally, serious concerns have been raised about the use of the NTI-tss device such as the

adverse effects of malocclusion, tooth mobility, swallowing, and aspiration (Jokstad et al 2005).

Conclusion

There is a strong overlap between TMD pain and the common primary headaches. It is likely that TMD are one of several peripheral triggers that may be involved in headache onset via direct neuronal excitation of the trigeminal pathway. Preliminary epidemiological data supports the clinical observations that TMD and primary headaches are co-morbid disorders. However causality cannot be inferred. From a clinical diagnostic perspective, patients presenting with headache need thorough neurological, cervical, myofascial, and TMD evaluation. Once TMJ or mastictatory muscle pathology is diagnosed either in isolation or in conjuction with primary headache appropriate treatment should be initiated. If no obvious pathology is found then the patient should be treated for a primary headache, which should be diagnosed utilizing current ICHD-II criteria.

References

Afari N, Wen Y, Buchwald D et al 2008 Are post-traumatic stress disorder symptoms and temporomandibular pain associated? Findings from a community-based twin registry. J Orofac Pain 22:41 49.

Al Quran FA, Kamal MS 2006 Anterior midline point stop device (AMPS) in the treatment of myogenous TMDs: comparison with the stabilization splint and control group. Oral Surg Oral Med Oral Pathol Oral Radiol Endod 101:741-747.

Allen JD, Rivera-Morales WC, Zwemer JD 1990 Occurrence of temporomandibular disorder symptoms in healthy young adults with and without evidence of bruxism. Cranio 8:312-318.

Ash MM, Ramfjord SP 1995 Occlusion, 4th edn. WB Saunders, Philadelphia.

Bader G, Lavigne G 2000 Sleep bruxism; an overview of an oromandibular sleep movement disorder. Sleep medicine reviews 4:27-43.

Bader GG, Kampe T, Tagdae T et al 1997 Descriptive physiological data on a sleep bruxism population. Sleep 20:982-990.

Balasubramaniam R, Ram S 2008 Orofacial movement disorders. Oral and maxillofacial surgery clinics of North America. 20:273-285.

Balasubramaniam R, de Leeuw R, Zhu H et al 2007 Prevalence of temporomandibular disorders in fibromyalgia and failed back syndrome patients: a blinded prospective comparison study. Oral

Surg Oral Med Oral Pathol Oral Radiol Endod 104:204-216.

Balasubramaniam R and Klasser G (eds) 2008 Orofacial Pain and Dysfunction. Oral and Maxillofacial Clinics of North America. 20(20):133-310.

Boering G 1966 Temporomandibular joint arthrosis: a clinical and radiographic investigation [thesis]. University of Groningen, The Netherlands.

Camparis CM, Siqueira JT 2006 Sleep bruxism: clinical aspects and characteristics in patients with and without chronic orofacial pain. Oral Surg Oral Med Oral Pathol Oral Radiol Endod 101:188-193.

Carroll LJ, Ferrari R, Cassidy JD 2007 Reduced or painful jaw movement after collision-related injuries: a population-based study. J Am Dent Assoc 138:86-93.

Ciancaglini R, Radaelli G 2001 The relationship between headache and symptoms of temporomandibular disorder in the general population. J Dent 29:93-98.

Clark GT, Beemsterboer PL, Solberg WK, Rugh JD 1979 Nocturnal electromyographic evaluation of myofascial pain dysfunction in patients undergoing occlusal splint therapy. J Am Dent Assoc 99: 607-611.

Clark GT, Tsukiyama Y, Baba K, Watanabe T 1999 Sixty-eight years of experimental occlusal interference studies: what have we learned? Journal of Prosthetic Dentistry 82:704-713.

Curran SL, Carlson CR, Okeson JP 1996 Emotional and physiologic responses to laboratory challenges: patients with temporomandibular disorders versus matched control subjects. J Orofac Pain 10:141-150.

Dao TT, Lund JP, Lavigne GJ 1994a Comparison of pain and quality of life in bruxers and patients with myofascial pain of the masticatory muscles. J Orofac Pain 8:350-356.

Dao TT, Lavigne GJ, Charbonneau A et al 1994b The efficacy of oral splints in the treatment of myofascial pain of the jaw muscles: a controlled clinical trial. Pain 56:85-94.

De Bont LG, Boering G, Liem RS, Havinga P 1985 Osteoarthritis of the temporomandibular joint: a light microscopic and scanning electron microscopic study of the articular cartilage of the mandibular condyle. J Oral Maxillofac Surg 43:481-488.

De Leeuw R (Ed) American Academy of Orofacial Pain 2008 Orofacial pain: guidelines for assessment, diagnosis, and management, 4th edn. Quintessence Publishing, Chicago.

De Rossi SS, Greenberg MS, Sollecito TP, Detre JA 2000 A prospective study evaluating the presence of temporomandibular disorders (TMD) in a cohort of patients referred to a neurology clinic for evaluation and treatment of

headache. Oral Surg Oral Med Oral Pathol Oral Radiol Endod 89:441.

Dworkin SF, LeResche L 1992 Research diagnostic criteria for temporomandibular disorders: review, criteria, examinations and specifications, critique. J Craniomandib Disord 6:301-355.

Dworkin SF, Huggins KH, Le Resche L 1990 Epidemiology of signs and symptoms in temporomandibular disorders: Clinical signs in cases and controls. J Am Dent Assoc 120: 273-281.

Egermark-Eriksson I, Carlsson GE, Ingervall B 1981 Prevalence of mandibular dysfunction and orofacial parafunction in 7-, 11- and 15-year-old Swedish children. European journal of Orthodontics 3:163-172.

Eriksson PO, Haggman-Henrikson B, Zafar H 2007 Jaw-neck dysfunction in whiplash-associated disorders. Archives of oral biology 52:404-408.

Farrar WB, McCarty VL 1983 A clinical outline of temporomandibular joint diagnosis and treatment, 7th edn. Normandie Study Group, Montgomery.

Fricton J 1990 Myofascial pain syndrome: Characteristics and epidemiology. In: Fricton J, Awad E (eds) Myofascial Pain and Fibromyalgia. Raven Press, New York.

Gerwin RD 2001 Classification, epidemiology, and natural history of myofascial pain syndrome. Curr Pain Headache Rep 5:412-420.

Glaros AG 1981 Incidence of diurnal and nocturnal bruxism. Journal of Prosthetic Dentistry 45:545-549.

Goulet JP, Lund JP, Montplaisir J, Lavigne G 1993 Daily clenching nocturnal bruxism, and stress and their association with TMD symptoms. J Orofac Pain 7:120.

Greene CS, Laskin DM 1988 Long-term status of TMJ clicking in patients with myofascial pain and dysfunction. J Am Dent Assoc 117:461-465.

Gross AJ, Rivera-Morales WC, Gale EN 1988 A prevalence study of symptoms associated with TM disorders. J Craniomandib Disord 2:191-195.

Guichet NE 1977 Occlusion: a teaching manual. The Denar Corporation, Anaheim.

Huang GJ, LeResche L, Critchlow CW et al 2002 Risk factors for diagnostic subgroups of painful temporomandibular disorders (TMD). J Dent Res 81:284-288.

ICHD 2004 International classification of headache disorders, 2nd edn. Cephalalgia 24(suppl 1): 9-160.

Isberg-Holm AM, Westesson PL 1982 Movement of disc and condyle in temporomandibular joints with clicking. An arthrographic and cineradiographic study on autopsy specimens. Acta Odontol Scand 40:151-164.

Jensen R, Olesen J 1996 Initiating mechanisms of experimentally induced tension-type headache. Cephalalgia 16:175-182; discussion 38-39.

John MT, Dworkin SF, Mancl LA 2005 Reliability of clinical temporomandibular disorder diagnoses. Pain 118:61-69.

Jokstad A, Mo A, Krogstad BS 2005 Clinical comparison between two different splint designs for temporomandibular disorder therapy. Acta Odontol Scand 63:218-226.

Kardachi BJ, Bailey JO, Ash MM 1978 A comparison of biofeedback and occlusal adjustment on bruxism. J Periodontol 49:367-372.

Kato T, Montplaisir JY, Blanchet PJ et al 1999 Idiopathic myoclonus in the oromandibular region during sleep: a possible source of confusion in sleep bruxism diagnosis. Mov Disord 14:865-871.

Kato T, Rompre P, Montplaisir JY et al 2001 Sleep bruxism: an oromotor activity secondary to micro-arousal. J Dent Res 80:1940-1944.

Kato T, Montplaisir JY, Guitard F et al 2003 Evidence that experimentally induced sleep bruxism is a consequence of transient arousal. J Dent Res 82:284-288.

Kavuncu V, Sahin S, Kamanli A et al 2006 The role of systemic hypermobility and condylar hypermobility in temporomandibular joint dysfunction syndrome. Rheumatol Int 26:257-260.

Kircos LT, Ortendahl DA, Mark AS, Arakawa M 1987 Magnetic resonance imaging of the TMJ disc in asymptomatic volunteers. J Oral Maxillofac Surg 45:852-854.

Klasser GD, Balasubramaniam R, Epstein J 2007 Topical review - connective tissue diseases: orofacial manifestations including pain. J Orofac Pain 21:171-184.

Koh H, Robinson PG 2004 Occlusal adjustment for treating and preventing temporomandibular joint disorders. J Oral Rehabil 31:287-292.

Laberge L, Tremblay RE, Vitaro F, Montplaisir J 2000 Development of parasomnias from childhood to early adolescence. Pediatrics. 106:67-74.

Larheim TA 2005 Role of magnetic resonance imaging in the clinical diagnosis of the temporomandibular joint. Cells, tissues, organs. 180:6-21.

Larheim TA, Westesson P, Sano T 2001 Temporomandibular joint disk displacement: comparison in asymptomatic volunteers and patients. Radiology 218:428-432.

Laskin DM, Greene CS, Hylander WL 2006 Temporomandibular disorders: an evidence-based approach to diagnosis and treatment. Quintessence Publishing, Hanover Park.

Lavigne GJ, Montplaisir JY 1994 Restless legs syndrome and sleep bruxism: prevalence and association among Canadians. Sleep 17:739-743.

Lavigne GJ, Rompre PH, Montplaisir JY 1996 Sleep bruxism: validity of clinical research diagnostic criteria in a controlled polysomnographic study. J Dent Res 75:546-552.

Lavigne GJ, Goulet JP, Zuconni M et al 1999 Sleep disorders and the dental patient: an overview. Oral Surg Oral Med Oral Pathol Oral Radiol Endod 88:257-272.

Lavigne GJ, Guitard F, Rompre PH, Montplaisir JY 2001 Variability in sleep bruxism activity over time. Journal of sleep research 10:237-244.

Lavigne GJ, Kato T, Kolta A, Sessle BJ 2003 Neurobiological mechanisms involved in sleep bruxism. Crit Rev Oral Biol Med 14:30-46.

Lavigne G, Manzini C, Kato T 2005 Sleep bruxism. In: Kryger M, Roth T, Dement WC (eds) Principles and practice of sleep medicine, 4th edn. Elsevier, Philadelphia.

Lieber RL, Friden J 2002 Morphologic and mechanical basis of delayed-onset muscle soreness. Journal of the American Academy of Orthopaedic Surgeons 10:67-73.

Lipton JA, Ship JA, Larach-Robinson D 1993 Estimated prevalence and distribution of reported orofacial pain in the United States. J Am Dent Assoc 124:115-121.

Luder HU 1993 Articular degeneration and remodeling in human temporomandibular joints with normal and abnormal disc position. J Orofac Pain 7:391-402.

Lund JP, Donga R, Widmer CG, Stohler CS 1991 The pain-adaptation model: a discussion of the relationship between chronic musculoskeletal pain and motor activity. Canadian Journal of Physiology and Pharmacology 69:683-694.

Macaluso GM, Guerra P, Di Giovanni G et al 1998 Sleep bruxism is a disorder related to periodic arousals during sleep. J Dent Res 77:565-573.

Magnusson T, Adiels AM, Nilsson HL, Helkimo M 2004 Treatment effect on signs and symptoms of temporomandibular disorders–comparison between stabilisation splint and a new type of splint (NTI). A pilot study. Swed Dent J 28:11-20.

Magnusson T, Egermarki I, Carlsson GE 2005 A prospective investigation over two decades on signs and symptoms of temporomandibular disorders and associated variables. A final summary. Acta Odontol Scand 63:99-109.

McNamara JA, Seligman DA, Okeson JP 1995 Occlusion, Orthodontic treatment, and temporomandibular disorders: a review. J Orofac Pain 9:73-90.

Medicine AAoS 2005 Sleep related bruxism. In: The International classification of sleep disorders: diagnostic and coding manual, 2nd edn. American Sleep Disorders Association, Westchester.

Minakuchi H, Kuboki T, Matsuka et al 2001 Randomized controlled evaluation of non-surgical treatments for temporomandibular joint anterior disk displacement without reduction. J Dent Res 80:924-928.

Ohayon MM, Li KK, Guilleminault C 2001 Risk factors for sleep bruxism in the general population. Chest 119:53-61.

Ohrbach R, Dworkin SF 1998 Five-year outcomes in TMD: relationship of changes in pain to changes in physical and psychological variables. Pain 74:315-326.

Okeson JP 2005 Bell's orofacial pains: the clinical management of orofacial pain, 6th edn. Quintessence Publishing, Chicago.

Okeson JP 2008 Management of temporomandibular disorders and occlusion, 6th edn. Elsevier Mosby, St Louis.

Okeson JP, Phillips BA, Berry DT et al 1990 Nocturnal bruxing events in healthy geriatric subjects. J Oral Rehabil 17:411-418.

Okeson JP, Phillips BA, Berry DT et al 1991 Nocturnal bruxing events in subjects with sleep-disordered breathing and control subjects. J Craniomandib Disord 5:258-264.

Okeson JP, Phillips BA, Berry DT, Baldwin RM 1994 Nocturnal bruxing events: a report of normative data and cardiovascular response. J Oral Rehabil 21:623-630.

Orofacial Pain and Dysfunction 2008 Elsevier, Philadelphia.

Pergamalian A, Rudy TE, Zaki HS, Greco CM 2003 The association between wear facets, bruxism, and severity of facial pain in patients with temporomandibular disorders. Journal of prosthetic dentistry 90:194-200.

Pierce CJ, Chrisman K, Bennett ME, Close JM 1995 Stress, anticipatory stress, and psychologic measures related to sleep bruxism. J Orofac Pain 9:51-56.

Pullinger AG, Seligman DA 1991 Trauma history in diagnostic groups of temporomandibular disorders.

Oral Surg Oral Med Oral Pathol 71:529-534.

Pullinger AG, Seligman DA, Gornbein JA 1993 A multiple logistic regression analysis of the risk and relative odds of temporomandibular disorders as a function of common occlusal features. J Dent Res 72: 968-979.

Ramfjord SP 1961 Bruxism, a clinical and electromyographic study. J Am Dent Assoc 62:21-44.

Randolph CS, Greene CS, Moretti R 1990 Conservative Management of temporomandibular disorders: A post treatment comparison between patients from a university clinic and from private practice. American Journal Orthod Dentofac Orthop 98:77-82.

Rasmussen BK, Jensen R, Schroll M, Olesen J 1991 Epidemiology of headache in a general population—a prevalence study. Journal of clinical epidemiology 44:1147-1157.

Reding GR, Rubright WC, Zimmerman SO 1966 Incidence of bruxism. J Dent Res 45:1198-1204.

Rugh JD, Solberg WK 1975 Electromyographic studies of bruxist behavior before and during treatment. J Calif Dent Assoc 3:56-59.

Rugh JD, Barghi N, Drago CJ 1984 Experimental occlusal discrepancies and nocturnal bruxism. Journal of prosthetic dentistry 51:548-553.

Salé H, Isberg A 2007 Delayed temporomandibular joint pain and dysfunction induced by whiplash trauma: a controlled prospective study. J Am Dent Assoc 138: 1084-1091.

Schiffman EL, Fricton JR, Haley DP, Shapiro BL 1990 The prevalence and treatment needs of subjects with temporomandibular disorders. J Am Dent Assoc 120:295-303.

Schille H 1986 Injuries of the temporomandibular joint: Classification, diagnosis and fundamental treatment. In: Kruger E, Schilli W (eds) Oral and maxillofacial traumatology. Quintessence Publishing, Chicago.

Schokker RP, Hansson TL, Ansink BJ 1990a Craniomandibular disorders in patients with different types of headache. J Craniomandib Disord 4:47-51.

Schokker RP, Hansson TL, Ansink BJ 1990b Differences in headache patients regarding response to treatment of the masticatory system. J Craniomandib Disord 4:228-232.

Sessle BJ 1999 The neural basis of temporomandibular joint and masticatory muscle pain. J Orofac Pain 13:238-245.

Shankland WE 2002 Nociceptive trigeminal inhibition - tension suppression system: a method of preventing migraine and tension headaches. Compend Contin Educ Dent 23:105-108, 110, 112-113; quiz 114.

Skeppar J, Nilner M 1993 Treatment of craniomandibular disorders in children and young adults. J Orofac Pain Fall 7:362-369.

Solberg WK, Clark GT, Rugh JD 1975 Nocturnal electromyographic evaluation of bruxism patients undergoing short term splint therapy. J Oral Rehabil 2:215-223.

Stegenga B, De Bont LG, Boering G 1989 A proposed classification of temporomandibular disorders based on synovial joint pathology. Cranio 7:107-118.

Stegenga B, de Bont LG, Boering G, van Willigen JD 1991 Tissue responses to degenerative changes in the temporomandibular joint: a review. J Oral Maxillofac Surg 49:1079-1088.

Stegenga B, de Bont LG, Dijkstra PU, Boering G 1993 Short-term outcome of arthroscopic surgery of temporomandibular joint osteoarthrosis and internal derangement: a randomized controlled clinical trial. Br J Oral Maxillofac Surg 31:3-14.

Stohler CS, Ash MM 1986 Excitatory response of jaw elevators associated with sudden discomfort during chewing. J Oral Rehabil 13:225-233.

Stohler CS, Ashton-Miller JA, Carlson DS 1988 The effects of pain from the mandibular joint and muscles on masticatory motor behaviour in man. Archives of Oral Biology 33:175-182.

Travell JG, Rinzler SH 1952 The myofascial genesis of pain. Postgrad Med J 11:425-434.

Tsukiyama Y, Baba K, Clark GT 2001 An evidence-based assessment of occlusal adjustment as a treatment for temporomandibular disorders. Journal of Prosthetic Dentistry 86:57-66.

Velly AM, Gornitsky M, Philippe P 2003 Contributing factors to chronic myofascial pain: a case-control study. Pain 104:491-499.

Von Korff M, Dworkin SF, Le Resche L, Kruger A 1988 An epidemiologic comparison of pain complaints. Pain 32:173-183.

Watanabe T, Ichikawa K, Clark GT 2003 Bruxism levels and daily behaviors: 3 weeks of measurement and correlation. J Orofac Pain 17:65-73.

Yatani II, Kaneshima T, Kuboki T et al 1997 Long-term follow-up study on drop-out TMD patients with self-administered questionnaires. J Orofac Pain 11:258-269.

8

Clinical features of cervicogenic and temporomandibular-related headache

Guy Zito

Differential diagnosis is one of the greatest challenges facing health practitioners who manage headache. Identifying cervicogenic headache and TMD-related headache so that treatment can be directed accurately is part of that challenge. In this chapter the author, a musculoskeletal physiotherapist, presents a system of examination to clarify the clinical overlap.

The lifetime prevalence of headache has been estimated at 96%, and the point prevalence at 16% (Rasmussen et al 1991). Whilst approximately 70% of persons with frequent intermittent headache report neck aching, pain or stiffness in association with their headache (Henry et al 1987), only about 18% of these headaches are considered to originate from the cervical region (Nilsson 1995, Pfaffenrath & Kaube 1990). On the other hand 50–75% of people have at least one sign of temporomandibular disorders (TMD) and 25–33% have at least one symptom, which may include TMD-related headache (Dworkin et al 1990, Gremillion & Mahan 2000). Thus, a significant number of patients will present for treatment with headache quite possibly related to cervical disorder or TMD, or both.

There are several reasons why the diagnostic process is so difficult. The close neuroanatomical

(Bogduk 1995, Drake et al 2005, Goadsby et al 1997, Sessle 1999, 2000, Svensson et al 2004) and biomechanical (Huggare & Raustia, 1992, Rocabado & Iglarsh 1991, Santander et al 2000) connections between the cervical and temporomandibular regions make the headaches arising from the two areas similar and difficult to distinguish. This process is compounded if there is sensitization in that part of the central nervous system that is involved in the processing and perception of head pain. Furthermore, the etiological link between the two regions results in cervical patients having signs or symptoms of TMD and jaw patients having cervical disorder (Ciancaglini et al 1999, Clark et al 1987, De Wijer et al 1996a & b, Fink et al 2002, Okeson 1996). Consequently, not only can the two headache forms have symptoms in common with each other, but they can often co-exist.

Treatment needs to be directed effectively and accurately towards the underlying cause to achieve the optimal outcome. To facilitate the diagnostic process, cues are needed to distinguish cervicogenic headache and TMD-related headache. They are also required to identify other common forms of headache not related to the musculoskeletal system with which they share symptoms, such as migraine and tension-type headache, (IHS 2004, Sjaastad & Stovner 1993). This chapter therefore addresses the relationship between the cervical and the temporomandibular region and the characteristic features of these two headache types in their pure form.

Neuroanatomical basis for pain referral

The cervical structures are innervated by C1–C3 while the masticatory muscles and the temporomandibular joint are innervated by branches of the mandibular division of the trigeminal nerve (Drake et al 2005). These structures are known to possess nociceptive afferents so it is reasonable to argue their potential for extensive pain referral patterns (Sessle 2006). As the cutaneous distribution of the upper three cervical spinal nerves extends only as far as the vertex and that of the trigeminal nerve covers the front half of the head (Drake et al 2005), the inference is that a neuro-anatomical mechanism is responsible for the spread of symptoms of cervicogenic headache to the front of the head (Bogduk 1995). The phenomenon results from the convergence of afferents of the trigeminal nerve and the first three cervical nerves onto the trigeminocervical nucleus (Goadsby et al 1997, Sessle 1999, 2000, Svensson et al 2004). The nociceptive nucleus receives afferent neurons from the two topographically different regions, with the result that noxious stimuli from the neck can be perceived as arising from the head (Bogduk 1992). Moreover, clinical investigators have reported that the ophthalmic branch of the trigeminal nerve is involved in the production of cervicogenic headache (Aprill et al 2002, Piovesan et al 2001).

Whilst there is little supportive anatomical evidence at this stage, it is not unreasonable to argue that this mechanism could be responsible for the referral of pain from the temporomandibular structures to the neck, making it difficult to distinguish between cervicogenic headache and TMD-related headache.

Biomechanical relationship

A biomechanical relationship of the craniocervical complex has also been proposed and several authors noted that zygapophyseal joint mobility may influence the rest position of the mandible (Passero et al 1985, Rocabado & Iglarsh 1991). Other studies have described a functional link between the muscles of the stomatognathic system and the cervical region (Rocabado & Iglarsh 1991, Santander et al 2000), whereby the masticatory muscles act with the cervical muscles to produce head movement and vice versa (Forsberg et al 1985) (Fig. 8.1). This may explain, in part, the incidence of cervical disorder in patients with TMD and vice-versa (Braun & Schiffman 1991, Burgess 1991, Clark et al 1987).

Clinical features of cervicogenic headache

Subjective characteristics

The subjective characteristics of cervicogenic headache have been well documented (Fredriksen & Sjaastad 1987, Sjaastad et al 1983, 1990, 1998, 1999). The symptoms typically extend anteriorly from the occipital and suboccipital areas through to the frontal and orbital regions (Sjaastad et al 1983). They were initially considered to be unilateral without sideshift, not changing from one side of the head to the other (Fredriksen & Sjaastad 1987, Sjaastad et al 1983, 1990). A subsequent review (Sjaastad et al 1998) of its characteristics resulted in

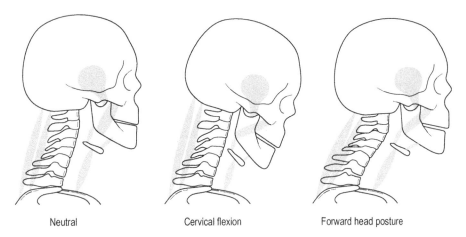

Neutral   Cervical flexion   Forward head posture

Figure 8.1 • Functional link between the muscles of the stomatognathic system and the cervical spine.

tempering of the initial rigid criterion of unilaterality and acknowledged the possibility of two unilateral cervicogenic headaches presenting concurrently as a bilateral headache.

Cervicogenic headache affects twice as many females as males. Sufferers are usually aged 6–40 years with a mean age of 30 years and they describe a moderate to severe, boring type of pain. Migraine medication is often ineffective, while non-steroidal anti-inflammatory medication may be of benefit. The symptoms tend to be worse in the morning and may continue to increase during the day. They may be provoked by neck movements or sustained postures including poor sleeping posture though the onset of the headache may be associated with physical or emotional trauma. The attacks are episodic, occurring 1–3 times per week and lasting from hours to days. In the chronic state the symptoms may be present continuously. Associated symptoms include dizziness, dysphagia, lacrimation, nausea or vomiting, phonophobia and photophobia, rhinorrhea, ipsilateral shoulder and arm symptoms, tinnitus, and visual disturbances (Fredriksen & Sjaastad 1987, Pfaffenrath & Kaube 1990, Sjaastad et al 1983, 1998).

Physical characteristics

The signs of impairment in the musculoskeletal system which are associated with cervicogenic headache include forward head posture, hyperalgesia, reduced mobility and disorders in the muscular system.

Forward head posture

Over the years authors have referred to the clinical significance of a forward head posture and its relationship to musculoskeletal dysfunction including headache. Whilst forward head posture is said to place undue load on the cervical structures (Braun & Amundson 1989, Mayoux-Benhamou et al 1994, Rocabado & Iglarsh 1991) there is still very little evidence to support the contention that it is a contributing factor to the pathological state (Haughie et al 1995, Refshauge et al 1995, Treleaven et al 1994, Zito et al 2006).

Hyperalgesia

Hyperalgesic areas, including myofascial trigger points (MTPs) and tender points, are poorly understood yet are often mentioned in the criteria for headaches (Fredriksen & Sjaastad, 1987, IHS 2004, Okifuji et al 1999, Pfaffenrath & Kaube 1990, Simons et al 1999, Sjaastad et al 1983, 1998). In the case of cervicogenic headache these MTPs are reported as being over the ipsilateral C2 root, greater occipital nerve, and the transverse process of C4 and C5 (Fredriksen & Sjaastad, 1987, Pfaffenrath & Kaube, 1990, Sjaastad et al 1983, 1998). It should be noted however that the presence of these MTPs is shared with other, non-specific diagnoses such as fibromyalgia and is considered of little diagnostic value with headache (Okifuji et al 1999).

Reduced mobility

Painful limitation of cervical movement is another feature of cervicogenic headache that is cited regularly (Fredriksen & Sjaastad 1987, Sjaastad et al 1983, 1990, 1998). Several studies, however, have shown that the difference in ranges of cervical movement between cervicogenic headache patients and other headache patients, as well as asymptomatic volunteers, did not reach significance levels in all directions of movement (Treleaven et al 1994, Zito et al 2006, Zwart 1997). Consequently findings of reduced mobility are of limited value in isolation of other clinical findings.

Evidence is mounting to support the use of manual examination as a diagnostic tool. A number of clinical trials have been able to demonstrate that upper cervical joint dysfunction in the form of reduced segmental mobility, in particular at C1–C2 and C2–C3, can assist in differentiating cervicogenic headache from other headache forms (Jull et al 1999, Jull & Niere, 2004, Watson & Trott, 1993, Zito et al 2006). In two studies on cervicogenic headache and migraine sufferers (Vincent & Luna, 1999, Zito et al 2006) the investigators were able to elicit either local or referred pain with pressure

over the upper cervical region of cervicogenic headache subjects. Such pain reproduction was not reported in migraine sufferers.

Dysfunction in the muscular system

A higher frequency of tightness of the cervical muscles has been noted in clinical trials on cervicogenic headache patients when compared to migraine with aura sufferers and asymptomatic volunteers (Jull et al 1999, Zito et al 2006). The most prevalent muscle was the upper trapezius, though the scalenes, levator scapulae, and deep cervical extensors were also found to be significantly less extensible (Zito et al 2006).

Cervical dysfunction patients including cervicogenic headache sufferers have a deficit in motor control of the deep neck flexor synergy. The impairment is characterized by a loss of endurance of the stabilizing muscles brought on by delayed onset and an altered pattern of activation. Endurance has been shown to be diminished in these patients when compared to the normal population (Falla 2004, Falla et al 2004, Jull et al 1999, Jull 2000, Watson & Trott, 1993, Zito et al 2006).

Clinical features of TMD-related headache

Unlike cervicogenic headache, TMD-related headache is not seen as a separate clinical entity but rather as a symptom of complex somatic pain, secondary to dysfunction in the temporomandibular region (IHS 2004, Okeson 2005). It has not received the same attention and the typical TMD-related headache is more difficult to define.

Current consensus is that TMD describes a multifactorial, biopsychosocial disorder which consists of a number of clinical problems arising from the masticatory muscles and/or the temporomandibular joint(s) and related structures (Greene 2006). The association between TMD and headache has been widely acknowledged for many years (Carlsson & Magnusson 1999, Ciancaglini & Radaelli 2001, Kemper & Okeson 1983, Okeson 1996, 2005, Pettengill 1999, Schokker et al 1990). Studies reported that between 70% and 86% of TMD patients suffer from headache (Bush & Harkins 1995, Ciancaglini & Radaelli 2001, Kemper & Okeson 1983, Nassif & Talic 2001, Reik & Hale 1981) and others reported that between 14% and 27% of headache patients also have TMD signs and/or symptoms (Reik & Hale 1981, Schokker et al 1990).

Subjective characteristics

The symptoms are more commonly felt in the temporal area, pre-auricular area, and along the mandibular region (Pettengill 1999, Rauhala et al 1999, Reik & Hale 1981) though there may be some radiation to the side of the neck (Reik & Hale 1981).

There is conjecture about the sidedness of the headache in the dental literature since the TMD related headache were not defined and were lumped together. More evidence supports a unilateral headache (Pettengill 1999, Reik & Hale 1981, Williamson 1990), though authors have suggested it can be either unilateral or bilateral (Lindsay 1980, Schokker et al 1990). In the absence of a central mechanism, the somatic referral along the path of the trigeminal nerve would support the contention that it is a unilateral headache. Similar to cervicogenic headache, an apparent bilateral headache might be the result of concurrent lesions in both jaws.

TMD-related headache affects about twice as many females as males (Goulet et al 1995, Svensson et al 2004); the age range is 19–83 years (Pettengill 1999). It occurs daily, is often worse on waking, and may be continuous from hours to days. Sufferers often describe a deep dull ache with a throbbing component (Pettengill 1999, Reik & Hale 1981, Schokker et al 1990) and may report associated symptoms including tinnitus, vertigo, and fullness in the ear (Pettengill 1999).

Mechanical precipitating factors include repetitive microtrauma or bruxism, though the clinical relationship between bruxism and TMD is a contentious topic (Lobbezoo & Lavigne, 1997, van der Meulen et al 2006). Macrotrauma to the region may result from overstretching, biting hard foods, prolonged or difficult dental procedures, or from a sports injury. Increased emotional stress and genetic predisposition are other, non mechanical factors cited (McCreary et al 1991, Schiffman et al 1992).

Physical characteristics

Unlike cervicogenic headache, there have been no controlled studies to validate the physical characteristics of TMD-related headache. The signs of impairment in the musculoskeletal system associated with TMD-related headache discussed include a forward head posture hyperalgesia, reduced mobility and muscular dysfunction.

Forward head posture

The clinical relevance of craniocervical posture and the temporomandibular region is contentious. A number of authors have reported the influence of craniocervical posture on the stomatognathic system (Makofsky 2000, Moya et al 1994, Rocabado & Iglarsh 1991) and in particular the rest position of the mandible (Gonzalez & Manns 1996, Moya et al 1994, Yamabe et al 1999). These altered states impact on joint mechanics (Visscher et al 2000) and affect the level of muscle activity

(Funakoshi et al 1976). The debate is just as intense with regard to abnormal craniocervical posture and whether it causes or predisposes the temporomandibular region to injury (Nicolakis et al 2000, Rocabado & Iglarsh 1991, Sonnesen et al 2001, Visscher et al 2000). A recent systematic review of the literature (Olivo et al 2006) highlighted the deficiencies in the research and confirmed that there is little evidence to support any of the contentions.

Hyperalgesia

Tender points and MTPs are often mentioned in the literature in association with TMD, particularly in the temporalis, masseter and pterygoid muscles (Merskey & Bogduk 1994, Okeson 2005, Saper et al 1999, Simons et al 1999). The anecdotal evidence can be quite convincing though inter-tester reliability in localizing MTPs in upper trapezius has been shown to be poor in specifying both the exact location and quantity of points (Lew et al 1997). Since hyperalgesic areas are associated with a number of musculoskeletal conditions they are of little assistance with respect to diagnosis.

Reduced mobility

Reduced mouth opening with or without deviation of the mandible is considered a sign of TMD (Carlsson & Magnusson 1999, Merskey & Bogduk 1994, Saper et al 1999). It may also be accompanied by noises in the temporomandibular joint such as clicking or popping (Carlsson & Magnusson 1999, Merskey & Bogduk 1994). It is hypothesized that opening without deviation is attributed to a myogenous cause of TMD, while a deviation, usually to the affected side, is suggestive of an arthrogenous cause, often associated with internal derangement of the disc (Carlsson & Magnusson 1999).

Dysfunction of the muscular system

Hyperactivity of the masticatory muscles and ensuing prolonged excessive pressure on the stomatognathic structures due to bruxism and other parafunctional habits can be noxious to muscle (Forssell et al 1986). It places undue forces on the teeth and jaws, reported to be greater than during chewing or mastication (Carlsson & Magnusson 1999) and may result in pain which propagates muscle dysfunction. The precise origin of the muscle pain is uncertain, though the suggestion is that it results from vasoconstriction and the accumulation of metabolic waste products (Okeson 2005). Co-contraction is a common phenomenon associated with myogenic pain and is able to affect neighboring muscles (Carlson et al 1993). The masticatory muscle symptoms may eventually overflow into the cervical musculature and it may be argued that they affect motor control (Svensson et al 2004) in much the same way that occurs in the cervical muscles of chronic neck pain sufferers (Falla 2004, Falla et al 2004). Based on this supposition, the finding of impairment in the muscular system may be of limited value in differentiating cervicogenic headache from TMD-related headache.

Differential diagnosis

When dealing with headache patients it is important to be cognizant of symptoms which are an indication of more serious or life-threatening brain pathology. As primary contact practitioners it is important to be aware of these more sinister conditions. It should never be assumed that headaches are emanating from the cervical region or temporomandibular region unless there is clinical evidence to support the diagnosis. The consequences of a misdiagnosis could be catastrophic, emphasizing the need for accurate diagnostic cues to distinguish the various forms of headache.

There appear to be no randomized controlled trials which draw distinction between cervicogenic headache and TMD-related headache. To facilitate the diagnostic process it is worth considering the salient features of the two forms of headache which are summarized in Tables 8.1 and 8.2.

Cervicogenic headache sufferers commonly complain of a unilateral headache which extends from the sub-occipital region anteriorly, into the area supplied by the ophthalmic branch of the trigeminal nerve. Increased neck stiffness and reduced segmental mobility in the upper cervical region may strengthen the hypothesis of a cervical cause for the headache, as would the finding of deficit in motor control.

Sjaastad and co-workers (Sjaastad et al 1998) described that the cervical contribution is confirmed if the headache is precipitated by neck movements, prolonged or awkward postures,

Table 8.1 Summary of the subjective characteristics of TMD-related headache and cervicogenic headache.

Characteristic	TMD-related headache	Cervicogenic headache
Sex ratio (females:males)	2:1	2:1
Age range	19–83 years	6–40 years
Area of pain	Spreads from the masticatory muscles/pre-auricular area into the temple and down into the jaw – the area supplied by the mandibular branch of the trigeminal nerve Can have referral into neck	Commences in sub-occipital and occipital region and extends anteriorly – more commonly in ophthalmic nerve distribution
Unilaterality	Unilateral headache. May present as bilateral	Unilateral headache, side-locked. Can be bilateral
Quality	Dull, deep ache Can be throbbing	Dull to boring pain Moderate to severe
Frequency, duration	Daily lasting hours to days May be continuous	1–3 per week, lasting hours Can be continuous if chronic
Behavior	Often worse in mornings	Often worse in mornings though may continue to increase during day
Precipitating mechanism	Trauma to the temporomandibular region due to parafunctional activity, e.g. bruxism, or a sports injury or a dental procedure Physical or emotional stress	Provoked by neck movements, sustained postures including poor sleeping posture Physical or emotional trauma
Reaction to medication	Can have good response to NSAIDs	Can have good response to NSAIDs Migraine medication ineffective
Associated symptoms	Tinnitus, vertigo, and fullness in the ear	Dizziness, dysphagia, lacrimation, nausea or vomiting, phonophobia, photophobia, rhinorrhea, shoulder or arm symptoms, tinnitus, visual disturbances

Table 8.2 Summary of the physical characteristics of TMD-related headache and cervicogenic headache.

Characteristic	Temporomandibular related headache	Cervicogenic headache
Posture	Forward head	Forward head
Hyperalgesia	Tenderness over TMJ MTPs in masticatory muscles, especially masseter and temporalis	Tenderness over the ipsilateral C2 root, the greater occipital nerve, and the transverse process of C4 and C5
Articular system	Reduced mouth opening with or without mandibular deviation May be accompanied by joint noises (clicking or popping)	Decreased neck mobility Reduced segmental mobility in upper cervical spine especially C1–C2 and C2–C3 and reproducing head pain
Muscular system	Hyperactivity of masticatory muscles – flow-on effect may influence motor control of cervical muscles	Loss of extensibility of cervical muscles Loss of endurance of neck flexor synergy

and/or external pressure over the upper cervical region. Other supporting characteristics include restriction of neck movement, and/or the presence of ipsilateral neck and/or shoulder pain. This correlates with a recent controlled study which investigated the physical characteristics of cervicogenic headache as well as the sensitivity of clinical signs to detect neuromusculoskeletal dysfunction (Zito et al 2006). The study was limited to a comparison of cervicogenic headache patients and migraine with aura patients and asymptomatic volunteers. The findings supported the contention that cervicogenic headache can be diagnosed through its physical impairment with tests of muscle extensibility, manual examination and muscle function, and to a lesser extent with tests of mobility.

Too much emphasis can be placed on restriction of ranges of movement however, and this latter finding should not be considered in isolation when it comes to differential diagnosis. In several comparative studies a significant difference in mobility of cervicogenic headache subjects was reported when compared to migraine, tension-type headache and asymptomatic controls (Vincent & Luna 1999, Zwart 1997).

Interestingly, decreased neck mobility was also found in migraine sufferers when compared to an asymptomatic control group (Kidd & Nelson 1993). Hence, cervical mobility on its own will not identify a particular disorder.

TMD-related headache sufferers commonly describe a unilateral headache which spreads from the masticatory muscles/pre-auricular area into the temple and down into the jaw – the area supplied by the mandibular branch of the trigeminal nerve. Another distinctive complaint may also be fullness in the ear (Pettengill 1999). These subjective findings, combined with reduced mouth opening with or without deviation, especially if accompanied by joint noises with pain, may serve to identify regional temporal headache as a symptom of temporomandibular dysfunction (Gobel 2005).

A study by Reik and Hale (Reik & Hale 1981) compared three headache forms: TMD-related headache, migraine and tension-type headache. It found that restricted movement and jaw deviation on opening as well as masticatory muscle tenderness are significantly more prevalent in TMD-related headache. Interestingly they found that jaw clicking, edentulous state and dental wear facets are equal in all groups, and that nausea, vomiting, photophobia and fatigue are unusual except for migraine headaches. Understandably posterior cervical tenderness was reported as being equal in those with temporomandibular related headache and tension-type headache, but less common in migraine which, in the pure form, does not have a cervical component.

In summary, with our current level of knowledge, the best cues to assist with differential diagnosis might arguably be as follows:

1. The cervicogenic headache patient complains of anterior spread of pain from the sub-occipital area to the front of the head while the TMD-related headache patient reports pain in the masticatory muscle/pre-auricular area radiating to the temple.

2. The TMD-related headache patient is more likely to complain of fullness in the ear associated with the headache.

3. Although not uncommon, precipitating factors such as bruxism and parafunctional activities may incriminate the temporomandibular region specifically.

4. Limitation of movement of the mandible with or without deviation or joint sounds would also suggest temporomandibular involvement.

5. Reduced segmental mobility in the upper cervical segments, reproducing head pain, would incriminate the cervical spine.

Conclusion

When diagnosing headache and facial pain it is necessary to take into account the clinical overlap of TMD-related headache and cervicogenic headache. A comprehensive history and a detailed physical examination are of paramount importance to establish the contribution of each structure to the symptomatology. It is only with an accurate diagnosis that an appropriate management plan can be formulated and an informed decision made about the limitations of a particular discipline. It is important to recognize the need to collaborate with other health practitioners to obtain the optimal result for the headache patient.

References

Aprill C, Axinn MJ, Bogduk N 2002 Occipital headaches stemming from the lateral atlanto-axial (C1-2) Joint. Cephalalgia 22:15-22.

Bogduk N 1992 The anatomical basis for cervicogenic headache. Journal of Manipulative and Physiological Therapeutics 15:67-70.

Bogduk N 1995 Anatomy and physiology of headache. Biomedicine and Pharmacotherapy 49:435-445.

Braun BL, Amundson LR 1989 Quantitative assessment of head and shoulder posture. Archives of Physical Medicine and Rehabilitation 70:322-329.

Braun BL, Schiffman EL 1991 The validity and predictive value of four assessment instruments for evaluation of the cervical and stomatognathic systems. Journal of Craniomandibular Disorders, Facial and Oral Pain 5:239-244.

Burgess J 1991 Symptom characteristics in TMD patients reporting blunt trauma and/or whiplash injury. Journal of Craniomandibular Disorders: Facial and Oral Pain 5:251-257.

Bush F, Harkins S 1995 Pain-related limitation in activities of daily living in patients with chronic orofacial pain: psychometric properties of a disability index. Journal of Orofacial Pain 9:57-63.

Carlson CR, Okeson JP, Falace DA et al 1993 Reduction of pain and EMG activity in the masseter region by trapezius trigger point injection. Pain 55:397-400.

Carlsson G, Magnusson T 1999 Management of temporomandibular disorders in the general dental practice. Quintessence Publishing, Chicago.

Ciancaglini R, Radaelli G 2001 The relationship between headache and symptoms of temporomandibular disorder in the general population. Journal of Dentistry 29:93-98.

Ciancaglini R, Testa M, Radaelli G 1999 Association of neck pain with symptoms of temporomandibular dysfunction in the general adult population. Scandinavian Journal of Rehabilitation Medicine 31:17-22.

Clark GT, Green EM, Dornan MR, Flack VF 1987 Craniocervical dysfunction levels in a patient sample from a temporomandibular joint clinic. Journal of the American Dental Association 115:251-256.

De Wijer A, Steenks MH, Bosman F et al 1996a Symptoms of the stomatognathic system in temporomandibular and cervical spine disorders. Journal of Oral Rehabilitation 23:733-741.

De Wijer A, Steenks MH, De Leeuw JRJ et al 1996b Symptoms of the cervical spine in temporomandibular and cervical spine disorders. Journal of Oral Rehabilitation 23:742-750.

Drake RL, Vogl W, Mitchell AWM 2005 Gray's anatomy for students. Philadelphia, Elsevier Churchill Livingstone.

Dworkin SF, Huggins KH, Leresche L et al 1990 Epidemiology of signs and symptoms in temporomandibular disorders: clinical signs in cases and controls. Journal of The American Dental Association 120:273-281.

Falla D 2004 Unravelling the complexity of muscle impairment in chronic neck pain. Manual Therapy 9: 125-133.

Falla D, Jull G, Hodges PW 2004 Feedforward activity of the cervical flexor muscles during voluntary arm movements is delayed in chronic neck pain. Experimental Brain Research 157:43-48.

Fink M, Tschernitschek H, Stiesch-Scholz M 2002 Asymptomatic cervical spine dysfunction (CSD) in patients with internal derangement of the temporomandibular joint. Journal of Craniomandibular Practice 20:192-197.

Forsberg CM, Hellsing E, Linder-Aronson S, Sheikholeslam A 1985 Emg activity in neck and masticatory muscles in relation to extension and flexion of the head. European Journal Of Orthodontics 7:177-183.

Forssell H, Kirveskari P, Kangasniemi P 1986 Distinguishing between headaches responsive and irresponsive to treatment of mandibular dysfunction. Proceedings of the Finnish Dental Society 82:219-222.

Fredriksen T, Sjaastad O 1987 Cervicogenic headache. A clinical entity. Cephalalgia 17:171-172.

Funakoshi M, Fujita N, Takehana S 1976 Relations between occlusal interference and jaw muscle activities in response to changes in head position. Journal of Dental Research 55:684-690.

Goadsby PJ, Knight YE, Hoskin KL 1997 Stimulation of the greater occipital nerve increases metabolic activity in the trigeminal nucleus caudalis and cervical dorsal horn of the cat. Pain 73:23-28.

Gobel H 2005 Headache or facial pain attributed to disorders of cranium, neck, eyes, ears, nose, sinuses, teeth, mouth, or other facial or cranial structures. In: Olesen J (ed.) Classification and diagnosis of headache disorders. Oxford University Press, Oxford.

Gonzalez HE, Manns A 1996 Forward head posture: its structural and functional influence on the stomatognathic system, a conceptual study. Cranio 14:71-80.

Goulet JP, Lavigne GJ, Lund JP 1995 Jaw pain prevalence among French speaking Canadians in Quèbec and related symptoms of temporomandibular disorder. Journal of Dental Research 74:1738-1744.

Greene CS 2006 Concepts of Tmd etiology: effects on diagnosis and treatment. In: Laskin DM, Greene CS, Hylander WL (eds) Temporomandibular disorders – an evidence-based approach to diagnosis and treatment. Quintessence Publishing, Chicago.

Gremillion HA, Mahan PE 2000 The prevalence and etiology of temporomandibular disorders and orofacial pain. Texas Dental Journal 117:30-39.

Haughie LJ, Fiebert IM, Roach KE 1995 Relationship of forward head posture and cervical backward bending neck pain. Journal of Manual and Manipulative Therapy 3:91-97.

Henry P, Dartigues JF, Puymirat E, Al E 1987 The association cervicalgia-headaches: an epidemiologic study. Cephalalgia 7:189-190.

Huggare J, Raustia A 1992 Head posture and craniovertebral and craniofacial morphology in patients with craniomandibular dysfunction. Cranio 10:173-177.

IHS 2004 Headache Classification Committee Of The International Headache Society – The International Classification Of Headaches Disorders. Cephalalgia 24:1-160.

Jull GA 2000 Deep cervical flexor muscle dysfunction in whiplash. Journal of Musculoskeletal Pain 8:143-154.

Jull GA, Niere KR 2004 Cervical headache: a review. In: Boyling G. Jull GA (eds) Grieve's modern manual therapy – the vertebral column, 3rd edn. Churchill Livingstone, Edinburgh.

Jull G, Barrett C, Magee R, Ho P 1999 Further clinical clarification of the muscle dysfunction in cervical headache. Cephalalgia 19:179-185.

Kemper JT, Okeson JP 1983 Craniomandibular disorders and headaches. Journal of Prosthetic Dentistry 49:702-709.

Kidd RF, Nelson R 1993 Musculoskeletal dysfunction of the neck in migraine and tension headache. Headache 33:566-569.

Lew PC, Lewis J, Story IH 1997 Inter-therapist reliability in locating latent myofascial trigger points using palpitation. Manual Therapy 2:87-90.

Lindsay B 1980 Muscular contraction headache and dental imbalance. Australian Family Physician 9: 513-522.

Lobbezoo F, Lavigne GJ 1997 Do bruxism and temporomandibular disorders have a cause-and-effect relationship? Journal of Orofacial Pain 11:15-23.

Makofsky HW 2000 The influence of forward head posture on dental occlusion. Cranio 18:30-39.

Mayoux-Benhamou MA, Revel M, Vallee C et al 1994 Longus colli has a postural function on cervical curvature. Surgical & Radiologic Anatomy 16:367-371.

Mccreary CP, Clark GT, Merril RL et al 1991 Psychological distress and diagnostic subgroups of temporomandibular disorder patients. Pain 44:29-34.

Merskey H, Bogduk N (eds) 1994 Classification of chronic pain. description of chronic pain syndromes and definitions of pain terms. Iasp Press, Seattle.

Moya H, Miralles R, Zuniga C et al 1994 Influence of stabilization occlusal splints on craniocervical relationships. Part 1: Cephalometric Analysis. Cranio 12:47-51.

Nassif N, Talic Y 2001 Classic symptoms in temporomandibular disorder patients: a comparative study. Journal of Craniomandibular Practice 19:33-41.

Nicolakis P, Nicolakis M, Piehslinger E, Al E 2000 Relationship between craniomandibular disorders and poor posture. Cranio 18:106-112.

Nilsson N 1995 The prevalence of cervicogenic headache in a random population sample of 20-59 year olds. Spine 20:1884-1888.

Okeson J 1996 Orofacial pain. Guidelines for assessment, diagnosis, and management. The American Academy of Orofacial Pain. Quintessence Publishing, Chicago.

Okeson J 2005 Bell's orofacial pain. The clinical management of orofacial pain. Quintessence Publishing, Chicago.

Okifuji A, Turk DC, Marcus DA 1999 Comparison of generalized and localized hyperalgesia in patients with recurrent headache and fibromyalgia. Psychosomatic Medicine 61:771-780.

Olivo S, Bravo J, Magee D 2006 The association between head and cervical posture and temporomandibular disorders: a systematic review. Journal of Orofacial Pain 20:9-23.

Passero PL, Wyman BS, Bell JW et al 1985 Temporomandibular joint dysfunction syndrome. A clinical report. Physical Therapy 65: 1203-1207.

Pettengill C 1999 A comparison of headache symptoms between two groups: a TMD group and a general dental practice group. Cranio 17: 64-69.

Pfaffenrath V, Kaube H 1990 Diagnostics of cervicogenic headache. Functional Neurology 5:159-164.

Piovesan EJ, Kowacs PA, Tatsui CE et al 2001 Referred pain after stimulation of the greater occipital nerve in humans: evidence of convergence of cervical afferences on trigeminal nuclei. Cephalalgia 21:107-109.

Rasmussen BK, Jensen R, Schroll M, Olesen J 1991 Epidemiology of headache in a general population—a prevalence study. Journal of Clinical Epidemiology 44:1147-1157.

Rauhala K, Oikarinen K, Raustia A 1999 Role of temporomandibular disorders (TMD) in facial pain: occlusion, muscle and TMJ pain. Journal of Craniomandibular Practice 17: 254-261.

Refshauge K, Bolst L, Goodsell M 1995 The relationship between cervicothoracic posture and the presence of pain. Journal of Manipulative and Physiological Therapeutics 21-24.

Reik L, Hale M 1981 The temporomandibular joint pain-dysfunction syndrome: a frequent cause of headache. Headache 21:151-156.

Rocabado M, Iglarsh ZA 1991 Musculoskeletal Approach to Maxillofacial Pain. JB Lippincott, Philadelphia.

Santander H, Miralles R, Perez J et al 2000 Effects of head and neck inclination on bilateral sternocleidomastoid EMG activity in healthy subjects and in patients with myogenic cranio-cervical-mandibular dysfunction. Journal of Craniomandibular Practice 18: 181-191.

Saper JR, Silberstein S, Gordon CD et al 1999 Handbook of headache management – a practical guide to diagnosis and treatment of head, neck and face pain. Lippincott Williams & Wilkins, Baltimore.

Schiffman EL, Fricton JR, Harley D 1992 The relationship of occlusion, parafunctional habits and recent life events to mandibular dysfunction in a non-patient population. Journal of Oral Rehabilitation 19:201-223.

Schokker RP, Hansson TL, Ansink BJ, Habets LL 1990 Craniomandibular asymmetry in headache patients. Journal of Craniomandibular Disorders 4:205-209.

Sessle BJ 1999 The neural basis of temporomandibular joint and masticatory muscle pain. Journal of Orofacial Pain 13:238-245.

Sessle BJ 2000 Acute and chronic craniofacial pain: brainstem mechanisms of nociceptive transmission and neuroplasticity, and their clinical correlates. Critical Reviews in Oral Biology & Medicine 11:57-91.

Sessle BJ 2006 Sensory and motor neurophysiology of the TMJ. In Laskin DM, Greene CS, Hylander WL (eds) Temporomandibular disorders. an evidence-based approach to diagnosis and treatment. Quintessence Publishing, Chicago.

Simons D, Travell J, Simons LS 1999 Travell and Simons' myofascial pain and dysfunction: the trigger point manual: upper half of body. Lippincott Williams and Wilkins, Philadelphia.

Sjaastad O, Stovner LJ 1993 The IHS classification for common migraine. Is it ideal? Headache 33:372-375.

Sjaastad O, Saunte C, Hovdahl H et al 1983 'Cervicogenic' headache. An hypothesis. Cephalalgia 3:249-256.

Sjaastad O, Fredriksen TA, Pfaffenrath V 1990 Cervicogenic headache: diagnostic criteria. Headache 30: 725-726.

Sjaastad O, Fredriksen TA, Pfaffenrath V 1998 Cervicogenic headache: diagnostic criteria. Headache 38: 442-445.

Sjaastad O, Fredriksen T, Pareja JA et al 1999 Coexistence of cervicogenic headache and migraine without aura(?). Functional Neurology 14: 209-218.

Sonnesen L, Bakke M, Solow B 2001 Temporomandibular disorders in relation to craniofacial dimensions, head posture and bite force in children selected for orthodontic treatment. *European* Journal of Orthodontics 23:179-192.

Svensson P, Wang K, Sessle BJ, Arendt-Nielsen L 2004 Associations between pain and neuromuscular activity in the human jaw and neck muscles. Pain 109:225-232.

Treleaven J, Jull G, Atkinson L 1994 Cervical musculoskeletal dysfunction in post-concussional headache. Cephalalgia 14:273-279.

van der Meulen MJ, Lobbezoo F, Aartman IHA, Naeije M 2006 Self-reported oral parafunctions and pain intensity in temporomandibular disorder patients. Journal of Orofacial Pain 20:31-35.

Vincent MB, Luna RA 1999 Cervicogenic headache: a comparison with migraine and tension-type headache. Cephalalgia 19:11-16.

Visscher CM, Huddleston Slater JJ, Lobbezo F, Naeije M 2000 Kinematics of the human mandible for different head postures. Journal of Oral Rehabilitation 27:299-305.

Wang K, Sessle BJ, Svensson P et al 2004 Glutamate evoked neck and jaw muscle pain facilitate the human jaw stretch reflex. Clin Neurophysiol. 115(6):1288-1295.

Watson DH, Trott PH 1993 Cervical headache: an investigation of natural head posture and upper cervical flexor muscle performance. Cephalalgia 13:272-284.

Williamson EH 1990 Interrelationship of internal derangements of the temporomandibular joint, headache, vertigo, and tinnitus: a survey of 25 patients. Cranio 8:301-306.

Yamabe Y, Yamashita R, Fujii H 1999 Head, neck and trunk movements accompanying jaw tapping. Journal of Oral Rehabilitation 26:900-905.

Zito G, Jull G, Story I 2006 Clinical tests of musculoskeletal dysfunction in the diagnosis of cervicogenic headache. Manual Therapy 11: 118-129.

Zwart JA 1997 Neck mobility in different headache disorders. Headache 37:6-11.

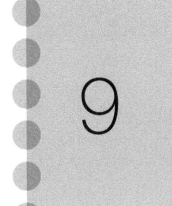

Chapter Nine

Central nervous system processing in cervicogenic headache

Ken Niere

Central nervous system processing is pivotal in the experience of cervicogenic headache. In this chapter the author, a musculoskeletal physiotherapist, presents a clinical approach to the identification of factors that might affect the sensitivity of key regions in the central nervous system thought to be involved in headache. Attention is given to the findings from the patient interview, physical examination, and evaluation of treatment response.

There is strong scientific evidence to suggest that physiotherapy is an effective treatment for cervical headache (Jull et al 2002). The diagnostic criteria for cervical or cervicogenic headache (CGH) according to the International Headache Society (2004) and Sjaastad et al (1998) are documented in Box 14.1. Both sets of criteria imply a predominantly peripheral or nociceptive mechanism of headache production caused by cervical spine pathology or impairment. However, many clinicians will have encountered patients with cervical headaches that do not respond as expected to treatment, often leading to frustration in both patient and therapist. It is the author's opinion, from over 20 years of assessing and providing physiotherapy for patients with headache, including cervical headache, that abnormally increased or maladaptive sensitivity within the central nervous system (CNS)

is often associated with poor outcome with treatment directed mainly at peripheral impairments. It is argued in this chapter that an appreciation of factors affecting sensitivity in areas of the CNS involved with headache processing must be considered for effective understanding and management of benign, recurrent headache, including cervical headache. In areas where evidence relating specifically to cervical headache is lacking, links are drawn from research relating to other headache types, most commonly tension-type headache and migraine.

CNS processing of cervical nociceptive input

In order to provide background information for the clinical recommendations of the chapter, this section describes pain referral from the neck to the head via the trigeminocervical nucleus (TCN) and explains the function of the TCN in relation to a broader model of pain processing and perception. The effect of nociceptive input to and descending control systems on the TCN is presented from the perspective of neurophysiology to facilitate understanding of the ways that physical, genetic, hormonal, psychological, and immune influences can affect headache processing.

The trigeminocervical nucleus and the neuromatrix theory of pain

Cervical headache occurs when the brain concludes that nociceptive input from the neck has arisen from somewhere in the head. The mechanism of pain referral from the neck to the head is generally accepted as being via convergence of primary afferent neurons from trigeminal and upper cervical receptive fields. This convergence occurs where the trigeminal pars caudalis overlaps with the dorsal horn gray matter of the upper cervical spinal cord (Goadsby et al 1997, Kerr 1961). This area of overlap has been termed the 'trigeminocervical nucleus' (TCN) and forms a common pathway for afferent input from the head and upper cervical regions (Bogduk 1992).

Clinicians should not assume that the TCN always relays nociceptive input to higher centers in a predictable manner that reflects a one-to-one relationship between peripheral injury and pain. The perception of pain in general and, by extension, headache, is dependent on interplay between numerous widely distributed neural networks and the effects of other body systems on these networks. This neural network or 'neuromatrix' theory of pain as described by Melzack (1999a) proposes that the sensation of pain is an output of a neural network that comprises somatosensory, limbic and thalamo-cortical components. The synaptic architecture of this neuromatrix is, theoretically, determined by genetic and sensory influences. Inputs to the matrix include:

(a) sensory, including somatic, visceral, visual and other sensory input

(b) cognitive and emotional inputs from other parts of the brain

(c) intrinsic neural inhibitory systems from other brain areas

(d) factors associated with stress regulation systems including endocrine, autonomic and immune systems.

The TCN is an integral part of the headache neuromatrix as it is the first region in the CNS that processing of afferent input from structures able to cause headache occurs. It is likely that sensitization of the TCN is pivotal in the pathophysiology and production of primary headaches such as migraine, chronic tension type headache and cluster headache (Goadsby 2006, Schmidt-Hansen et al 2007, Schoenen & Sandor 1999, Schoenen 2006). It has also been suggested that cervical headache in its chronic form is maintained by central mechanisms (Schoenen & Maertens de Noordhout 1994). If the TCN is in a sensitized state, incoming nociceptive input is likely to be amplified or facilitated. If the TCN is in a suppressed state, then nociceptive input may be reduced or even completely blocked. Therefore, an understanding of the factors affecting sensitivity of the TCN is important for clinicians involved in the management of patients with primary headache and benign secondary headaches, including cervical headache.

Nociceptive input and trigeminocervical nucleus sensitivity

Primary sensory neurons from trigeminal and upper cervical fields terminate in the TCN where synaptic connections are made with ascending projection neurons and local inter-neurons. In healthy individuals where the TCN is in a state of normal transmission, innocuous stimuli such as pressure, light touch and non-injurious heat or cold will be interpreted as such. High intensity stimuli that activate high threshold receptors without causing tissue injury will produce a transient, localized pain. Nociceptive information carried by myelinated A delta and unmyelinated C fibers induces release of substance P and excitatory amino acids (EAAs) such as glutamate in proportion to the peripheral nociceptive stimulus. This results in activation of neurokinin1 and AMPA (α-amino-3-hydroxyl-5-methyl-isoxazolepropionic acid) receptors and subsequent depolarization of second order TCN neurons (Doubell et al 1999, Watkins & Maier 2005). This state enables a clear distinction to be made between damaging and non-damaging stimuli and enables prompt and appropriate reactions (Doubell et al 1999).

Nociceptive input associated with tissue damage and peripheral inflammation is likely to cause increased excitability in second order TCN neurons (Hu et al 1992, Woolf & Salter 2000). It appears that substance P, calcitonin gene-related peptide (CGRP) and glutamate are key neurotransmitters in dorsal horn and TCN nociception processing (Bird et al 2006, Doubell et al, 1999, Oshinsky & Luo 2006). The n-methyl-d-aspartate (NMDA) receptor, in particular, is considered integral in the induction and maintenance of central sensitization (Woolf & Salter 2000, Woolf & Thompson 1991). Persistent depolarization of the post synaptic membrane of TCN neurons enables glutamate and other agents to remove the magnesium molecule that normally blocks the activation of pre and post synaptic NMDA receptors. This initiates a cascade of biochemical changes including nitric oxide (NO) release that increases pre-synaptic substance P and EAA release, resulting in further excitation of the post synaptic membrane (Watkins & Maier 2005). Sensitivity can be further enhanced by presynaptic augmentation of neurotransmitter release, and decreased pre- and postsynaptic inhibition.

The role of glia in CNS sensitivity

There has been increasing interest and research into the role of glial cells in the production and maintenance of increased central sensitivity, including that of the TCN (Watkins et al 2007, Xie et al 2007). Glia (mainly microglia and astrocytes) have historically been regarded housekeepers for neurons, performing roles such as debris removal, regulation of extracellular ion concentration and provision of energy and neurochemical precursors (Watkins et al 2007, Wieseler-Frank et al 2005). Neuronal release of substance P, EAAs and NO has been shown to activate spinal cord glia, leading to production and release of the inflammatory cytokines interleukin 1β (IL-1 β, interleukin 6 (IL-6) and tumor necrosis factor alpha (TNFα), as well as NO and prostaglandins (Holguin et al 2004, Milligan et al 2001, Watkins et al 2007). The glial release of these substances further sensitizes pre- and postsynaptic TCN neurons. Based on these mechanisms, it has been proposed that glia can act as a 'volume control' for nociception (Wieseler-Frank et al 2005). Central nervous system glia can also be activated by factors such as psychological stress, bacterial or viral infection, peripheral nerve injury, or trauma (Steptoe et al 2007, Watkins & Maier 2000, 2005). The pathways thought to underlie peripherally mediated glial activation include blood-borne signaling and neural signaling where cytokine stimulation of the vagus and possibly the hypoglossal nerves conveys information to the medullary nucleus tractus solarius and on to other brain areas (Watkins & Maier 2000, 2005). It is likely that even after the stimulation or challenge has ceased (for example cessation of the nociceptive input or resolution of the infection), astrocytes and microglia remain 'primed', allowing for increased speed and magnitude of reaction the next time they are activated (Pasti et al 1995, 1997).

Descending control systems and TCN sensitivity

Sensitivity of the TCN can be modulated by local and descending inhibitory systems that act pre-synaptically and/or post-synaptically (Thompson 2006). Nociceptive activity in the

TCN is strongly influenced by descending pathways originating from the midbrain, most notably the dorsal and ventral peri-aqueductal gray (PAG) and rostroventromedial medulla (RVM) (Heinricher 2005) (Fig. 9.1). Once thought to be an exclusively antinociceptive system it is likely that the PAG/RVM system exerts significant bidirectional control over nociceptive transmission from the TCN and dorsal horn (Heinricher 2005,

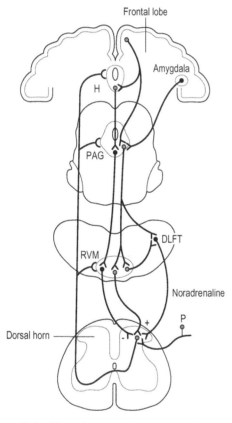

Ren & Dubner 2002). The main pathways principally use serotonin as a neurotransmitter (Fields et al 2006). Dysregulation of central serotonergic function has been proposed as a key step in the onset of migraine (Hamel 2007, Joseph et al 1989, Marcus 1993) cluster headache (D'Andrea et al 1998) and a likely factor in the development of chronic tension type headache (Marcus 1995). However, close links and connections with noradrenergic centers in the locus ceruleus and dorsolateral pontine tegmentum would indicate a degree of synergy between serotonergic and noradrenergic systems (Joseph et al 1989, Lance et al 1983, Malmgren 1990). The PAG/RVM system receives ascending input from the dorsal horn, particularly from the cervical region and TCN. There are also substantial inputs from the limbic forebrain including frontal lobe, prefrontal and anterior cingulate cortices, amygdala and hypothalamus. These connections indicate that the PAG/RVM system is integral in the coordination of cortical and limbic inputs for a 'top-down' regulation of nociception processing. Corrive & Morgan (2004) describe the PAG as being the crossroads of an ascending sensory system relaying noxious input and a descending limbic system organizing emotional responses. Thus, due to the connections of the PAG/RVM system, top-down regulation of TCN activity is likely to be influenced by a number of factors. These include psychosocial factors such as stress and anxiety, circadian rhythm, as well as endocrinological, hormonal and autonomic influences (Fields et al 2006).

Hyperalgesia and allodynia in TCN sensitization

Through combinations of nociceptive input, possible glial activation and impaired descending control, sensitization of the TCN has the effect of amplifying nociceptive input from areas of tissue damage or inflammation. One clinical

Figure 9.1 ● The main connections of the PAG/RVM system of descending control of the TCN. The figure shows a diagrammatic representation of a major pain modulating pathway with major links in the midbrain periaqueductal gray (PAG) and rostral ventromedial medulla (RVM). Regions of the frontal lobe and amygdala project directly and via the hypothalamus (H) to the PAG. The PAG in turn controls spinal nociceptive neurons through relays in the RVM and the dorsolateral pontine tegmentum (DLPT). The RVM, which projects directly and via the DLPT to the dorsal horn, exerts bidirectional control over nociceptive transmission. The control by RVM and DLPT involves both inhibitory and excitatory interneurons.

manifestation of this process is primary hyperalgesia or tenderness at the site of tissue damage or inflammation. Nociception from other areas that have inputs into the sensitized areas of the TCN will also be amplified, resulting in secondary hyperalgesia or tenderness/increased pain response in areas outside the site of tissue damage/inflammation. Additionally, with a sufficient increase in sensitization, even non nociceptive input such as light touch, or non-noxious heat and cold may be interpreted as painful (allodynia). As a cardinal sign of central sensitization, allodynia has been demonstrated in animal models of headache (Hu et al 1992) and in humans with some forms of migraine (Cooke et al 2007, Kitaj & Klink 2005), cluster headache (Ashkenazi & Young 2004), chronic daily headache, and chronic tension type headache (Bendtsen 2000). The clinical relevance of this knowledge is that in patients where TCN sensitization is likely, there may be areas of increased tenderness in trigeminal or cervical fields remote from any peripheral source of nociception or tissue damage. This is addressed in the discussion of physical examination. However it should be noted that detailed studies of hyperalgesia and allodynia in populations with cervical headache are lacking. Figure 9.2 shows some of the inputs

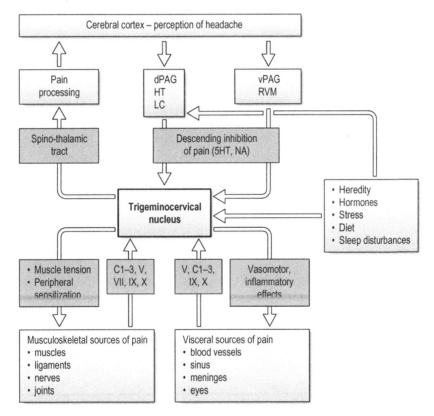

Figure 9.2 ● Transmission of nociceptive impulses from the trigeminocervical nucleus (TCN) will be dependent on the level of afferent input from either musculoskeletal or visceral sources as well as the level of descending inhibition. Sensitization of the TCN could also lead to peripheral changes in both musculoskeletal and visceral structures. dPAG = dorsal periacqueductal grey matter, HT = hypothalamus, LC = locus ceruleus, vPAG = ventral periacqueductal grey matter, RVM = rostro ventromedial medulla, 5HT = 5hydroxytryptamine (serotonin), NA = noradrenaline.

and outputs of the TCN. It should be remembered that visceral nociception from structures supplied by the trigeminal nerve can also contribute to sensitization of the TCN and that TCN sensitization can lead to peripheral changes in both visceral and somatic (musculoskeletal) structures.

Patient interview and history

Information gained from the patient interview can alert the clinician to the possibility that there may be factors other than cervical nociceptive input that are contributing to a patient's headaches. It is beyond the scope of this chapter to give a detailed overview of an appropriate interview for patients presenting with possible cervical headache; see Jull & Niere (2004) and Chapter 14 for more detail. This section addresses precipitating and triggering factors of headaches and attempts to describe how these might be related to peripheral nociceptive input and/or affect TCN processing of this input.

Do specific neck movements or postures trigger or exacerbate the headache?

This is a criterion for cervicogenic headache (CGH) as described by Sjaastad et al (1998) and would suggest cervical causation where the TCN is in a normal mode of transmission. If the TCN is in a sensitized state, non-nociceptive input from cervical spine motion or strain receptors that travel in large diameter afferents could be interpreted as painful and may be enough to trigger and maintain a headache. The absence of precipitating factors involving the neck does not exclude the cervical spine as a source or major contributor to the headache. For example, in a clinical trial involving 200 participants with CGH, 40% did not relate the onset of their headaches to neck movements or sustained postures; yet, during physical examination, all reported pain associated with one or more cervical active movements (Jull et al 2002). In addition, some patients may not appreciate or be aware of links between their headaches and neck postures or movements until their attention is drawn to the possibility by appropriate questioning.

What is the effect of medication?

These may include analgesics, anti-inflammatory, antimigraine preparations (prophylactic or for acute episodes), membrane stabilizers or tricyclic antidepressants (see Chapter 3). Patient reports of benefit from steroidal or nonsteroidal anti-inflammatory medication may indicate a significant inflammatory component. This may be associated with local tissue damage or be associated with a systemic condition such as rheumatoid arthritis or polymyalgia rheumatica. Benefit from medication that decreases CNS sensitivity, either directly or indirectly (e.g. triptans or tricyclic antidepressants) could suggest that central sensitization is a significant contributing mechanism to the patient's headache.

Medication overuse from repeated or heavy use of analgesics (including opiates) and/or triptans can lead to increased headache activity and has been proposed as a mechanism by which relatively infrequent headaches can transform into frequent or chronic daily headaches. Proposed mechanisms include 'upregulation' of pro-nociceptive systems or 'mini-withdrawals' caused by the cessation of the medication (Meng & Cao 2007). Spinal cord or TCN glial activation may also be partly responsible for increased CNS sensitivity and decreased symptom relief with repeated medication use. Watkins et al (Watkins et al 2007) proposed that while opioids inhibit neuronal nociceptive transmission within the CNS, concurrent opioid activation of glia leads to prolonged cytokine release within the CNS and subsequent increased sensitivity that may become apparent clinically once the neuronal analgesic effects of the opioids diminish. The role of glial involvement in analgesic tolerance, dependence and withdrawal has been demonstrated experimentally (Johnston & Westbrook 2005, Raghavendra et al 2004, Shavit et al 2005) and is providing potential options for pharmacological management of neuropathic and chronic pain conditions (Watkins et al 2007).

Is there a family history of headaches?

Strong genetic links have been demonstrated for migraine (Russell 2001, Sandor et al 2000) and tension type headache (Russell 2001). It would follow that a family history of either of these headache types in a patient presenting with possible cervical headache would increase the possibility that the patient has that headache type or at least a familial tendency for increased TCN sensitivity or reactivity in association with any musculoskeletal impairment associated with the headache. Although there does not appear to be any experimental evidence of a genetic contribution to cervical headache it is this author's clinical impression that patterns of clinical presentation for cervical headache can be very similar between immediate family members or between generations.

What is the effect of hormonal changes?

The role of ovarian hormones in the precipitation or maintenance of different headache types is well documented, although most of this literature relates to migraines (MacGregor 1996, Marcus 1995, 2004, Martin & Behbehani 2006, Welch 1997). Hormonal changes can influence headaches and TCN sensitivity might be affected by these changes. There are three times when hormonal changes are more likely to influence a woman's headaches. These are during the menstrual cycle, pregnancy, and menopause.

Menstrual cycle

Table 9.1 shows the percentages of women in each of the selected studies who indicated that menstruation precipitated their headaches. It is interesting to note the lower percentage in patients referred for physiotherapy (2%) as opposed those presenting for physiotherapy (23%), suggesting that the role of hormonal changes is low in confirmed cervical headache. This has been reinforced in studies by Jull et al (2002) and Sjaastad & Fredriksen (2002), suggesting that in patients where hormonal changes are a significant headache precipitant, cervical headache is unlikely. However Niere (1998) found that hormonal changes as a precipitant were not a predictor of physiotherapy treatment outcome. More research is required to clarify the role of hormonal changes in female patients with a cervical cause or component.

The phases of the menstrual cycle and the associated serum estrogen and progesterone levels at each phase are shown in Figure 9.3. Fioroni et al (1996) found increased serotonin catabolism and decreased serotonin levels in the luteal phase in migraine sufferers. A meta-analysis by Riley et al (1999) found that thresholds to experimentally produced pain in women were highest in the follicular phase and lowest in the luteal phase or pre-menstrually, corresponding to the time in the menstrual cycle when there is likely to be increased headache

Table 9.1 Headache precipitants for different populations.

Author/year	Population	N	Hormonal (%) (of females)	Stress (%)	Diet (%)
Van den Bergh et al (1987)	Migraine with aura	217	48	49	45
Drummond (1985)	Non cluster	317	39	61	43
Drummond (1985)	Cluster	58	14	27	61
Scharff et al (1995)	Migraine and tension type	172	62	72	22 (chocolate) 33 (alcohol)
Rasmussen (1993)	Tension-type	167	39	70	5–11
Rasmussen (1993)	Migraine	119	24	44	10
Rothrock et al (1996)	Chronic Daily headache	132	29	56	27 33 (alcohol)
Rothrock et al (1996)	Episodic migraine	243	44	57	24
Niere (1998)	Presenting to physio	112	23	53	7
Jull (1986)	Referred to physio	96	2	30	0

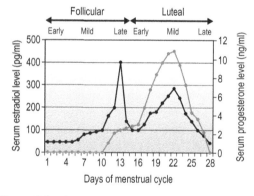

Figure 9.3 • Changes in serum levels of estrogen (-o-) and progesterone (-■-) during the menstrual cycle. Increased activity is relative to the activity experienced during other phases of the menstrual cycle. Headaches are more likely in the late luteal phase when estrogen levels are falling.

activity. Gazerani et al (2005) demonstrated that healthy females showed greater levels of capsaicin induced trigeminal sensitization than healthy males in both the luteal and menstrual phases of the menstrual cycle.

Martin & Behbehani (2006) proposed the following mechanisms by which hormonal changes can affect headache activity:

(i) prostaglandin release

(ii) magnesium deficiency

(iii) effects on neurotransmitter systems.

Prostaglandin release into the circulation by the shedding endometrium during menstruation has been shown to be associated with migraine activity (Silberstein & Merriam 1991) although this mechanism does not explain migraines and headaches occurring premenstrually or consistently at other times in the cycle, for example at ovulation.

Magnesium is important in regulation of the tone of the cerebral arteries and blocks activation of NMDA receptors in the TCN (Altura & Altura 1996). Magnesium, along with calcium and vitamin B6 are cofactors in neurotransmitter synthesis including the conversion of tryptophan to serotonin (O'Brien 1993) implying that disturbances in magnesium levels could affect CNS sensitivity, possibly at the level of the TCN or via alterations in descending pain inhibition via PAG/RVM serotonergic pathways. Mauskop and Altura (2002) demonstrated a high incidence of magnesium deficiency and elevated calcium/magnesium ratio in a sample of 61 women with menstrual migraine, while magnesium supplements have been shown to be effective in the prevention of menstrual migraine (Facchinetti et al 1991) and migrainous headache in children (Wang et al 2003). Although these results may not be generalizable to patients with cervical headache, altered magnesium levels may be significant in some women whose headaches are affected by hormonal changes.

The most likely mechanism by which changes in ovarian hormones can affect headache behavior is through their effect on the neurotransmitter systems that play a significant role in the production and processing of headache pain. These systems are likely to include those involving serotonin, glutamate, noradrenaline, gamma amino butyric acid (GABA) and opiates (Fioroni et al 1996, Marcus 2004, Martin & Behbehani 2006). Although altered progesterone levels can either trigger or prevent migraine in certain populations (Martin & Behbehani 2006), the most likely mechanism of hormonal influence on TCN sensitivity and headache activity is via estrogen withdrawal, usually in the late luteal and early menstrual phases of the menstrual cycle (Martin & Behbehani 2006, Martin et al 2007). It is likely that increased estrogen levels are associated with increased levels of serotonergic function in the CNS, increased beta endorphin levels and decreased noradrenergic responses (Marcus 1995, Martin & Behbehani 2006). From this information it can be postulated that reduction in estrogen levels may cause a decrease in CNS serotonergic function, increased sensitivity of the trigeminocervical nucleus and, therefore increased likelihood of headache production.

Pregnancy and menopause

Pregnancy is usually associated with a sustained increase in estrogen levels (Fig. 9.4) and migraine sufferers appear to be more likely than sufferers of tension type headache to experience a reduction in their levels of headache (Rasmussen 1993). Women with cervicogenic headache are less likely than those with migraine to have an improvement in their headaches associated with pregnancy. Sjaastad and Fredriksen (2002) found that of 14 women with cervicogenic headache only one reported complete relief of her headaches during pregnancy, as opposed to 32 (65%) of 49 women with migraine who experienced complete relief. In some women headache may increase or begin during pregnancy, particularly in the first trimester when estrogen levels are lower or less stable. Similar variability exists with oral contraceptive use and during menopause where existing headaches may be exacerbated or ameliorated, or new headaches generated (Silberstein & Merriam 1991). After delivery,

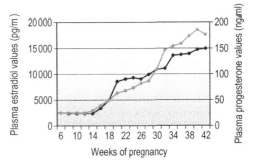

Figure 9.4 • Mean plasma estradiol and progesterone levels during pregnancy. Plasma estradiol (-♦-) and progesterone (-■-) levels rise abruptly during the second and third trimesters (weeks 14 to 40) of pregnancy.

estrogen levels usually drop dramatically and many women suffer from increased headaches in the first week post delivery (Sances et al 2003, Stein 1981). Breast feeding has been shown to be associated with decreased migraine recurrence after delivery, possibly because hormone levels are more likely to be maintained (Sances et al 2003).

Clinical observation suggests that headache activity may increase during menopause, possibly associated with falling or fluctuating estrogen levels. Headaches associated with this mechanism are often relieved with hormone replacement therapy and may be exacerbated if this therapy is interrupted or if hormone levels fall towards the end of any period of use of implants or patches.

Are there dietary triggers or symptoms of food intolerances?

The Diet column in Table 9.1, representing the percentages of subjects whose headaches were precipitated by diet, shows that there is great variability between the studies and different headache types. Sufferers of migraine with aura (Van den Bergh et al 1987) and cluster headache (Drummond 1985) appear to be more likely to have their headaches precipitated by diet than sufferers of other headache types. The classic food triggers of migraine are chocolate, oranges, red wine, and cheese – particularly camembert, cheddar, and parmesan (Marcus et al 1997, Wöber et al 2007). Glutamates (e.g., MSG), aspartame (artificial sweetener), and coffee have also been associated with the onset of migraines and other headache types (Koehler & Glaros 1988, Scharff et al 1995). Despite the strong reported association between dietary factors and headache production, double blind studies are often inconclusive (Marcus et al 1997). This has led some authors to propose a strong

psychological or expectation effect (Kohlenberg 1981, Marcus et al 1997). Patients who report that their headaches are precipitated by specific foods are less likely to achieve a favorable outcome with physiotherapy treatment (Niere 1998), implying that there is unlikely to be a significant cervical contribution to their headaches or that the dietary factors are somehow perpetuating the cervical headaches despite the effects of the treatment.

Caffeine

The degree of caffeine consumption and the reaction when caffeine is withdrawn is worth ascertaining in patients with headache. Caffeine alone may have an analgesic effect in headache (Ward et al 1991) and has been shown to enhance the analgesic effect of aspirin, paracetamol, and ibuprofen (McQuay et al 1996). Silverman et al (1992) reported headaches in over 50% of 62 subjects who were withdrawn from low to moderate coffee consumption (average 2.5 cups per day). It should be remembered that caffeine is also present in tea, chocolate, and cola drinks.

Mechanism of dietary effect on headaches

The mechanism by which dietary factors can affect headaches is unclear. It has been proposed that dietary aggravation or precipitation of headache is often due to an allergic response involving the release of histamines and other inflammatory mediators from mast cells (Egger et al 1983, Monro et al 1980). Another proposed mechanism is through alteration of neural function by modulation of neurotransmitter levels, including serotonin, noradrenaline, dopamine and acetylcholine (Millichap & Yee 2003, Seltzer et al 1981). Wine, in particular, appears to have the potential to affect both peripheral and central nociceptive transmission by inhibiting the binding of serotonin to serotonin receptors and facilitating the release of serotonin from platelets. Caffeine, as an adenosine receptor antagonist (Bell 2007), enhances dopaminergic and glutaminergic function within the CNS which may affect the sensitivity of the TCN in susceptible individuals.

Identification of dietary factors

The identification of a dietary component to a patient's headaches may be difficult. The onset of headache may be substantially delayed after the ingestion of the offending food. Sandler et al (1995) reported a lag between ingestion and headache onset of three hours for red wine and 22 hours for chocolate in study participants with migraine. It is also possible that dietary substances alone may not necessarily trigger a headache but predispose the sufferer to an attack when other factors are present (Scharff et al 1995). The patient may therefore be unaware of the contribution of diet to their headaches unless there is clear causation. Chapter 18 provides further information regarding the identification and management of dietary factors in headache production.

What is the effect of psychosocial factors?

Psychological stress has a possible effect on headache processing and perception. All patient assessments should incorporate a biopsychosocial approach. Where relevant, psychological, social, and biological factors are ascertained during the examination and are considered when formulating treatment and management plans. It has been proposed that psychosocial factors can play a significant role in the production and maintenance of headaches, particularly in the transformation of episodic to chronic headaches (Holroyd & Lipchik 1999). In particular, patients with chronic, high frequency headaches such as chronic daily headache and chronic tension-type headache are more likely to have higher levels of psychological distress when compared to patients with episodic headaches or matched controls (Barton-Donovan & Blanchard 2005, Holroyd et al 2000). A study by Schmidt-Hansen et al (2007) showed that central sensitization associated with headache is likely to be more pronounced in patients with high frequency headaches. However, it is not known whether psychological factors in patients with high frequency headaches are causative of the headaches or caused by the headache pain and associated disability. Space does not permit a detailed discussion of psychosocial influences on headache. However, it is acknowledged that factors such as patient attitudes and beliefs about their pain, behaviors such as fear avoidance, medication overuse, decreased physical function and level of social, familial and work support may be pivotal in the production or maintenance of some headaches, although there does not appear to be any research addressing the role of these factors in cervical headaches. Additionally, indicators of psychological distress such as depression, exaggerated attention to bodily symptoms, anxiety and anger may also be associated with maladaptive pain processing (Fernandez 2002, Watson 1999). Identification of psychosocial factors that could be contributing to a patient's headaches may be achieved during the examination/treatment process, through the use of patient completed questionnaires such as the General Health Questionnaire 28 (Goldberg & Hillier 1979) or the Distress and Risk Assessment Method (DRAM) (Main et al 1992), or with the assistance of psychological or psychiatric referral.

Nash and Thebarge (2006) defined psychological stress as an imbalance between perceived demands and perceived resources resulting in demands or strain in the biological system. They indicated four ways that psychological stress could be related to headaches:

(i) as a predisposing factor contributing to the onset of headaches

(ii) as a factor that accelerates or exacerbates the progression of the headaches

(iii) as a precipitant or aggravating factor of individual headaches

(iv) as a contributor to impaired quality of life by leading to avoidance of particular activities, situations or foods that may be associated with headache production.

Stress as a trigger of headaches

Table 9.1 shows that stress may be a significant contributor to or causative factor of a variety of headache types. Reynolds & Hovanitz (2000) demonstrated a positive relationship between negative life event stress and headache frequency in 1289 college students. A common clinical observation is that some patients do not have increased headache activity during stressful times, but suffer from attacks once the stress is relieved. Typically, this may occur on the weekends, once holidays start, or after exams. Patients may be oblivious to or may not acknowledge the role of stress on precipitating or maintaining headaches. The ability to cope with stressful situations varies enormously between individuals and even within individuals, depending on the situation, degree of available support, and coping strategies utilized. Clinically, a key to the recognition that psychological stress may be affecting a patient's headaches is whether the patient feels unable to cope with the perceived demands placed upon them or whether they feel that they are not in control of a particular situation. In addition to acting as a trigger factor for headaches, changes in

stress levels can impact upon treatment outcome. Niere & Robinson (1997) surveyed 91 headache patients two months after their initial physiotherapy consultation. Twenty reported that changes in stress levels had affected their headaches. Of these, 10 felt that reduced stress levels had improved their headaches, 6 felt that increased stress had exacerbated their headaches, while 4 did not indicate the effect of changed stress levels.

Effects of experimentally-induced stress on headache

It is has been shown that experimentally-induced stress leads to increased headache activity in patients with headache, indicating greater reactivity in one or both of central and peripheral pathways (Leistad et al 2006). Bansevicius & Sjaastad (1996) measured EMG of shoulder-neck and facial muscles as well as pain levels in cervical headache patients and group-matched controls before, during, and after a stressful reaction time test. They found that in the cervical headache patients, pain values for the shoulder increased markedly during the test, while pain values for the temple and neck increased in the post-test period. There were no significant changes in pain levels for the controls. Similarly, trapezius EMG in headache patients increased significantly during the test while the increase in trapezius EMG for the controls was not significant. Farella et al (2000) found that dental students undergoing academic examinations had higher stress levels and decreased pressure pain thresholds in jaw muscles and achilles tendons compared to students not undertaking examinations. These findings support a causative link between stress and CNS sensitization, particularly affecting the TCN if the individual already experiences headache.

Mechanism of stress affecting headaches

The typical physiological reaction in healthy individuals to stressful situations is activation of the hypothalamic-pituitary-adrenal (HPA) axis (Bomholt et al 2004) and locus coeruleus-noradrenaline (LC-NA) systems (Melzack 1999b). Activation of the HPA axis ultimately leads to increased cortisol, noradrenaline and adrenaline levels necessary for the 'fight/flight' response, comprising increased heart rate, blood pressure and glucose levels for energy release (Foy et al 2006, Melzack 1999b). Acute stress is often associated with decreased pain responses, probably due to beta endorphin release and enhanced inhibitory action of the LC-NA system in suppressing spinal cord and TCN nociception (Melzack 1999b, Meng & Cao 2007). However, ongoing or repeated stress can lead to increased pain sensitivity, possibly as a result of dysregulation of the normal (predominantly serotonergic) descending pain inhibitory systems by a shift towards enhanced noradrenergic/sympathetic systems. Another possible mechanism for stress-associated pain sensitivity is through cortisol mediated NMDA and glial activation within the CNS, with glial activation leading to production of pro-inflammatory cytokines and further CNS or TCN sensitization (Nair & Bonneau 2006).

Stress, pain, and the immune system

It is now widely held that the CNS and immune systems form a bi-directional communication network with the CNS receiving signals from the periphery, then coordinating appropriate behavioral and neuroendocrine responses (Maier 2003, Watkins & Maier 2005). In healthy individuals acute stress leads to various forms of immune system activation, depending on the nature and duration of the stressor and the immune factor being measured (Connor et al 2005, Kemeny & Schedlowski 2007). Stress is likely to be associated with increased levels of both central and peripheral pro-inflammatory mediators such as tumor necrosis factor alpha (TNFα), interleukins 1B and 6, and nitrous oxide (NO), potentially having the effect of increasing both central and peripheral sensitivity (Maier 2003). In a meta-analysis of the effects of acute psychological stress on circulating cytokine levels in humans Steptoe et al (2007) found that acute stress was significantly associated with increased levels of the pro-inflammatory cytokines Interleukin 6 and Interleukin 1β. The relationship between immune and pain systems has been reviewed by Watkins and Maier (2005) who described the pivotal role of the pro-inflammatory cytokines in acting at the site of the peripheral immune challenge and within the CNS. A common example of pain facilitation as a consequence of immune system activation is the generalized hyperalgesia or allodynia often experienced with viral infections such as influenza. Clinically, it is a common observation that patients' headaches can be exacerbated or triggered by immune system challenges from viral infections such as colds or influenza and by bacterial infections affecting other body regions. Clinicians should be mindful of the likely state of the headache patient's immune system and the possible interactions between stress, immune activation and peripheral and TCN sensitivity.

Physical examination

For a detailed account of the physical examination appropriate for patients with cervical headache the reader is referred to Chapter 14. This section will briefly describe the main physical examination findings associated with cervical headache and the findings that might be associated with increased TCN sensitivity.

Identification of patterns of musculoskeletal impairment consistent with headache production is essential to justify physical treatment. In a study of 73 subjects with single headache types and 57 non-headache controls, Jull et al (2007a) found that cervicogenic headache could be differentiated from tension-type headache and migraine by a pattern of musculoskeletal impairment that included: i) restricted neck motion, ii) upper cervical joint dysfunction, and iii) impaired muscle function. Although isolated musculoskeletal impairment may exist in patients with migraine and tension-type headache, studies have shown that the incidence of these findings is not significantly different to populations of headache-free controls (Amiri et al 2007, Marcus et al 1999, Zwart 1997).

Musculoskeletal nociceptive input and trigeminocervical sensitivity

Physical examination findings must be interpreted in the light of the likely degree of TCN sensitivity. Pain, local or referred, elicited by neck movement or palpation might, in some cases, be due to hyperalgesia or allodynia caused by a sensitized TCN, effectively comprising a false positive. That is, the pain may lead the clinician to believe that there is impairment of the underlying tissues where no impairment exists. Signs of increased CNS sensitivity have been demonstrated in populations with chronic neck pain (Sheather-Reid & Cohen 1998) and whiplash (Curatolo et al 2001, Johansen et al 1999, Sterling et al 2002), indicating that nociceptive input from the cervical spine can be associated with central sensitization, particularly if the pain is persistent or severe. Bartsch & Goadsby (2002)

stimulated the greater occipital nerve (C2) in rats for five minutes which led to increases in response to supratentorial dural stimulation that lasted for more than one hour. They concluded that the cervical nociceptive input led to sensitization of second order TCN neurons. Similar effects were demonstrated by dural stimulation, also in rats (Bartsch & Goadsby 2003). Jensen and Olesen (1996) subjected 58 subjects with TTH and 30 matched controls to 30 minutes of sustained tooth clenching. They found that 69% of the TTH group and 17% of the controls developed headache. The authors concluded that in the TTH group, peripheral nociception acted as a trigger for increased central sensitivity. This knowledge is clinically important because it indicates that cervical nociceptive input, for example from musculoskeletal impairment can produce or enhance TCN sensitization.

Physical examination findings suggestive of increased TCN sensitivity

In this author's clinical experience the following physical examination findings might alert the clinician to the likelihood of increased TCN sensitivity in a patient with headache:

- Allodynia or hyperalgesia on palpation of the cervical and upper thoracic areas, particularly areas not directly supplied by the upper cervical nerves.
- Excessive pain production on active or passive motion testing
- A physical or emotional reaction out of proportion to the nature and type of, or symptoms produced by an examination procedure
- Progressive exacerbation of headache during the examination or significant flare-up after the examination.

It should be noted that these findings rely on the clinician's interpretation of what is an appropriate or excessive response. They may also be due to peripheral mechanisms or a combination of peripheral and central processes. A higher index of suspicion of increased TCN sensitivity is warranted when these examination findings are accompanied by one or more of the factors outlined in the history/interview. On the other hand, a peripheral dominant mechanism is more likely when there is a predictable and consistent stimulus-response behavior to physical examination procedures.

Management and treatment

Different aspects of physiotherapy can affect peripheral and central processes in cervical headache. The reader is referred to Chapters 15, 16, 17, and 19 for an account of contemporary physiotherapy, chiropractic, and osteopathic treatment of headaches. Management of cervical headache usually focuses on musculoskeletal impairment thought to be causative or contributing to the patient's headaches. This should be performed as part of a biopsychosocial approach with appreciation of and, if appropriate, management of relevant psychosocial factors as well as consideration of the degree of sensitization of the TCN. If factors such as hormonal changes, stress or dietary intolerances are considered to be significant contributors to a patient's headaches then referral to other health care practitioners for management may be warranted. Chronic, refractory headaches may respond well to behavioral approaches (Holroyd & Lipchik 1999), particularly if there has been an over-reliance on and lack of long term results with passive therapies.

One of the IHS diagnostic criteria is that the headaches resolve within three months after successful treatment of the causative disorder or lesion (IHS 2004). If a patient's headaches resolve with treatment aimed at musculoskeletal impairment then it might be reasonable to assume that the headache source lay in the periphery and that central processes were not dominant or significant in the headache production. However, there is increasing evidence to suggest that spinal manual therapy and certain types of spinal muscle system retraining can exert significant effects on the central nervous system, see Souvlis et al (2004) for a review. Research by Ashkenazi & Young (2004) supports the concept of altered cervical input affecting CNS/TCN sensitivity. They demonstrated that blockades of the greater occipital nerve in humans caused significant decreases in both pain and associated allodynia associated with migraine attacks. Therefore it could be hypothesized that interruption of cervical nociceptive input with physiotherapy can decrease TCN sensitivity, even in cases of primary headache where central sensitization is the likely predominant mechanism. However, it is this author's clinical experience that such changes are often short-lived unless peripheral nociception is the main driver of the central changes.

Treating therapists should also be reminded that positive responses may be caused by altered psychological processes inherent in the patient-therapist interaction. This may include placebo or expectation responses. Other psychological or cognitive-behavioral strategies often associated with physiotherapy treatment include education, goal setting, reinforcement of attitudes and behaviors conducive to recovery and extinguishing or modifying behaviors and attitudes detrimental to recovery. Examples of this include relieving fear and anxiety with appropriate education and encouragement, or employing strategies to aid adherence to an exercise or postural correction program.

Physical treatment to address the musculo-skeletal impairments found with cervical headache should achieve a good result in the majority of patients. In a randomized trial Jull et al (2002) investigated the effects of either low load exercises, manual therapy, a combination of low load exercises and manual therapy, and GP managed 'control' on a population of 200 chronic cervical headache sufferers. They found that all treatment groups were superior to the control group with 81% of the exercise therapy/manual therapy group achieving a 50% reduction in headache frequency at 12 month follow up and 41% of this group achieving compete headache resolution at 12 months. Interestingly, in this trial, 28% of participants with cervical headache failed to achieve a 50% reduction in headache frequency with treatment. It is tempting to speculate that persistent TCN sensitivity for whatever reason may have been a factor in the lack of treatment response. Unfortunately, there have been no studies performed where treatment outcome for cervical headache has been analyzed in regard to signs of central sensitivity such as mechanical or thermal hyperalgesia. Recent research into whiplash injuries indicates that participants with signs of central sensitization (widespread mechanical or cold hyperalgesia) are less likely to respond to physical treatment and have delayed recovery (Jull et al 2007b). It is this author's opinion that patients with cervical headache and associated maladaptive or CNS driven central sensitization are less likely to respond favorably to physical treatment than those where peripheral nociception is the primary symptom mechanism.

Conclusion

Health care professionals involved in the management of patients with cervical headache should be aware of factors that can alter the sensitivity of central nervous system areas involved in the processing of nociceptive input from the head and neck. These factors may include persistent or severe pain, dietary factors, psychological or immune system stress, and hormonal changes. A patient interview needs to consider triggers and contributing factors in conjunction with physical examination findings and an evaluation of the effect of any physical treatment. This can help the clinician to determine whether these factors are having a significant impact on the patient's headaches.

References

Altura BM, Altura BT 1996 Role of magnesium in patho-physiological processes and the clinical utility of magnesium ion selective electrodes. Scandinavian Journal of Clinical and Laboratory Investigation 224 (suppl):211-234.

Amiri M, Jull GA, Bullock-Saxton J et al 2007 Cervical musculoskeletal impairment in frequent intermittent headache. Part 2: Subjects with concurrent headache types. Cephalalgia 27:891-898.

Ashkenazi A, Young WB 2004 Dynamic mechanical (brush) allodynia in cluster headache. Headache 44:1010-1012.

Bansevicius D, Sjaastad O 1996 Cervicogenic headache: the influence of mental load on pain level and EMG of shoulder-neck and facial muscles. Headache 36:372-378.

Barton-Donovan K, Blanchard EB 2005 Psychosocial aspects of chronic daily headache. Journal of Headache Pain 6:30-39.

Bartsch T, Goadsby PJ 2002 Stimulation of the greater occipital nerve induces increased central excitability of dural afferent input. Brain 125:1496-1509.

Bartsch T, Goadsby PJ 2003 Increased responses in trigeminocervical nociceptive neurons to cervical input after stimulation of the dura mater. Brain 126:1801-1813.

Bell RF 2007 Food and pain: should we be more interested in what our patients eat? Pain 129:5-7.

Bendtsen L 2000 Central sensitization in tension-type headache-possible mechanisms. Cephalalgia 20:486-508.

Bird GC, Han JS, Fu Y et al 2006 Pain-related synaptic plasticity in spinal horn neurons: role of CGRP. Molecular Pain 2:31-43.

Bogduk N 1992 The anatomical basis for cervicogenic headache. Journal of Manipulative and Physiological Therapeutics 15:67-70.

Bomholt SF, Harbuz MS, Blackburn-Munro G, Blackburn-Munro RE 2004 Involvement and role of the hypothalamo-pituitary-adrenal (HPA) stress axis in animal models of chronic pain and inflammation. Stress 7:1-14.

Connor TJ, Brewer C, Kelly JP, Harkin A 2005 Acute stress supresses pro-inflammatory cytokines TNFA and Il-1b independent of a catecholamine-driven increase in Il-10 production. Journal Neuroimmunology 159: 119-128.

Cooke L, Eliasziw M, Becker WB 2007 Cutaneous allodynia in transformed migraine patients. Headache 47:531-539.

Corrive P, Morgan MM 2004 Periaqueductal gray. In: Paxinos G, Mai JK (eds) The Human Nervous System, 2nd edn. Elsevier Academic Press, Amsterdam.

Curatolo M, Arendt-Nielsen L, Petersen-Felix S 2001 Central sensitivity in chronic pain after whiplash injury. Clinical Journal Of Pain 17:306-315.

D'andrea G, Granella F, Alecci M, Manzoni GC 1998 Serotonin metabolism in cluster headache. Cephalalgia 18:94-96.

Doubell TP, Mannion RJ, Woolf CJ 1999 The dorsal horn: state dependent sensory processing, plasticity and the generation of pain. In: Wall PD, Melzack R (eds) Textbook of pain, 4th edn. Churchill Livingstone, Edinburgh.

Drummond PD 1985 Predisposing, precipitating and relieving factors in different categories of headache. Headache 25:16-22.

Egger J, Carter CM, Wilson J et al 1983 Is migraine food allergy? A double blind trial of oligoantigenic diet treatment. Lancet 14:865-868.

Facchinetti F, Sances G, Borella P et al 1991 Magnesium prophylaxis of menstrual migraine: effects on intracellular magnesium. Headache 31:298-301.

Farella MA, Cimino TA, Martina R 2000 Changes in pressure-pain thresholds of the jaw muscles during a natural stressful condition in a group of symptom-free subjects. Journal of Orofacial Pain 14:279-285.

Fernandez E 2002 Anxiety, depression and anger in pain. Advanced Psychological Resources, Dallas.

Fields HL, Basbaum AI, Heinricher MM 2006 Central nervous system mechanisms of pain modulation. In: McMahon SB, Koltzenburg S (eds) Wall and Melzack's textbook of pain, 5th edn. Elsevier/Churchill Livingstone, Philadelphia.

Fioroni L, Andrea GD, Alecci M et al 1996 Platelet serotonin pathway in menstrual migraine. Cephalalgia 16:427-430.

Foy MR, Kim JJ, Shors TJ, Thompson R 2006 Neurobiological foundations of stress. In: Yehuda S, Mostofsky DI (eds) Nutrients, stress and medical disorders. Humana Press, Totawa New Jersey.

Gazerani P, Andersen OK, Arendt-Nielsen L 2005 A human experimental capsaicin model for trigeminal sensitisation. Gender-specific differences. Pain 118:155-163.

Goadsby PJ 2006 Primary neurovascular headache. In: McMahon SB, Koltzenburg S (eds) Wall and Melzack's Textbook of Pain, 5th edn. Elsevier/Churchill Livingstone, Philadelphia.

Goadsby PJ, Knight YE, Hoskin KL 1997 Stimulation of the greater occipital nerve increases metabolic activity in the trigeminal nucleus caudalis and cervical dorsal horn of the cat. Pain 73:23-28.

Goldberg DP, Hillier VF 1979 A scaled version of the general health questionnaire. Psychological Medicine 9:139-145.

Hamel E 2007 Serotonin and migraine: biology and clinical implications. Cephalalgia 27:1295-1300.

Heinricher MM 2005 Central processing of pain: modulation of nociception. In: Justins DM (ed) Pain 2005 – An updated review: Refresher Course Syllabus. IASP Press, Seattle.

Holguin A, O'connor KA, Biedenkapp J et al 2004 Hiv-1 Gp120 stimulates proinflammatory cytokine-mediated pain facilitation via activation of nitric oxide synthase-I (NOS). Pain 110:517-530.

Holroyd KA, Lipchik GL 1999 Psychological management of recurrent headache disorders: progress and prospects. In: Gatchel RJ, Turk D (eds) Psychosocial factors in pain. Guilford Press, New York.

Holroyd KA, Stensland M, Lipchik GL et al 2000 Psychosocial correlates and impact of chronic tension-type headaches. Headache 40:3-16.

Hu JW, Sessle BJ, Raboisson P et al 1992 Stimulation of craniofacial muscle afferents induces prolonged facilitatory effects in trigeminal nociceptive brain-stem neurones. Pain 48:53-60.

International Headache Society 2004 The International Classification Of Headache Disorders 2nd edn. Cephalalgia 24(suppl 1).

Jensen R, Olesen J 1996 Initiating mechanisms of experimentally induced tension-type headache. Cephalalgia 16:175-182.

Johansen MK, Graven-Nielsen TG, Olesen S, Arendt-Nielsen L 1999 Generalised muscular hyperalgesia in chronic whiplash syndrome. Pain 83:229-234.

Johnston IN, Westbrook RF 2005 Inhibition of morphine analgesia by LPS: role of opioid and nmda receptors and spinal glia. Behavioural Brain Research 156:75-83.

Joseph R, Welch KMA, D'andrea G 1989 Serotonergic hypofunction in migraine: a synthesis of evidence based on platelet dense body dysfunction. Cephalalgia 9:293-299.

Jull GA 1986 Headaches associated with the cervical spine – a clinical review. In: Grieve GP (ed) Modern Manual Therapy of the Vertebral Column. Edinburgh, Churchill Livingstone.

Jull GA, Niere KR 2004 The cervical spine and headache. In: Boyling JD, Jull GA (eds) Grieve's modern manual therapy of the vertebral column, 3rd edn. Churchill Livingstone, Edinburgh.

Jull G, Trott P, Potter H et al 2002 A randomized controlled trial of exercise and manipulative therapy for cervicogenic headache. Spine 27:1835-1843.

Jull GA, Amiri M, Bullock-Saxton J et al 2007a Cervical musculoskeletal impairment in frequent intermittent headache. Part 1: Subjects with single headaches. Cephalalgia 27:793-802.

Jull GA, Sterling M, Kenardy J, Bellar E 2007b Does the presence of sensory hypersensitivity influence outcomes of physical rehabilitation for chronic whiplash? – a preliminary RCT. Pain 129:28-34.

Kemeny ME, Schedlowski M 2007 Understanding the connection between psychological stress and immune-related diseases: a stepwise progression. Brain, Behaviour And Immunity 21:1009-1018.

Kerr FWL 1961 Mechanisms, diagnosis and treatment of some cranial and facial pain syndromes. Surgical Clinics Of North America 43:951-961.

Kitaj MB, Klink M 2005 Pain thresholds in daily transformed migraine versus episodic migraine headache patients. Headache 45:992-998.

Koehler SM, Glaros A 1988 The effect of aspartame on migraine headaches. Headache 28:10-13.

Kohlenberg RJ 1981 Tyramine sensitivity in dietary migraine: a critical review. Headache 22:30-34.

Lance JW, Lambert GA, Goadsby PJ, Duckworth JW 1983 Brainstem influences on the cephalic circulation: experimental data from cat and monkey of relevance to the mechanism of migraine. Headache 23:258-265.

Leistad RB, Sand T, Westgaard RH et al 2006 Stress-induced pain and muscle activity in patients with migraine and tension-type headache. Cephalalgia 26:64-73.

Macgregor EA 1996 'Menstrual' migraine: towards a definition. Cephalalgia 16:11-21.

Maier SF 2003 Bi-directional immune-brain communication: implications for understanding stress, pain and cognition. Brain, Behaviour And Immunity 17:67-85.

Main CJ, Wood PL, Hollis S et al 1992 The distress and risk assessment method: a simple patient classification to identify distress and evaluate the risk of poor outcome. Spine 17:42-52.

Malmgren R 1990 The central serotonergic system. Cephalalgia 10:199-204.

Marcus DA 1993 Serotonin and its role in headache pathogenesis and treatment. Clinical Journal of Pain 9:159-167.

Marcus DA 1995 Interrelationships of neurochemicals, estrogen, and recurring headache. Pain 62:129-139.

Marcus DA 2004 Estrogen and chronic daily headache. Current Pain and Headache Reports 8:66-70.

Marcus DA, Scharff L, Mercer S, Turk DC 1999 Musculoskeletal abnormalities in chronic headache: a controlled comparison of headache diagnostic groups. Headache 39:21-27.

Marcus DA, Scharff L, Turk D, Gourley LM 1997 A double-blind provocative study of chocolate as a trigger of headache. Cephalalgia 17:855-862.

Martin VT, Behbehani M 2006 Ovarian hormones and migraine headache: understanding mechanisms and pathogenesis. Part 1. Headache 46:3-23.

Martin VT, Lee J, Behbehani MM 2007 Sensitization of the trigeminal sensory system during different stages of the rat estrous cycle: implications for menstrual migraine. Headache 47:552-563.

Mauskop A, Altura BT 2002 Serum ionized magnesium levels and serum ionized calcium/ionized magnesium ratios in women with menstrual migraine. Headache 42:242-248.

Mcquay HJ, Angell K, Carroll D et al 1996 Ibuprofen compared with ibuprofen plus caffeine after third molar surgery. Pain 66:247-251.

Melzack R 1999a From the gate to the neuromatrix. Pain (suppl)6: S121–S126.

Melzack R 1999b Pain and stress: a new perspective. In: Gatchel RJ, Turk DC (eds) Psychosocial factors in pain. Guilford Press, New York.

Meng ID, Cao L 2007 From migraine to chronic daily headache: the biological basis of headache transformation. Headache 47:1251-1258.

Millichap JG, Yee MM 2003 The diet factor in pediatric and adolescent migraine. Pediatric Neurology 28:9-15.

Milligan ED, O'Connor KA, Nguyen KT et al 2001 Intrathecal Hiv-1 envelope glycoprotein Gp120 induces enhanced pain states mediated by spinal cord proinflammatory cytokines. Journal of Neuroscience 21:2808-2819.

Monro J, Brastoff J, Carmine C, Zilkha K 1980 Food allergy in migraine – a study of dietary exclusion and fast. Lancet 11:1-4.

Nair A, Bonneau RH 2006 Stress-induced elevation of glucocorticoids increases microglia proliferation through NMDA receptor activation. Journal of Neuroimmunology 171:72-85.

Nash JM, Thebarge RW 2006 Understanding psychological stress, its biological processes and impact on primary headache. Headache 46:1377-1386.

Niere KR 1998 Can characteristics of benign headache predict manipulative physiotherapy treatment outcome? Australian Journal of Physiotherapy 44:87-93.

Niere KR, Robinson PM 1997 Determination of manipulative physiotherapy treatment outcome in headache patients. Manual Therapy 2:199-205.

O'Brien PMS, 1993 Helping women with premenstrual syndrome. British Medical Journal 307:1471-1475.

Oshinsky ML, Luo J 2006 Neurochemistry of trigeminal activation in an animal model of migraine. Headache 46(suppl 1):S39–S44.

Pasti L, Pozzan T, Carmignoto G 1995 Long-lasting changes of calcium oscillations in astrocytes. A new form of glutamate-mediated plasticity.

Journal of Biological Chemistry 270:15203-15210.

Pasti L, Volterra A, Pozzan T, Carmignoto G 1997 Intracellular calcium oscillations in astrocytes: a highly plastic, bidirectional form of communication between neurons and astrocytes in situ. Journal of Neuroscience 17:817-830.

Raghavendra V, Tanga FY, Deleo JA 2004 Attenuation of morphine tolerance, withdrawal-induced hyperalgesia and associated spinal inflammatory immune responses by propentophylline in rats. Neuropsychopharmacology 29:327-334.

Rasmussen BK, 1993 Migraine and tension-type headache in a general population: precipitating factors, female hormones, sleep pattern and relation to lifestyle. Pain 53:65-72.

Ren K, Dubner R 2002 Descending modulation in persistent pain: an update. Pain 100:1-6.

Reynolds DJ, Hovanitz CA 2000 Life event stress and headache frequency revisited. Headache 40:111-118.

Riley JL, Robinson ME, Wise EA, Price DD 1999 A meta-analytic review of pain perception across the menstrual cycle. Pain 81:225-235.

Rothrock J, Patel M, Jackson C 1996 Demographic and clinical characteristics of patients with episodic migraine versus chronic daily headache. Cephalalgia 16:44-49.

Russell MB 2001 Genetics of migraine without aura, migraine with aura, migrainous disorder, head trauma, migraine without aura and tension-type headache. Cephalalgia 21:778-780.

Sances G, Granella F, Nappi RE et al 2003 Course of migraine during pregnancy and postpartum: a prospective study. Cephalalgia 23:197-205.

Sandler M, Li N-Y, Jarrett N, Glover V 1995 Dietary migraine: recent progress in the red (and white) wine story. Cephalalgia 15:101-103.

Sandor PS, Afra J, Albert A, Schoenen J 2000 From neurophysiology to genetics: cortical information processing in migraine underlies

familial influences – a novel approach. Functional Neurology 15 (suppl 3):68-72.

Scharff L, Turk D, Marcus DA 1995 Triggers of headache episodes and coping responses of headache diagnostic groups. Headache 35:397-403.

Schmidt-Hansen PT, Svensson P, Bendtsen L et al 2007 Increased muscle pain sensitivity in patients with tension-type headache. Pain 129:113-121.

Schoenen J 2006 Tension-type headache. In: Mcmahon SB, Koltzenburg S (eds) Wall and Melzack's textbook of pain, 5th edn. Elsevier/Churchill Livingstone, Philadelphia.

Schoenen J, Maertens De Noordhout A 1994 Headache. In: Wall PD, Melzack R (eds) Textbook of pain, 3rd edn. Churchill Livingstone, Edinburgh.

Schoenen J, Sandor PS 1999 Headache. In Wall PD, Melzack R (eds) Textbook of pain, 4th edn. Churchill Livingstone, Edinburgh.

Seltzer S, Marcus R, Stoch R 1981 Perspectives in the control of chronic pain by nutritional manipulation. Pain 11:141-148.

Shavit Y, Woolf G, Goshen I et al 2005 Interleukin 1 antagonizes morphine analgesia and underlies morphine tolerance. Pain 115:50-59.

Sheather-Reid RB, Cohen ML 1998 Psychophysical evidence for a neuropathic component of chronic neck pain. Pain 75:341-347.

Silberstein SD, Merriam GR 1991 Estrogens, progestins and headache. Neurology 41:786-793.

Silverman K, Evans SM, Strain EC, Griffiths RR 1992 Withdrawal syndrome after the double blind cessation of caffeine consumption. New England Journal of Medicine 327:1109-1114.

Sjaastad O, Fredriksen TA 2002 Cervicogenic headache: lack of influence of pregnancy. Cephalalgia 22:667-671.

Sjaastad O, Fredriksen T, Pfaffenrath V 1998 Cervicogenic headache: diagnostic criteria. Headache 38:442-445.

Souvlis T, Vicenzino B, Wright A 2004 Neurophysiological effects of spinal manual therapy. In: Boyling JD, Jull GA (eds) Grieve's modern manual therapy of the vertebral column, 3rd edn. Elsevier Churchill Livingstone, Edinburgh.

Stein GS 1981 Headaches in the first week post partum and their relationship to migraine. Headache 21:201-205.

Steptoe A, Hamer M, Chida Y 2007 The effects of acute psychological stress on circulating inflammatory factors in humans: a review and meta-analysis. Brain, Behaviour And Immunity 21:900-912.

Sterling M, Treleaven J, Edwards S 2002 Pressure pain thresholds in chronic whiplash associated disorder: further evidence of altered central pain processing. Journal of Musculoskeletal Pain 10:69-81.

Thompson S 2006 Clinical pain, experimental evidence: molecular mechanisms within the spinal cord. In: Gifford L (ed) Topical issues in pain 5. Kestrel, CNS Press.

Van Den Bergh V, Amery WK, Waelkens J 1987 Trigger factors in migraine: a study conducted by The Belgian Migraine Society. Headache 27:191-196.

Wang F, Vandeneeden SK, Ackerson LM et al 2003 Oral magnesium oxide prophylaxis of frequent migrainous headache in children: a randomized, double-blind, placebo-controlled trial. Headache 46:601-610.

Ward N, Whitney C, Avery D, Dunner D 1991 The analgesic effect of caffeine in headache. Pain 44:151-155.

Watkins LR, Maier SF 2000 The pain of being sick: implications of immune to brain communication for understanding of pain. Annual Review of Psychology 51.

Watkins LR, Maier SF 2005 Immune regulation of central nervous system functions: from sickness responses to pathological pain. Journal of Internal Medicine 257:139-155.

Watkins LR, Hutchinson MR, Ledeboer A et al 2007 Glia as the 'bad guys'; implications for improving clinical pain control and the clinical utility of opioids. Brain, Behavior And Immunity 21:131-146.

Watson P 1999 Psychosocial predictors of outcome from low back pain. In: Gifford L (ed) Topical issues in pain 2. Kestrel, CNS Press.

Welch KMA, 1997 Migraine and ovarian steroid hormones. Cephalalgia 20:12-16.

Wieseler-Frank J, Maier SF, Watkins LR 2005 Immune to brain communication dynamically modulates pain: physiological and pathological

consequences. Brain, Behaviour And Immunity 19:104-111.

Wöber C, Brannath W, Schmidt K et al 2007 Prospective analysis of factors related to migraine attacks: the Pamina study. Cephalalgia 27:304-314.

Woolf CJ, Salter MW 2000 Neuronal plasticity: increasing the gain in pain. Science 288:1765-1768.

Woolf CJ, Thompson SW 1991 The induction and maintenance of central sensitization is dependent on N-methyl-D-aspartic acid receptor

activation; implications for the treatment of postinjury pain hypersensitivity states. Pain 44:293-299.

Xie YF, Zhang S, Chiang CY et al 2007 Involvement of glia in central sensitization in trigeminal subnucleus caudalis (trigeminal dorsal horn). Brain, Behaviour And Immunity 21:634-641.

Zwart JA 1997 Neck mobility in different headache disorders. Headache 37:6-11.

ENT causes of orofacial pain

Stephen O'Leary

ENT pathology, temporomandibular disorders, and conditions referred for otolaryngology-head and neck surgery share a common constellation of symptoms, particularly facial pain. Therefore, a patient with an ENT problem may present to a range of health care professionals. In this chapter the author, an ENT surgeon, highlights the differential diagnosis and management of ENT-related orofacial symptoms.

The ear nose throat (ENT) region can contribute to headache and orofacial symptoms. A major diagnostic challenge in the assessment and management of headache and orofacial pain is the interpretation of patterns of symptoms as they relate to specific disease conditions. Ear pain, for example, may be caused by otologic infection but could as easily derive from disorder of the temporomandibular joint (TMJ), a neoplasm from the oropharynx or laryngopharynx, or be referred from the cervical region.

There are several reasons why head and neck symptoms may not point to specific organs or diseases. The most obvious is the anatomical proximity of structures within the head and neck. Second, the innervation of the head and neck can result in the referral of pain to sites remote from the primary pathology, e.g., overlap of the trigeminal and upper cervical afferent information in the trigeminocervical nucleus

(as described in Ch. 5). Finally, the middle ear, nose, and throat are linked by mucosa, and are in continuity via the post-nasal space and eustachian tube.

The clinician needs to bear in mind that the low specificity of head and neck symptoms increases the chances of misdiagnosis. It is not uncommon for patients to arrive for a consultation with a diagnostic label that fails to stand up to closer scrutiny. Similarly, the clinician is often left with a degree of diagnostic uncertainty, and may need to work through the possible etiologies before an optimal treatment is found.

This chapter focuses on presenting symptoms, with particular emphasis on establishing a clinical diagnosis in relation to otalgia, facial pain, and tinnitus. Information relating to management is provided for diseases usually treated by otolaryngology-head and neck surgery (OHNS) specialists. When referring to conditions usually treated by disciplines such as physical therapy or dentistry, the focus will be on differential diagnosis rather than treatment.

Otalgia

Most medical practitioners have been faced with the perplexing situation of seeing a patient suffering from severe earache (otalgia) and having a normal looking ear canal and drum. Often the patient is convinced that there is something very wrong with their ear and the doctor faces a diagnostic dilemma. However, not all otalgia results from ear disease and the medical practitioner must assess for alternative diagnoses (Box 10.1).

The following section describes the otological and non-otological causes of ear pain, the latter due to referred pain from another area of the body.

Box 10.1

Differential diagnosis of otalgia.

1. Otological
   Pinna
   - perichondritis
   - trauma
   - neoplasia (uncommon cause)
   External ear canal
   - otitis externa
   - skull base osteitis (malignant otitis externa)
   - bullous meningitis
   - herpes zoster
   - neoplasia
   Middle ear
   - acute otitis media
   - chronic otitis media
   - barotrauma
2. Non-otological
   Dental disease
   Temporomandibular disorder
   Neck
   - zygapophyseal joint
   - myofascial pain
   Parotid gland infection
   Nasopharynx
   Oropharynx
   - post tonsillectomy
   - foreign body in tonsils
   - carcinoma in tonsils
   Laryngopharynx
   - vocal cord granuloma
   - cancer of larynx
   - cancer of piriform fossa

Otological causes

Ear infection is a common and potentially serious cause of otalgia (Gross et al 2008). Infection can affect the pinna, the ear canal, or the ear drum.

Inflammation of the pinna

Inflammatory disease of the pinna typically causes a throbbing otalgia. Diagnosis is usually made relatively easily due to the readily apparent pathology of the pinna. The classical viral cause is reactivation of the varicella zoster virus (herpes zoster) (Crabtree, 1968). This condition presents with ear pain, and transient blistering of the conchal bowl, ear canal or the lower half of the pinna.

Herpes zoster affects the lower cranial nerves, and the extent of the disease is dependent upon the sensory and motor distribution of the nerves affected. If confined to the trigeminal nerve, the presenting sign will be the vesiculation described. When the auditory-vestibular nerve is affected, the patient will present with acute dysequilibrium and/or a sensorineural hearing loss. Involvement of the facial nerve causes a partial or complete facial paralysis, severe ear ache, vertigo and tinnitus and described as the Ramsay-Hunt Syndrome (Gross et al 2008, Sweeney et al 2001). Glossopharyngeal nerve involvement may present with vesicles on the soft palate, within the sensory distribution of the nerve (Sachs et al 1956).

In the early phase of the disease, the diagnosis may be confirmed by viral culture from the vesicles (Kowalski et al 1993). The primary treatment is the systemic administration of antiviral agents and glucocorticoid steroids, although the benefit of the antiviral agents has not yet been confirmed in randomized controlled trials. Secondary infections of the skin are treated with oral antibiotics.

A detailed description of the management of hearing loss, vestibular dysfunction and facial nerve paralysis is beyond the scope of this chapter. Even with aggressive medical treatment, the sensory and motor deficits frequently do not fully recover (Yeo et al 2007). The same applies for vestibular dysfunction, but central compensation for the peripheral deficit will usually lead to a good resolution of the clinical symptoms of dizziness. The vestibular management may need to be supplemented by vestibular rehabilitation by a physical therapist if the central compensation is not complete. Vestibular rehabilitation is described in Chapter 12.

Perichondritis

Perichondritis is inflammation of the cartilage that gives the ear its shape, so adequate and appropriate treatment is required to maintain cosmesis of the ear. Most perichondritis is due to bacterial infection, usually as a complication of aural trauma, surgery, or ear piercing. Compound lacerations pose the greatest risk. The perichondritis will usually have a delayed presentation, becoming clinically apparent through swelling, pain and tenderness of the pinna up to two weeks following the trauma. The causative organism is usually *pseudomonas aeruginosa* (Prasad et al 2007) and occasionally *staphylococcus aureus*. The treatment of choice is a quinolone antibiotic, such as ciprofloxacin. Bacterial infections of the pinna can be distinguished from autoimmune inflammation because the latter do not respond to antibiotic therapy and relapses, which is why it is often known as 'relapsing perichondritis'.

Inflammatory disease of the pinna is usually apparent upon inspection of the ear. The ear will be painful when palpated or moved. Disease of the external ear canal should be considered if the ear is painful upon movement but there is no disease of the pinna.

Neoplastic disease of the pinna or external ear is an uncommon cause of pain. It should always be considered with otalgia and unhealing cutaneous lesions, and deep persistent pain of unknown origin.

Otitis externa

Acute otitis externa is a bacterial (Dibb 1991) infection of the external ear canal. Fungal infection is usually associated with chronic otitis externa. Acute otitis externa is characterized by otalgia and aural discharge, sometimes leading on to cellulitis of the pinna and/or peri-auricular skin. This condition is usually secondary to excessive moisture within the ear canal (Osguthorpe et al 2006) and hence its colloquial name 'swimmer's ear'. Water entrapment is more likely when there is wax retention, narrowness, or tortuosity of the ear canal. Unclean water predisposes to infection, as does an underlying dermatitis of the ear canal or high humidity. The latter may help to explain why people who wear hearing aids are more prone to otitis externa (Ahmad et al 2007); hearing aids raise humidity by occluding the external ear canal. Patients who complain of 'itchy' ears due to seborrheic or eczematous dermatitis of the ear canal are more prone to experiencing recurrent external ear infections (Osguthorpe et al 2006). The diagnosis is confirmed by the presence of inflammation and debris, and discharge in the external ear canal but an intact tympanic membrane. Treatment involves a thorough aural toilet, the topical application of antibiotics via drops, either directly into the ear, or via wicks or packs, and when cellulitis is present, the prescription of oral quinolone antibiotics.

A rare, but potentially life-threatening form of otitis externa is malignant otitis externa (also referred to as invasive osteitis or skull base osteitis). This condition occurs in diabetic or immunocompromised patients. If left untreated it can lead to a fulminant necrotizing inflammation of the skull base (Bhandary et al 2002). It is usually caused by *Pseudomonas aeruginosa*. The treatment involves intravenous, followed by a prolonged course of oral, antibiotic therapy (e.g., ciprofloxacin) in consultation with infection disease specialists.

Ear wax within the external auditory canal is usually not painful, but may be under some circumstances. Ear wax may become very hard, especially when impacted, and cause otalgia at its point of impaction. Water trapped behind impacted wax not uncommonly leads to an infection, again causing a painful otitis externa. Syringing of wax or removal of wax usually reduces the risk of, but may be complicated by, otitis externa.

Otitis media

Acute otitis media is the classical earache of the young child in the first few years of life (Leibovitz 2006). It presents also with constitutional symptoms such as fever, lethargy, malaise, hearing loss, irritability, and disturbed sleep pattern (Gross et al 2008). The condition occasionally occurs in adults. The diagnosis is made by the presence of a red and swollen tympanic membrane. Should the eardrum perforate there will be mucus in the ear canal. Usually the pain decreases when the tympanic membrane perforates. This condition is treated with antibiotics, decongestants, and analgesia. There is a consensus that antibiotics are indicated when the symptoms persist for more than 24 hours or when there is a complication of the otitis media such as facial nerve palsy or intracranial infection (Ganiats et al 2004).

Acute otitis media should be differentiated from an otitis media with effusion ('glue ear'), in which case the drum is immobile due to the presence of the middle ear fluid, but not inflamed, and there is rarely any pain. Acute otitis media can be difficult to differentiate from inflammation localized to the tympanic

membrane, a condition known as 'bullous myringitis'. This is more often viral, but can be bacterial infection (McCormick et al 2003) that presents as otalgia with blood-filled blisters on the tympanic membrane with bullous blebs. It is sometimes associated with sensorineural hearing loss (Hariri 1990), and is treated symptomatically with analgesics.

Eustachian tube dysfunction

Otalgia, in the absence of any obvious signs of disease of the pinna, the external ear canal, or the tympanic membrane is unlikely to be due to ear disease, with the exception of eustachian tube dysfunction. This condition can be difficult to diagnose clinically. In eustachian tube dysfunction, there is an obstruction of air flow from the nasopharynx to the middle ear. The middle ear is therefore unable to equalize to atmospheric pressure. The dysfunction frequently follows upper respiratory tract infection and this blockage of the ear and partial hearing loss sometimes occurs with the common cold.

Eustachian tube dysfunction may become clinically manifest when there is a rapid change of atmospheric pressure, particularly when the pressure increases (Mirza & Richardson 2005). The classic example is the young child with immature eustachian tube function who develops severe otalgia upon descent during an aeroplane flight. This severe otalgia also occurs with acute barometric otitis media and may be associated with hemorrhages on the tympanic membrane.

Non-otological causes

Pain can be referred to the ear from other structures due to the sensory innervation of the ear. The sensory branches of the trigeminal, facial, glossopharyngeal, vagus, the lesser occipital and the greater occipital nerves all innervate the ear (Gross et al 2008). It is reported that in 50% of patients non-otological otalgia is due to dental dysfunction and in the other 50% it is due to referred pain from non-otological related conditions (Gross et al 2008, Yanagisawa & Kveton 1992).

Temporomandibular disorders

If the cause for the otalgia is not found within the ear, or the throat, the clinician should turn attention to evaluate for the presence or absence of temporomandibular disorders (TMD), described in Chapter 7.

Many patients presenting to the ENT surgeon with otalgia have TMD as their primary diagnosis. It is a diagnosis of exclusion in that patients have a normal ear canal, normal tympanic membrane, normal hearing and tympanogram, and absence of pharyngeal pathology such as carcinoma of the tonsil or a granuloma of the vocal cord through laryngeal reflux disease (Devaney et al 2005).

That TMD can cause otalgia is probably a reflection of the close proximity between the temporomandibular joint (TMJ) and the ear. The posterior aspect of the joint is separated from the anterior wall of the external ear canal by a relatively thin plate of bone, and both structures receive a common innervation from branches of the trigeminal nerve, such as the auriculotemporal nerve (Hollinshead 1982). So close is the proximity of these structures that an otologist can easily encounter the joint when drilling the anterior wall of the external ear canal. A fractured or inflamed joint can be displaced backwards into the ear canal following trauma (Selesnick et al 1995), and an absence of bone can occur between the two. If so, movement of the anterior canal wall may be observed during speech or mastication.

Otalgia from TMD is usually described as originating deep within the ear. It may be constant and often radiates to the angle of the jaw or temporal region and is exacerbated by sleep bruxism. Specific questioning will lead some patients to volunteer that the pain is in fact pre-auricular. A history of sleep bruxism, or recent orthodontic or dental work should heighten clinical suspicion of TMD. Tenderness of the TMJ is localized to its cutaneous landmark – anterior to the tragus. Direct palpation will not always elicit pain, but palpation during jaw movement may reproduce pain. Direct palpation of the muscles of mastication, either externally or peri-orally, will usually elicit tenderness. Furthermore, since temporomandibular pain frequently radiates to the angle of the jaw and temporal area, these regions should be assessed for the presence of any referred pain (Okeson 2005).

Most causes of temporomandibular pain and tenderness are treated by dental and oral medicine specialists, but a few rare conditions are the shared domain of these specialists and the ENT surgeon. One is a posterior fracture of the temporomandibular joint that has been displaced into the external ear canal. Here the role of the otologist is to exclude an injury to the tympanic membrane, ossicles or hearing and to ensure that the fracture is reduced sufficiently to maintain the patency of the external ear canal. This may necessitate packing of the external ear canal until the fracture heals.

Another shared management problem is neoplasia traversing from or invading the TMJ (Selesnick et al 1995). Tumors invading the joint usually arise from the external ear canal, and squamous cell carcinoma is the most common type. Surgical resection of these tumors may also necessitate resection encompassing both the TMJ and the lateral petrous temporal bone.

Pharyngeal pathology

When there is no obvious otological cause for ear pain the clinician must look beyond the ear. The most important region to examine is the pharynx (nasopharynx, oropharynx, and laryngopharynx). Pain from pathology within the region of the palantine tonsils, the lateral pharyngeal wall or the larynx may be referred to the ears and is frequently precipitated by swallowing. Referral of pain from the throat to the ear is due to the common innervation of both regions by branches of the trigeminal, glossopharyngeal, and vagus nerves.

The disease to exclude is neoplasia (Charlett & Coatesworth 2007). The otalgia from neoplasia of the tonsils, pharynx or larynx is usually a constant, deep-seated ache in the TMJ region and needs to be differentiated from TMJ pain. Throat pain, dysphagia and breathing difficulties may also be experienced (Wazen 1989). Ulceration of the pharynx because of carcinoma or more benign causes such as trauma, foreign body impaction, or viral infection may cause an otalgia that worsens transiently upon swallowing. This explains the cause and nature of the severe otalgia that some patients suffer following tonsillectomy (Johnson et al 2002). Exclusion of a pharyngeal cause for otalgia demands a thorough examination of the upper airways as the pathology can be subtle. An infiltrative carcinoma of the tonsil may present with little apparent mucosal ulceration, and only be diagnosed upon palpation, imaging or excision biopsy (Schmalbach & Miller 2007).

The examination is not complete without an examination of the neck to exclude lymphadenopathy that may point to occult neoplasm of the throat (Schmalbach & Miller 2007). This should include a bimanual examination of the floor of the mouth and lateral pharynx with the soft tissue palpated between a gloved finger in the oropharynx and a hand on the anterior aspect of the neck, to exclude masses within the tonsil, tongue base, upper neck near the angle of the jaw, or the floor of the mouth.

Neck

As mentioned earlier when discussing neoplasia of the throat, a clinical investigation of otalgia is not complete without examination of the neck.

In addition, non-neoplastic pain and/or tenderness of any peri-auricular muscle can present as otalgia, with the sternocleidomastoid most often involved (Simons et al 1999). The sternocleidomastoid inserts into the mastoid process, so it is in intimate contact with the inferior margin of the conchal bowl (i.e. the cartilaginous floor of the pinna). The otalgia that may arise from muscle pain is often described by patients as aural 'fullness' or 'pressure'. This description may assist in differentiating other conditions that may derive from the neck, such as headache. Otologic causes of aural 'fullness', such as that associated with Meniere's disease should also be considered.

The causes of neck pain are numerous, the most common being cervical zygapophyseal joint dysfunction (Govind et al 2005), spondylosis and/or muscle dysfunction (Simons et al 1999). These are described in Chapters 5 and 14. Less often the pain is a result of inflammatory disease along the course of a muscle, such as infection of a cervical lymph node or within a deep neck space. Muscle tension, arising from emotional stress may also cause neck discomfort and aural fullness. Headaches may also be associated with neck pain, TMD, dental disease, nasal disease or neurological disease (Okeson 2005, Gross et al 2008).

Facial pain

It is useful to classify facial pain as rhinological or non-rhinological. Box 10.2 lists the causes of facial pain in both these categories.

Rhinological

Rhinosinusitis

The facial pain of rhinosinusitis is usually localized to the affected sinus(es); the maxillary to the infraorbital region (malar region) of the

Box 10.2

Differential diagnosis of facial pain.

1. Rhinological
   Rhinitis
   Sinusitis
   Barotrauma
   Neuralgia (Sluder's syndrome)
   Malignancies
   – nose
   – sinus
2. Non-rhinological
   Dental
   Temporomandibular disorders
   Mid-facial segment pain (atypical facial
      neuralgia)
   – migraine
   – cluster headaches
   – tension-type headache
   Temporal arteritis
   – unilateral facial pain

face, the ethmoidal sinuses to the lateral wall of the nose, the frontal sinuses to the medial supra-orbital region, and the sphenoid sinuses to the vertex or bitemporal regions. Sinus pain is described as constant (Salman & Rebeiz 1994), with a 'pounding' character during exacerbations or on flexing the neck or coughing. Sinus pain is typically worse when the head is in a dependent position, for example, when lying down. The severity of sinus pain ranges from mild to severe, depending upon the severity of the disease.

The pressure within the sinuses should equal atmospheric levels. The ostia between the nose and the sinuses are the route by which 'equalization' of air pressure (between the atmosphere and the sinuses) occurs. 'Barotrauma' of the sinuses (sinus squeeze) may occur when there is a sudden change in atmospheric pressure that exceeds the rate at which the sinus pressure can adjust. Descent during scuba diving (Klingmann et al 2007), or descent from altitude in an airplane (Weitzel et al 2008) are

the usual causes of sinus squeeze. The less severe 'sinus pressure' that many people experience during an upper respiratory tract infection is also due to poor pressure equalization, but here the etiology is infection causing mucosal swelling which narrows the ostia. Like the sinus pain caused by infection, sinus squeeze and 'pressure' are worsened by a dependent head position, coughing and sneezing.

Sinus pain is frequently associated with the nasal symptoms of infection, such as nasal obstruction and coryza. Interestingly, in acute rhinosinusitis, the pain is worst before there is substantial nasal discharge. This phenomenon is because the pain is caused by the build-up of infected mucus (mucopus) within the sinus, while drainage of the mucopus (into the nose) relieves the pain. In this respect, the symptomatic relief achieved by drainage of mucopus from a sinus is analogous to that experienced when an abscess is drained.

Non-rhinological

Dental

Dental disease may cause facial pain that resembles either rhinosinusitis or TMD, depending upon the teeth affected. If the bony floor of the maxillary sinus is thin, tooth roots may be present within the antrum, and a dental abscess may cause sinusitis (Mehra & Murad 2004). More often, facial pain originates from the vicinity of the abscessed tooth root. Rarely, dental infections spread to the deep facial spaces.

Temporomandibular disorders

Temporomandibular disorders are frequently confused with rhinosinusitis since they often presents as a facial pain, typically in the infraorbital region. However, the character of TMD-related pain, and its radiation, is different. Because pain arising from TMD may radiate along muscles of mastication or in the distribution of the branches of the trigeminal nerve (Okeson 2005), it may be considered to originate in the peri-auricular region and radiate to the face. If the temporalis muscle is involved frontal pain may occur, but this will be located in the fronto-temporal region, lateral to the site associated with rhinosinusitis (Simons 1999). TMD-related pain may be exacerbated by chewing, but not sinus pain.

Cervical dysfunction

Mid-facial segment pain, with or without a headache, is thought sometimes to be referred from the upper cervical region of the neck (Armijo et al 2006). Although systematic reviews of the literature support this association, the quality of the literature is not of the highest grade, and physiological basis by which the pain may arise is subject to debate (Armijo et al 2006). From a clinical perspective, until better evidence is available it is prudent to bear in mind that any muscle dysfunction or degenerative change within the neck may cause facial pain and the latter could be confused with rhinosinusitis.

Headache

Facial pain may be a prominent feature of neurological conditions involving the head and neck. The clinician needs to be aware of the possible diagnoses when faced with a patient who presents with 'sinusitis'. Neurological causes of mid-facial neuralgias include trigeminal or post-herpetic neuralgia (Burchiel 2003). Tension-type headache may cause mid-facial segment pain that mimics rhinosinusitis (Jones 2004). It is characterized by pressure or pain involving the nose and ethmoidal regions (between the eye and the nose), much like sinusitis and is described to be often associated in women with a family history of headache and or migraine. Nasal obstruction and stuffiness

may be a feature of this condition, making it difficult to distinguish from true rhinosinusitis. Migraine too, may be associated with facial pain (Nixdorf et al 2008) with symptoms such as photophobia, nausea and vomiting pointing towards this diagnosis. A notable feature of these neurological causes for facial pain and pain associated with TMD or the neck is the absence of sinus pathology on CT scans of the sinuses.

Tinnitus

Tinnitus may accompany disease of the ear, TMD or cervical dysfunction but often there is no clearly identifiable cause (Box 10.3).

Box 10.3

Differential diagnosis of tinnitus.

1. **Otological**
   Conductive hearing loss
     Impacted wax (Cerumen)
     Otitis media
     Eustachian tube dysfunction
     Barotrauma
     Serous and mucoid otitis media
     Cholesteatoma
     Otosclerosis
   Sensorineural hearing loss
     Age-related hearing loss
     Noise exposure
     Meniere's disease
     Acoustic neuroma
     Ototoxic drugs
       – gentamicin
       – salicylic acid
       – cytotoxic drugs
2. **Non-otological**
   Intracranial vascular anomalies
     Pulsatile tinnitus
   Benign intracranial hypertension
   Glomus tumors
   Temporomandibular disorders
   Dental pathology
   Neck pathology
   Anemia

The most common cause of tinnitus is age (presbyacusis). Tinnitus may also be related to drugs such as high doses of salicylic acid, aminoglycoside drugs used for treatment of septicemia, and cytotoxic drugs used in the treatment of neoplastic cancers and lymphomas.

The patient experience of tinnitus is usually similar, irrespective of the cause, so it is useful to appreciate the natural history of this condition, before discussing the causes and management. At first the ringing in the ears is usually very loud and intrusive and may keep the patient awake at night. Tinnitus may interfere with hearing, as the patient struggles to differentiate between sounds in the external environment and the 'internal' noise. The person who has 'overcome' tinnitus will not be aware of the ringing most of the time, but the tinnitus will still be there if they are reminded of it or if they are distressed or fatigued.

It is essential that the natural history of tinnitus is explained to patients early on, as many people are under the misapprehension that their initial distress will be ongoing. Counseling (Henry et al 2007), reassuring the patient that the tinnitus is likely to fade with time, is probably the best way of ensuring a good outcome as it allays the patient's fears and promotes the adoption of a positive attitude towards this condition. When an individual is having difficulty coping with tinnitus active therapeutic intervention (beyond counseling) may be required. Sound-based treatments provide acoustic stimulation that will either compete with, or alternatively mask, the tinnitus. Competing sounds aim to distract the patient's attention away from the tinnitus (i.e. give the patient something more interesting, or 'useful' to listen to). Examples include the prescription of a hearing aid for the hearing impaired (Trotter et al 2008), or the introduction of ambient environmental sounds or music. The alternative is to deliver a sound that will mask out the tinnitus (Jastreboff 2007). One

recent development is a device that interleaves short (subliminal) bursts of masking noise with music (Davis et al 2007).

Otological conditions causing tinnitus include wax impaction within the external ear canal, especially if it obstructs the ear canal and causes hearing loss. Tinnitus usually accompanies the temporary hearing loss that follows acoustic shock or exposure to loud noise or music. Fortunately, the tinnitus usually settles as the hearing returns. A permanent sensorineural hearing loss from any cause may be accompanied by tinnitus.

Tinnitus is usually bilateral and difficult to localize to one ear. Unilateral tinnitus may be a sign of a vestibular schwannoma ('acoustic neuroma'), a benign tumor within the cerebellopontine angle. An MRI scan is recommended for all patients presenting with unilateral tinnitus, especially when associated with asymmetrical hearing loss.

Another cause of unilateral tinnitus is Meniere's disease. The condition is characterized by episodic aural pressure, reduced hearing in one ear associated with tinnitus followed by prostrating vertigo that may last hours (Minor et al 2004). The patient may experience recurrent episodes over days or a week, each episode lasting for a few hours. The pathophysiology of Meniere's disease is increased pressure within the endolymphatic space. It is usually idiopathic, but may be precipitated by trauma to the ear, autoimmune disease, or surgery. Early in this disease the hearing fluctuates, decreasing during an attack and then recovering, but with repeated attacks a permanent sensorineural hearing loss develops. End-stage Meniere's disease is characterized by a severe sensorineural hearing loss without further 'attacks' but often with a sense of chronic imbalance and/or 'drop' attacks.

Meniere's disease is one of the most over-diagnosed conditions in otology. Over-diagnosis occurs because all of the symptoms are frequently encountered and all have multiple potential causes. Therefore, some clinicians have a tendency to cluster these symptoms, arriving at a diagnosis of Meniere's disease even when the history does not fit the 'classical' description. The diagnosis is frequently termed 'atypical' Meniere's disease. In clinical practice, it is better to categorize the likelihood that a patient may have Meniere's disease, using an accepted scale, such as that recommended by the American Academy of Otolaryngology Head and Neck Surgery (Committee on Hearing and Equilibrium 1995). This categorization helps both the patient and the doctor to understand the degree of confidence that should be given to the diagnosis of Meniere's disease – and therefore to what extent other diagnoses should be considered.

A pulsatile tinnitus is either the awareness of blood passing through the great vessels of the temporal bone or neck (a vascular anomaly or tumor), or alternatively a type of increased intracranial pressure known as benign intracranial hypertension (Mattox et al 2008). This condition is usually investigated with imaging of the head and neck (MRI, MRA, MRV or alternatively a CT scan with intravenous contrast). Pulsatile tinnitus via this mechanism is usually heard on the right, because the right jugular vein (known as the 'sigmoid sinus' within the temporal bone) is dominant in most people and passes very close to the ear. If no cause for pulsatile tinnitus can be found within the neck a neurological consultation is indicated to exclude benign intracranial hypertension

Conclusion

For each of the head and neck symptoms discussed there are numerous causes. Differential diagnosis may be difficult, and is the essence of 'clinical acumen'. The following principles are suggested: first, exclude potentially serious disease from either local or remote regions; second, examine all regions of the head and neck that may cause the presenting symptom; third, treat any obvious disease that could have caused the symptom, such as neck dysfunction that may co-exist with other causes of otalgia and/or facial pain. Finally, accept that there may be some uncertainty with the diagnosis.

References

Ahmad N, Etheridge C et al 2007 Prospective study of the microbiological flora of hearing aid moulds and the efficacy of current cleaning techniques. J Laryngol Otol 121(2):110-113.

Armijo Olivo S, Magee D et al 2006 The association between the cervical spine, the stomatognathic system, and craniofacial pain: a critical review. J Orofac Pain 20(4):271-287.

Bhandary S, Karki P et al 2002 Malignant otitis externa: a review. Pac Health Dialog 9(1):64-67.

Burchiel KJ 2003 A new classification for facial pain. Neurosurgery 53(5):1164-1166; discussion 1166-1167.

Bylander A 1984 Upper respiratory tract infection and eustachian tube function in children. Acta Otolaryngol 97(3-4):343-349.

Charlett SD, Coatesworth AP 2007 Referred otalgia: a structured approach to diagnosis and treatment. Int J Clin Pract 61(6):1015-1021.

Committee on Hearing and Equilibrium 1995 Committee on Hearing and Equilibrium guidelines for the diagnosis and evaluation of therapy in Meniere's disease. American Academy of Otolaryngology-Head and Neck Foundation, Inc. Otolaryngol Head Neck Surg 113(3):181-185.

Crabtree JA 1968 Herpes zoster oticus. Laryngoscope 78(11):853-878.

Davis PB, Paki B et al 2007 Neuromonics Tinnitus Treatment: third clinical trial. Ear Hear 28(2):242-259.

Devaney KO, Rinaldo A et al 2005 Vocal process granuloma of the larynx-recognition, differential diagnosis and treatment. Oral Oncol 41(7):666-669.

Dibb WL 1991 Microbial aetiology of otitis externa. J Infect 22(3):233-239.

Ganiats TG, Lieberthal AS, Culpepper L et al 2004 A joint clinical practice guideline for acute otitis media. Am Fam Physician 69(11):2537-2538, 2540.

Govind J, King W, Giles P et al 2005 'Headache and the cervical zygapophyseal joints (Cervicogenic Headache) Orthopaedic Proceedings' J Bone Joint Surg, 87B:399-340.

Gross M, Eliashar R 2008 Otolaryngological aspects of orofacial pain. In: Orofacial pain and headache. Eds: Sharav Y, Benoliel R (eds) Elsevier, Edinburgh, p 91-107.

Hariri MA 1990 Sensorineural hearing loss in bullous myringitis. A prospective study of eighteen patients. Clin Otolaryngol Allied Sci 15(4):351-353.

Henry JA, Loovis C et al 2007 Randomized clinical trial: group counseling based on tinnitus retraining therapy. J Rehabil Res Dev 44(1):21-32.

Hollinshead WH 1982 Anatomy for surgeons: the head and neck. JB Lippincott, Philadelphia.

Jastreboff MM 2007 Sound therapies for tinnitus management. Prog Brain Res 166:435-440.

Johnson LB, Elluru RG et al 2002 Complications of adeno-tonsillectomy. Laryngoscope 112(8 pt 2, suppl 100):35-36.

Jones NS 2004 Midfacial segment pain: implications for rhinitis and sinusitis. Curr Allergy Asthma Rep 4(3):187-192.

Klingmann C, Praetorius M et al 2007 Otorhinolaryngologic disorders and diving accidents: an analysis of 306 divers. Eur Arch Otorhinolaryngol 264(10):1243-1251.

Kowalski RP, Gordon YJ et al 1993 A comparison of enzyme immunoassay and polymerase chain reaction with the clinical examination for diagnosing ocular herpetic disease. Ophthalmology 100(4):530-533.

Leibovitz E 2006 Acute otitis media in children aged less than 2 years: drug treatment issues. Paediatr Drugs 8(6):337-346.

Mattox DE, Hudgins P 2008 Algorithm for evaluation of pulsatile tinnitus. Acta Otolaryngol 128(4):427-431.

McCormick DP, Saeed KA et al 2003 Bullous myringitis: a case-control study. Pediatrics 112(4):982-986.

Mehra P, Murad H 2004 Maxillary sinus disease of odontogenic origin. Otolaryngol Clin North Am 37(2):347-364.

Minor LB, Schessel DA et al 2004 Meniere's disease. Curr Opin Neurol 17(1):9-16.

Mirza S, Richardson H 2005 Otic barotrauma from air travel. J Laryngol Otol 119(5):366-370.

Nixdorf DR, Velly AM et al 2008 Neurovascular pains: implications of migraine for the oral and maxillofacial surgeon. Oral Maxillofac Surg Clin North Am 20(2):221-235, vi-vii.

Okeson J 2005 Bell's orofacial pain. The clinical management of orofacial pain, Quintessence Pub. Co. Inc., Chicago.

Osguthorpe JD, Nielsen DR 2006 Otitis externa: Review and clinical update. Am Fam Physician 74(9):1510-1516.

Prasad HK, Sreedharan S et al 2007 Perichondritis of the auricle and its management. J Laryngol Otol 121(6):530-534.

Sachs E Jr, House RK 1956 The Ramsay Hunt syndrome, geniculate herpes. Neurology 6(4):262-268.

Salman SD, Rebeiz EE 1994 Sinusitis and headache. J Med Liban 42(4):200-202.

Schmalbach CE, Miller FR 2007 Occult primary head and neck carcinoma. Curr Oncol Rep 9(2):139-146.

Selesnick SH, Carew JF et al 1995 Herniation of the temporo-mandibular joint into the external auditory canal: a complication of otologic surgery. Am J Otol 16(6):751-757.

Simons D, Travell J, Simons L 1999 Travell and Simons' myofascial pain and dysfunction: the trigger point manual. Upper half of the body, Lippincott Williams and Wilkins, Philadelphia.

Sweeney CJ, Gilden DH 2001 Ramsay Hunt syndrome. J Neurol Neurosurg Psychiatry 71:149-154.

Trotter MI, Donaldson I 2008 Hearing aids and tinnitus therapy: a 25-year experience. J Laryngol Otol 1-5.

Wazen JJ 1989 Referred Otalgia. Otolaryngol Clin N Am 22(6):1205-1215.

Weitzel EK, McMains KC et al 2008 Aerosinusitis: pathophysiology, prophylaxis, and management in passengers and aircrew. Aviat Space Environ Med 79(1):50-53.

Yanagisawa K, Kveton JF 1992 Referred otalgia. Am J Otolaryngol 13(6):323-327.

Yeo SW, Lee DH et al 2007 Analysis of prognostic factors in Bell's palsy and Ramsay Hunt syndrome. Auris Nasus Larynx 34(2):159-164.

Chapter **Eleven**

11

Ocular causes of headache

Julian Rait

Ocular dysfunction, including myopia and hyperopia, can cause tension in the orbicularis oculi muscle and the muscles controlling the eye, thus triggering headaches. Tumors within the eye and involvement of the optic and abducent nerves may also cause headache. In this chapter the author, an ophthalmologist, highlights ocular causes of headache and management strategies.

Although headaches are most frequently due to migraine or muscle tension, the list of the possible causes of headache is extensive. While 80% of the population is affected by headache at some time (Phillips 1977), the types of headache that can affect vision and/or produce pain in and around the eye or orbital region of the face will be discussed in this chapter. The ocular diseases that can be responsible for headache, the ocular manifestations of migraine, and the referred pain of neck disease will also be considered. However, from an ophthalmology perspective, ocular diseases are frequently quite painful and concerning and include several conditions that can be sight threatening if missed or misdiagnosed. These are listed in Table 11.1 with their usual corresponding symptoms.

Headache, facial pain and eye disease

It is widely believed that uncorrected refractive errors are an important cause of headaches. However, the importance of these conditions in the etiology of headaches is widely over-estimated. Refractive error and headache are common disorders that can co-exist but are not causally connected. Other common ocular and orbital pathologies can produce headache and pain in and around the eyes by virtue of stimulation of the nerves connected to the first division of the trigeminal nerve.

Detailed anatomic research has revealed that there is little sensory innervation of the choroid and ciliary body, with minimal innervation of the iris. The base of the iris, and particularly the trabecular meshwork, is intensely innervated by both afferent and efferent nerve fibers, reflecting perhaps some regulation of fluid outflow by the nervous system. Nonetheless, Bergmanson (1977) has found that there are no proprioceptors in the eye at all and thus pain, temperature, and tactile stimulation (particularly stretch) are the only sensations that can be felt by the eye.

Table 11.1 Conditions that may threaten sight.

Disease	Common symptoms
Acute angle closure glaucoma	Halos around lights
Giant cell arteritis	Transient obscurations of vision
Diplopia (ophthalmoplegia)
Sudden visual loss in either eye
Herpes zoster ophthalmicus	Burning pain with later vesicular rash
Acute optic neuritis	Painful unilateral visual loss or pain on eye movement
Headache associated with history of neurological loss (especially motor or sensory impairment)

Table 11.2 Classification and symptoms of ocular and orbital conditions.

Condition	Symptoms
Superficial corneal disease	Pain may be recurrent, sharp almost like a needle
Scleritis	Severe pain often described as a dull ache
Iritis	Moderately severe dull aching pain with photophobia
Glaucoma	Severe throbbing pain in acute angle closure, often associated with nausea and vomiting
Optic nerve disease	A dull aching or throbbing pain, mainly on ocular movements
Orbital lesions	Throbbing dull aching pain, worse when lying down
Refractive errors	Vague, heavy feeling in and around the eyes
Herpes zoster	Severe sharp unilateral headache, beginning with few clinical signs

Pain sensations from the eye can be generated in the eye by direct mechanical effects of tissue distortion, raised intraocular pressure, heat, and chemoreceptor stimulation by inflammatory mediators. Furthermore, the clinical ocular and orbital conditions that can cause pain from the eye can be classified according to the anatomic classification proposed by Hitchings (1980). Table 11.2 presents the classification of ocular and orbital conditions and the usual types of pain produced.

Superficial corneal disease

Ulceration of the cornea from infection, trauma, or a foreign body can directly irritate the superficial corneal nerves and produce pain. Because of neural reflexes arising from the nasociliary nerves, such irritation will almost invariably produce vasodilatation of the conjunctival vessels, photophobia, blepharospasm, and watering from the eye. Initially the sensations differ from the deeper, aching pain of iritis and iridocyclitis; however, such pain can evolve from corneal disease as inflammatory mediators (especially substance P) are released from the iris and ciliary body.

One of the most troubling superficial conditions is recurrent erosion syndrome. This can produce severe uniocular pain that can awaken a patient at night. Such pain can be temporarily relieved by topical anesthesia; however the patient should be referred to an ophthalmologist immediately for definitive treatment.

On initial examination, this diagnosis may be suspected on history alone, even in the absence of obvious signs of corneal erosions. Referral for slit lamp examination is necessary as frequently there are other signs, including microcysts in the cornea, which are evident between episodes.

Scleritis

Anterior scleritis may produce a dull aching pain from tissue distortion and release of inflammatory mediators. The pain of scleritis is often severe and disturbs sleep, whereas episcleritis will be associated with a milder ache or discomfort. Symptoms of scleritis may include local or diffuse conjuctival injection (increase in redness from prominent blood vessels) or tenderness of the affected eye. As there are few sensory nerves in the posterior sclera, posterior scleritis can produce pain from irritation of the posterior ciliary nerves and/or the adjacent orbital structures. This is a dull ache with few signs and forms a continuum with other inflammatory orbital diseases, such as orbital pseudotumor.

Iritis

The pain of anterior uveitis can be severe and evolve to become a widespread pain including earache, pain in the upper teeth and/or pain over the frontal, ethmoid or maxillary sinuses. It is often associated with blurred vision, lacrimation, and photophobia which may be the dominant symptom.

Blepharospasm, miosis, and tenderness of the globe may also be observed with the symptoms being worse at night. The pain of uveitis derives from the release of inflammatory mediators such as bradykinin, prostaglandin E1 and prostaglandin E2, and substance P. Iritis is often a recurrent syndrome in patients with sarcoidosis, juvenile rheumatoid arthritis, and those who are HLA-B27 positive, including those with ankylosing spondylitis.

Acute angle closure glaucoma

The most severe type of ocular pain that can occur is associated with primary angle closure glaucoma. It can easily be confused with ocular migraine but unlike most cases of migraine, the visual loss of angle closure glaucoma can rapidly become irreversible. Symptoms may include a vague and poorly localized pain around the face and upper jaw, but most patients describe severe and excruciating headache localized to the orbit and forehead. Pain is constant and often pulsating, frequently associated with nausea, vomiting, and abdominal pain by virtue of the spread of neural impulses from the trigeminal nuclei to other brain stem nuclei, especially the nucleus of the vagus nerve. Exploratory laparotomies have even been performed because of the abdominal symptoms, but most patients have pain referred to the eye. Similarly bradycardia and diaphoresis are often also observed due to parasympathetic activation.

Intermittent angle closure glaucoma is defined as repeated brief episodes of angle closure with normal ocular function between attacks. It can occur for months or years in patients with shallow anterior chambers or plateau iris syndrome, and may occur prior to a full blown attack of acute angle closure glaucoma. Episodes are commonly associated with fatigue, dim light, and using the eyes for near work. They usually occur about the same time of day or night, last for one-half to one hour, and may be relieved by sleep, probably from sleep-induced miosis and reduced aqueous humor production.

Haloes around lights or blurred vision are often reported by patients with raised eye pressure. Initially such attacks occur with intervals of weeks to months but eventually the episodes occur almost nightly. Usually one eye is involved but rare cases of bilateral angle closure glaucoma have been reported, especially in association with some drug reactions.

Unfortunately, the eye appears normal between attacks of angle closure glaucoma except for the presence of a narrow anterior chamber angle. Ocular (or retinal) migraine is a diagnosis of exclusion. Painful unilateral visual loss requires a slit lamp examination and gonioscopy to exclude angle closure glaucoma.

Patient self-diagnosis or health professional misdiagnosis of migraine, sinusitis, or eyestrain can add complexity to assessment and management. Laser iridotomy produced complete and dramatic relief from years of suffering in most of these patients. Some patients also have a history that is characterized as 'painful amaurosis fugax'. Again the pain and unilateral visual loss can easily be confused with ocular (retinal) migraine so this diagnosis should only be made after an ophthalmologic examination has excluded a shallow anterior chamber.

Laser iridotomy is the definitive treatment for intermittent and acute angle closure glaucoma. Provided the angle is not occluded by a mechanism other than pupil block, early referral to an ophthalmologist will be curative and the patient's symptoms will subside and usually not recur.

Optic nerve disease

Of patients with acute optic neuritis, 90% have pain in and around the eye (Chan & Lam 2004). While usually mild and aggravated by eye movement, it can be extremely severe and more debilitating than any associated loss of vision. It is believed that pain in optic neuritis is caused by inflammation and swelling of the optic nerve sheaths that are innervated by small branches of the Trigeminal nerve. The pain usually lasts for several days before subsiding and may be moderated by systemic corticosteroids.

Optic neuritis is frequently due to multiple sclerosis so patients with suspicious symptoms and signs should be referred to a neurologist for further investigation including magnetic resonance imaging (MRI).

Orbital and/or sinus lesions

Orbital infection or idiopathic orbital inflammation, (so-called orbital pseudotumor) are generally associated with moderate to severe pain by virtue of direct irritation of the major trigeminal sensory nerves in the orbit.

Ocular and facial pain can also occur with various types of sinus disease; however neither acute nor chronic inflammation of the sinuses will usually produce pain (Schor 1993). Indeed, when such patients have headache they usually have migraine or tension-type headaches independent of their sinus disease. When the ethmoid or sphenoid sinus is involved, pain can be referred to the back of the eyes, while frontal sinusitis produces pain over the brows and forehead and antral disease is most marked over the maxillary area. When sinus disease is suspected as a cause of headache, this can be further investigated by CT or MRI.

Aspirin, codeine and other simple analgesics can be effective and diminish the headache caused by disease of the nasal and paranasal sinuses. Orbital tumors however, are rarely painful unless they involve the orbital apex or cavernous sinus. Chronic severe burning orbital pain is suggestive of perineural infiltration by neoplastic cells usually from basal cell, squamous cell, or nasopharyngeal carcinoma at the orbital apex.

Refractive errors and 'eyestrain'

The headache associated with so-called 'eyestrain' is usually characterized by a sensation of 'heaviness' in and around the eyes. It often represents a tension-type headache arising from efforts to overcome refractive error or ocular misalignment. In children, such headaches may explain poor school performance, or in adults, difficulties at work or boredom with prolonged use of computer screens. Nonetheless, psychological stress and tension headaches frequently co-exist so it is often difficult to discriminate eye strain as a discrete diagnosis.

Those patients with hypermetropia and those of presbyopic age may complain of fatigue or vague eye ache as they struggle to focus without glasses. However, these conditions rarely produce true headache.

Pain without obvious ocular or orbital disease

Ophthalmologists often encounter patients who complain of mild, localized ocular or retro-bulbar pain who have no obvious pathology found on thorough examination and CT or MRI. In some cases mild symptoms may be magnified by anxiety and the irrational belief that they are likely go blind from undiagnosed glaucoma or die from a brain tumor. Investigation may yield little other than mild eye dryness or signs of blepharitis. Minor epithelial changes on slit-lamp examination can often be managed with lubrication or lid cleansing.

Some patients have a more periodic and severe type of pain called 'ophthalmodynia periodica', which was described by Lansche (1964). The pain is an intermittent single stab or jab of local ocular that strikes without warning. While Lansche had no explanation for these symptoms, many suspect that this may be a variant of recurrent erosion syndrome or dry eye. A trial of ocular lubricants should be used first in an effort to reduce symptoms.

It should also be remembered to exclude involvement of structures in the cervical region of the spine in patients who suffer from unexplained frontal or peri-orbital pain. Inquiry about neck soreness or upper cervical tenderness may reveal the true origin of the pain and lead to more appropriate treatment.

Specific ophthalmic pain syndromes

Herpes zoster ophthalmicus

Herpes zoster and post-herpetic neuralgia most commonly affects the ophthalmic division of the trigeminal nerve. The infection reactivates through the peripheral branches of this nerve and spreads to affect arteries and the surrounding tissues. It is increasingly common with age and commonly begins with an acute herpetic neuritis characterized by a sustained burning pain in and around one orbit. Some days later, often as the pain is subsiding, a typical erythema and vesicular rash follows and is associated with abnormal hyperesthesia, hypoesthesia, or paresthesia. The pain usually settles over several weeks unless it is replaced by post-herpetic neuralgia. Provided systemic antiviral medication can be commenced within several days of the onset of the rash, much of the pain can be moderated and the risk of post-herpetic neuralgia minimized.

Post-herpetic neuralgia is a severe and quite debilitating condition that can bring misery to the elderly. It is lancinating or aching in nature, often associated with altered skin sensation and light touch may even precipitate severe exacerbation of the pain.

While younger patients may recover in months, patients over 70 years may require a prolonged period of recovery, sometimes even years. Therapy is mainly symptomatic; however, the use of gabapentin and/or a transcutaneous electrical nerve stimulation (TENS) machine can be helpful for some patients.

Indeed, gabapentin for the treatment of post-herpetic neuralgia in adults has been assessed in two randomised, double blind, parallel group, placebo controlled, multicentre studies (Witten et al 2005). Results from both studies demonstrated that gabapentin provided statistically significantly improvement in neuropathic pain. Gabapentin was significantly better than placebo in controlling pain ($p < 0.001$), and reducing interference with sleep while some of the quality of life measures showed significant differences in favor of gabapentin. It has been suggested that gabapentin reduces neuropathic pain by inhibiting the spinal release of glutamate (Coderre et al 2005).

Painful ophthalmoplegia

Painful ophthalmoplegia is a weakness of the muscles that control eye movement, which can be of muscular or neurogenic origin. Generally all these conditions will require referral to an ophthalmologist for specialist diagnosis and care. The major causes were summarized from the case reports of the Massachusetts General Hospital (1993), and are presented in Table 11.3.

Tolosa-Hunt syndrome

Severe retrobulbar or supraorbital pain followed by progressive impairment of cranial nerves III, IV, and VI, and the corneal reflexes, suggest Tolosa-Hunt syndrome. First observed by Tolosa in 1954 and further described by Hunt (1976), it is characterized by a steady, boring pain behind the eye or brow. The oculomotor, trochlear and abducens nerves may also become involved in a non-specific inflammatory process that can also effect the first and second divisions of the trigeminal nerve and even the optic nerve. The syndrome lasts weeks or months without treatment but responds dramatically to systemic corticosteroids. Recurrent episodes, months or years later, can occur and frequently findings of investigations are normal.

Tolosa-Hunt syndrome often shows an abnormal thickening of the wall of the

Table 11.3 Differential diagnosis of painful ophthalmoplegia.

Region	Type	Cause	Condition
Orbital	Inflammatory		
		Infection	Bacterial: sinusitis
			Viral: Herpes zoster ophthalmicus
			Fungal: Mucormycosis
		Other	Thyroid ophthalmopathy
	Idiopathic	Orbital pseudotumor	
	Vascular	Orbital hemorrhage	
	A-V malformation		
	Neoplastic	Direct extension of sinus/intra-cranial lesions	
		Remote metastasis	Breast, prostate, lung
Non-orbital	Neoplastic	Pituitary adenoma or Craniopharyngioma	
		Meningioma	
		Chordroma	
		Multiple myeloma	
		Lymphoma	
		Nasopharngeal carcinoma	
		Breast, prostate, lung adenocarcinoma	
	Infectious	Primary; Herpes zoster ophthalmicus	
	Inflammatory	Giant cell arteritis	
		Tolosa-Hunt syndrome	
		Wegener's granulomatosis	
		Sarcoidosis	
	Vascular	Aneurysm	
		Carotico-cavernous fistula	
		Dural cavernous fistula	
		Cavernous sinus thrombosis	

cavernous sinus on MRI. There is frequently high signal intensity on T1 weighted images enhanced with gadolinium. The abnormalities on CT scanning are more subtle although multislice imaging often can reveal thickening of the same tissues with similar contrast enhancement. An aneurysm of the carotid sinus or a neoplastic infiltration of the orbital apex are important differential diagnoses that are usually also clarified by CT or MRI.

Tolosa-Hunt syndrome is quite sensitive to low dose systemic steroids (25–30 mg/day). However, some cases require much higher doses and the ophthalmoplegia may take many months to resolve and in some cases, may never resolve completely.

Grandenigo's syndrome

Suppurative otitis media and ipsilateral paralysis of the abducens nerve was described in 1904 by Grandenigo. It occurs due to apex petrositis whereby inflammation spreads from the middle ear to the apex of the petrous temporal bone. Infection can involve cranial nerve VI and produce paresis of the ipsilateral lateral rectus muscle.

The pain of Grandenigo's syndrome is usually localized to the ear and is aggravated by movement of the jaw, tragus, or auricle. The pain may, however, radiate to the parietal or frontal region particularly when there is involvement of the adjacent ganglion of the trigeminal nerve, within the middle cranial fossa.

Fortunately, Grandenigo's syndrome is rare. The prompt use of modern antibiotic treatment for ear infections makes spreading suppuration unlikely.

Trigeminal neuralgia

Trigeminal neuralgia occurs in the fifth to seventh decades and is characterized by unilateral and severe facial pains described as being 'shock-like' and evoked by trivial cutaneous stimuli, such as shaving or brushing teeth. The pain may last for only a few seconds and usually begins in one division of the trigeminal nerve and may then spread to the others. The ophthalmic division is usually the least often affected and more rarely it is affected alone. Trigeminal neuralgia can also be marked by remission that lasts from days to years during which time little pain is experienced.

The etiology of trigeminal neuralgia can be unclear. MRI should always be performed to exclude tumor, A-V malformation, or intracranial aneurysm, particularly of the anterior cerebellar artery that may cause vascular compression of the sensory roots of the trigeminal nerve (Janetta 1977).

Trigeminal neuralgia is usually treated with medical or surgical therapy. Carbemazepine has long been regarded as the most useful medication to treat trigeminal neuralgia and has been found to be 60–80% effective (Blom 1962), but adverse reactions are not uncommon. Secondary drug choices are baclofen, lamotrigine, oxcarbazepine, phenytoin, gabapentin, sodium valproate, and botulinum toxin (Turk et al 2005). Controlled trials testing the effect of some of these drugs, and especially the newer drugs, and drug combinations are needed (Sindrup & Jensen 2002).

Some form of neurosurgery is required when medication fails. Posterior fossa microvascular decompression of the trigeminal nerve (Mullan & Brown 1996) has been found to have a 70% success rate for this condition (Barker et al 1996), and this is the preferred initial surgical technique. The other main technique is percutaneous radiofrequency trigeminal rhizotomy (PRTR).

Atypical facial neuralgia

Chronic, deep facial pain that spreads across the zones of several cranial nerves or to both sides of the face and which does not seem to be precipitated by touch may be atypical facial neuralgia. Onset may commence after trauma or surgery to the orbit or paranasal sinuses, with pain frequently localized to within or between the eyes.

The etiology of atypical facial neuralgia is obscure, although it seems likely to be central in origin. Lascelles has reported that many patients also have an atypical depression with irritability, agitation and sleep disturbance (Lascelles 1966) and this may certainly be a contributing factor.

Fortunately, atypical facial neuralgia is usually a self-limiting condition and will subside over several years regardless of the outcome of any symptomatic treatment.

Raeder's paratrigeminal neuralgia or 'cluster' migraine

Raeder's syndrome is described as a severe unilateral headache most frequently localized to the ophthalmic division of the trigeminal nerve and is associated with an oculosympathetic palsy with nasal stuffiness and increased sweating on the affected side. This condition affects middle or old age males almost exclusively. It usually begins as a throbbing headache behind, within or above one or other eye, beginning in the morning after awakening or even disturbing sleep. It gradually subsides into the afternoon occurring daily over a number of weeks or months before spontaneous resolution.

Patients observed during an attack are seen to have drooping of the ipsilateral eyelid with miosis of the pupil on that side, which becomes more obvious in a darkened room.

In the absence of any associated cranial nerve palsies, Ford and Walsh have suggested that Raeder's syndrome is a benign disorder and probably a variant of classic migraine (Ford & Walsh 1958). Nonetheless, any atypical features, including neuropathies involving cranial nerves II, III, IV, V or VI should be investigated by MRI.

SUNCT syndrome

Short-lasting unilateral neuralgia with conjunctival injection and tearing has been described by the acronym SUNCT syndrome. It is characterized by brief pain in the periocular area associated with autonomic symptoms such as temporary conjunctival injection, nasal stuffiness, and forehead sweating. SUNCT syndrome seems likely to be a variant of cluster headache localized to the eye and may have some features suggestive of trigeminal neuralgia but coming in clusters of attacks lasting days to months.

Ocular manifestations of migraine

Migraine without aura

Migraine headache without aura (previously known as common migraine) accounts for two-thirds of migraine-type headaches. The International Headache Society (2004) diagnostic criteria for migraine without aura are presented in Box 11.1.

Most migraine headaches last from one to two days although they can range from four hours to (rarely) several weeks in duration. One-third of migraine headaches are bilateral but more usually migraine without aura is unilateral and located in a frontal, temporal, or retro-orbital location. The migraine begins as a dull ache and usually evolves into a moderate to severe throbbing pain that can be relieved by direct pressure on the superficial scalp arteries in the region of the pain (Selby & Lance 1960).

The frequency of migraine without aura varies from one or two attacks per month to a

Box 11.1

Revised IHS criteria for migraine without aura (International Headache Society 2004)

A. Headache descriptions (at least two)
- Unilateral
- Pulsatile quality
- Moderate to severe (moderate generally defined as inhibiting daily activities, severe as prohibiting daily activities) pain intensity
- Aggravation by or causing avoidance of routine physical activity

Associated symptoms (one or both)
- Nausea and/or vomiting
- Photophobia and phonophobia

B. The headaches last 4–72 hours (untreated or treated unsuccessfully)

C. Must have 5 attacks fulfilling the above criteria and not attributed to another disorder.

Box 11.2

Revised IHS criteria for migraine with typical aura (International Headache Society 2004).

At least two attacks fulfilling criteria A–C.

A. Aura consisting of at least one of the following, but no motor weakness:
- fully reversible visual symptoms including positive features (e.g. flickering lights, spots or lines) and/or negative features (i.e. loss of vision)
- fully reversible sensory symptoms including positive features (i.e. pins and needles) and/or negative features (i.e. numbness)
- fully reversible dysphasic speech disturbance

B. At least two of the following:
- Homonymous visual symptoms and/or unilateral sensory symptoms
- At least one aura symptom develops gradually over $\geq$ 5 minutes and/or different aura symptoms occur in succession over $\geq$ 5 minutes
- Each symptom lasts $\geq$ 5 and $\leq$ 60 minutes

C. Headache fulfilling criteria A & B for migraine without aura begins during the aura or follows aura within 60 minutes

D. Not attributed to another disorder.

headache every few days. Bright lights, loud noises and physical activity often increase the intensity of migraine, with nausea and vomiting accompanying the more severe episodes, especially in children (Bille 1964).

The differential diagnosis of migraine without aura includes the previously described syndrome of cluster headache. This primary form of headache is sometimes termed Horton's headache or ciliary neuralgia. It is much less common than migraine with a prevalence of 5 per 10 000 of the adult population and is 3–4 times more prevalent in men. The headaches are brief, intense and debilitating and localized to distribution of the trigeminal nerve. They cluster in time over a period of some weeks with attack free months following (McGeeney 2005).

Migraine with aura

Approximately one-fifth of migraine sufferers experience an aura. Migraine with aura has three distinct phases: the aura, the headache, and the post-headache phase. There must be at least two episodes to confirm the diagnosis and, like common migraine, there must be no evidence of neurological abnormality between attacks. Box 11.2 details the International Headache Society (2004) diagnostic criteria for migraine with aura.

The aura begins as a transient visual or neurological disturbance that lasts up to sixty minutes and often terminates before the headache begins and gradually gets worse. The characteristic of the visual aura varies widely between patients and can arise in any part of the visual field, corresponding to the site of origin in the visual cortex, retina, optic nerve, or optic chiasm. Differential diagnosis of migraine with visual aura is given in Box 11.3. The aura is usually binocular, hemianopic, and invariably

Box 11.3

Differential diagnosis of migraine with visual aura.

1. Disorders of the retina and vitreous: Acute posterior vitreous or retinal detachment can produce sparks or bright flashes of white light. Unlike migraine, it is always uniocular and lacks colored lights or fortification spectra.

2. Occipital lobe lesions: Cerebral tumors of the visual cortex occasionally produce scintillating scotomas like classic migraine.

3. Migraine headaches with aura can also be seen as a complication of cerebral arteriovenous malformations in the occipital cortex.

begins centrally and moves peripherally as a shimmering wave-like arc or as a zig-zag fortification pattern with bright, glittering edges. As the scotoma spreads, the border of the field defect often seems to flicker and undulate and can have a distinct cross-hatched pattern (Manzoni et al 1985).

While the characteristic partial scotoma can have bright or colorful edges, one of the most dramatic and frightening forms of migrainous aura is total blindness. Fortunately, recovery occurs within 10–15 minutes. These episodes begin as a gradual contraction from the nasal and temporal periphery until a vague faint central light remains. The recovery follows as the fields widen again from the centre outwards.

While the most common auras of migraine are visual, transient neurological deficits can also occur including vertigo, paresthesias, aphasia, and more complicated syndromes. Sensory disturbances are the most common transient neurological disturbances and usually recur in a stereotyped fashion but unlike visual auras the sensory disturbance does not spread. Transient aphasia can be another frightening variant where the patient cannot speak at all for some minutes even though the patient can clearly

understand questions and respond in other ways. Interestingly, right-handed paresthesia can occur with the onset of aphasia. Transient paralysis with migraine was first described by the pioneering french neurologist Jean-Martin Charcot in 1892 and, while rare, can persist for days and recover gradually (Charcot 1892).

Vascular syndromes

Ophthalmoplegic migraine

Ophthalmoplegic migraine is a form of paralysis affecting the vasculature of the nerves controlling the extra-ocular muscles. It has three major diagnostic criteria:

1. History of typical migraine headache that is severe, throbbing and predominantly unilateral.

2. An obvious unilateral ophthalmoplegia that may include one or more nerves to the extra-ocular muscles of the eye and may affect alternate sides with subsequent attacks.

3. Exclusion of other causes by arteriography digital subtraction angiography (DSA) and/or magnetic resonance angiography (MRA).

Ophthalmoplegic migraine is always unilateral and most frequently affects the oculomotor nerve. Therefore it is characterized by ptosis and limited eye movements affecting adduction, elevation, and depression of the globe. The pupil is almost always affected to some degree, with mild dilatation and a poor response to both light and accommodation (Loewenfeld 1980). Complete and rapid resolution usually occurs with the lid recovering first. Isolated trochlear or abducens palsies are less common and can occur in combination with oculomotor palsies.

Basilar artery migraine

Basilar artery migraine is another vascular syndrome that occurs more frequently in children and is often associated with attacks of extreme unsteadiness and nystagmus. Visual dysfunction, including transient blindness has also been reported (Gowers 1907) in association with such symptoms prior to the onset of a typical migraine headache.

Ocular (retinal) migraine

Ocular migraine typically presents with repeated attacks of a monocular scotoma or unilateral blindness lasting less than one hour with associated headache. It occurs in as many as 1 in 200 migraine sufferers (Troost 1996), and usually presents as a transient monocular visual loss in young adults. Altitudinal or concentric field defects can also occur. During such attacks the retinal vasculature appears constricted to ophthalmoscopy and the prognosis, like migraine with aura, is generally very good.

Permanent visual defects can arise, as they can with any patient who experiences a visual aura. It has been observed that in more than half of reported cases of retinal migraine, permanent scotomas can arise with signs of retinal infarction or ischemic optic neuropathy (Grosberg et al 2005). However most clinicians believe that only a small proportion of ocular migraine sufferers develop permanent infarction and visual field defects. It is important, to distinguish ocular migraine from intermittent angle closure glaucoma (Maggioni et al 2005) and giant cell arteritis when considering differential diagnosis.

Headache referred from the neck

Headache in the region of the eye could suggest a cervicogenic origin for many headaches. This is a significant class of headache and of all chronic headaches, as many as 14–18% may fall into this category (International Headache Society 2004). The reader is directed to Chapters 14 and 15 for detailed description and discussion of etiology, mechanism of referral of pain from the neck, clinical assessment and management of cervicogenic headache.

Conclusion

This chapter has provided a comprehensive account of the differential diagnosis of eye pain and associated headache. It has discussed headache and facial pain associated with eye disease as well as specific ophthalmic pain syndromes. The ocular manifestations of migraine have been presented with particular emphasis on the description and differential diagnosis of visual auras.

References

Barker FG, Jannetta PJ, Bissonette DJ, Jho HD 1996 The long term outcome of microvascular decompression for trigeminal neuralgia. New Eng J Med 334:1077-1083.

Bergmanson JP 1977 The ophthalmic innervation of the uvea in monkeys. Exp Eye Research 24:225-240.

Bille BO 1964 Migraine in school children. Acta Paediatrica 64:499-508.

Blom S 1962 Trigeminal neuralgia: its treatment with a new anti-convulsive drug. Lancet 1:839-840.

Chan C, Lam D 2004 Optic neuritis treatment trial: 10-year follow-up results. Am J Ophthalmol 138:695.

Charcot JM 1892 Cliniques des Maladies des Systeme Nerveux. Veuve Babeet Cie, Paris.

Coderre TJ, Kumar N, Lefebvre CD, Yu JS 2005 Evidence that gabapentin reduces neuropathic pain by inhibiting the spinal release of glutamate. J Neurochem 94:1131-1139.

Ford FR, Walsh FB 1958 Reader's paratrigeminal syndrome. A benign disorder, possibly a complication of migraine. Bull Johns Hopkins Hosp 103:296-298.

Gowers WR 1907 The Borderlands of Epilepsy: Faints, Vagal Attacks, Vertigo, Migraine, Sleep

Symptoms and their Treatment. Churchill, London.

Grosberg BM, Solomon S, Lipton RB 2005 Retinal migraine. Curr Pain Headache Rep 9:268-271.

Hitchings RA 1980 The symptom of ocular pain. Trans Ophthalmol Soc UK 100:257-259.

Hunt WE 1976 Tolosa–Hunt syndrome. One cause of painful ophthalmoplegia. J Neurosurg 44:544-549.

International Headache Society 2004 The international classification of headache disorders, 2nd edn. Cephalalgia 24 (suppl 1):1-160.

Janetta PJ 1977 Observation of the aetiology of trigeminal neuralgia, hemifacial spasm and gloss-pharyngeal neuralgia. Definitive microsurgical treatment and results in 117 patients. Neurochiurgica 20:145-154.

Lansche RK 1964 Ophthalmodynia Periodica. Headache 4:247-249.

Lascelles RG 1966 Atypical facial pain and depression. Br J Psychiatry 112:651-659.

Loewenfeld IE 1980 Pupillary defect in "ophthalmoplegic migraine". Symposium of the Bascom Palmer Eye Institute and the University of Miami 10:180-200.

Maggioni F, Dainese F, Mainardi F et al 2005 Intermittent angle-closure glaucoma in the presence of a white eye, posing as retinal migraine. Cephalgia 25:622-626.

Manzoni GC, Farina S, Lanfranchi M et al 1985 Classic Migraine - Clinical findings in 164 patients. Eur Neurol 24:163-169.

Massachusetts General Hospital 1993 Case reports of the Massachusetts General Hospital Case 4-1993. N Eng J Med 328:266-275.

McGeeney BE 2005 Cluster headache pharmacotherapy. A J Ther 12:351-358.

Mullan S, Brown JA 1996 Trigeminal Neuralgia. Neurosurg Quant 6:267-288.

Phillips C 1977 Headache in general practice. Headache 16:322.

Schor DI 1993 Headache and facial pain – the role of the paranasal sinuses: a literature review. Cranio 11:36-47.

Selby G, Lance JW 1960 Observations on 500 cases of migraine and allied vascular headache. J Neurol Neurosurg and Psychiatry 23:23-32.

Sindrup SH, Jensen TS 2002 Pharmacotherapy of trigeminal neuralgia. Clin J Pain 18:22-27.

Troost BT 1996 Migraine and other headaches. In: Tasman W, Jaeger EA (eds) Duane's Clinical Ophthalmology, vol 3. JB Lippincott, Philadelphia.

Turk U, Ilhan S, Alp R, Sur H 2005 Botulinum toxin and intractable trigeminal neuralgia. Clin Neuropharmacol 28:161-162.

Wiffen P, McQuay H, Edwards J, Moore R 2005 Gabapentin for acute and chronic pain. Cochrane Database Syst Rev 20:CD005452.

12

Vestibular dysfunction

Keith Hill, Kate Murray and John Waterston

Vestibular dysfunction can result in symptoms such as dizziness, nausea, neck pain, and headache. There is considerable overlap between symptoms associated with vestibular dysfunction and cervical impairment. In this chapter the authors, two neurophysiotherapists and a neurologist, present the etiology, clinical findings, and management of symptoms associated with vestibular dysfunction.

The vestibular system is a complex system that includes the balance component of the inner ear and central nervous system structures. Its primary functions are to sense linear and angular accelerations of the head, coordinate head and eye movements, and assist with the maintenance of equilibrium. Primary symptoms often associated with vestibular dysfunction include dizziness, true vertigo, disequilibrium, and nausea (Curthoys et al 1995). In addition, secondary symptoms can include headache, neck and shoulder pain, and anxiety. Vestibular dysfunction originating in the inner ear or central nervous system (CNS) therefore needs to be considered as a potential differential diagnosis for patients presenting with these symptoms, along with other causes such as cardiovascular disease, cervical pathology, temporomandibular disorders, and bruxism.

Many people with vestibular symptoms, particularly dizziness, do not seek medical assistance. This is particularly true for older people, who may perceive the symptoms to be age-related. Of those who do seek health professional advice, assessment and management may be inadequate. Health professional advice has often included rest, the avoidance of aggravating movements, or prescription of vestibular suppressant medication. In the majority of vestibular disorders, these management strategies may actually impede recovery (Curthoys et al 1995). It is important to recognize when it is appropriate to refer on to health professionals with specific expertise in vestibular assessment and management (e.g. neurologists, otologists, or physiotherapists with specific training or experience in vestibular dysfunction).

This chapter focuses on the assessment and management of vestibular disorders, and should be read in conjunction with other chapters in this book to provide the clinician with a global perspective of the importance of accurate diagnosis and management of vestibular dysfunction within the context of assessment and management of headaches and bruxism.

Epidemiology

Up to one-third of people aged over 60 have experienced at least one moderate episode of dizziness severe enough for them to see a doctor, take medication, or to limit their daily activities (Colledge et al 1994). Up to 24% of this age group have experienced these symptoms in the preceding 12 months (Tinetti et al 2000), with the average duration of symptoms being three years (Sloane et al 1989). Involvement of the peripheral vestibular system has been identified in approximately half of cases (Sloane et al 1989), with the single most common diagnosis being benign paroxysmal positional vertigo (BPPV). This common vestibular disorder appears to be highly prevalent, but largely under-recognized in older patients, and may contribute to falls risk in this population (Oghalai et al 2000).

Anatomy, physiology and pathology

The vestibular, somatosensory and visual systems are the three primary sensory systems responsible for effective balance. Each sensory system contributes unique information for central integration and processing to determine the most appropriate response for a specific threat to balance. There is considerable adaptability within these systems, with the potential for increased reliance on an intact system (e.g. the visual system) when another sensory system (e.g. the vestibular system) is impaired.

The peripheral vestibular apparatus

The peripheral vestibular apparatus is located in the inner ear within a bony labyrinth in each temporal bone. Within each bony labyrinth is a membranous labyrinth, in which the sensory organs of the vestibular apparatus are contained (Fig. 12.1).

The sensory organs of the vestibular apparatus are:

* the semicircular canals. These three ducts are aligned at right angles to each other, and are filled with endolymph fluid (the posterior, anterior, and horizontal semicircular canals) (Honrubia et al 1993). When the head is stationary, intact vestibular nuclei have a symmetrical resting firing rate. Head acceleration in

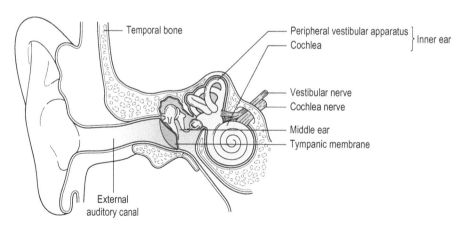

Figure 12.1 • The peripheral vestibular apparatus and surrounding structures.

any direction causes endolymph flow in one or more of the semicircular canals in each ear. The resultant mechanical deflection of hair cells in the cupula (the basic sensory component) is translated into electrical nerve impulses. Because of the orthogonal alignment of the semicircular canals and the mirrored structure bilaterally, endolymph will flow in the paired canals (those that are in the plane/s of movement), resulting in an increase in the firing rate on one side, and a concomitant reduction in the firing rate on the opposite side (Honrubia et al 1993).

* the otoliths (the saccule and the utricle). These two structures are also part of the membranous labyrinth (Fig 12.2), with connections to the semicircular canals that enable endolymph flow. Both contain a sensory region called the macula, which is lined with receptor hair cells linked to a gelatinous membrane embedded with small calcium carbonate crystals called otoconia. These hair cells are sensitive to linear acceleration, including the influence of gravity (Honrubia et al 1993).

The cochlea (the primary sensory organ for hearing) is in close proximity to the sensory structures of the peripheral vestibular apparatus, but is not considered part of the vestibular system, and is not discussed here.

The central vestibular system

Information from the inner ear travels via the vestibular nerve (cranial nerve VIII) to the vestibular nuclear complex within the brainstem, and the cerebellum. This information is processed in conjunction with auditory, somatosensory and visual input, as well as input from the reticular formation, the cervical spine, and the contralateral vestibular nuclei. Connections from the vestibular nuclei project widely to the parietal and temporal cortex, the extra-ocular muscles (vestibulo-ocular reflex) and the spinal cord (vestibulospinal reflex) (Honrubia et al 1993).

Vestibular dysfunction

Unilateral vestibular pathology often causes an alteration in the resting firing rates of the vestibular neuron, and a resultant mismatch in the changes in firing rates with head acceleration, contributing to the sensation of vertigo. A sudden unilateral loss of vestibular function usually causes acute, severe vertigo and nystagmus that persists for hours or days. The severe spontaneous vertigo gradually settles as a result of restoration of the symmetrical firing rates in the brainstem vestibular nuclei. However it is usually followed by a period during which vertigo continues to be induced by head or body motion. Natural resolution of the resting and motion-induced symptoms is achieved through a complex neuronal process known as 'compensation' which can occur in the absence of recovery of peripheral vestibular function.

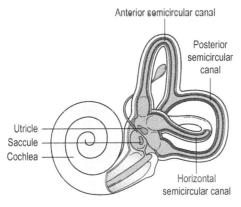

Anterior semicircular canal

Posterior semicircular canal

Utricle
Saccule
Cochlea

Horizontal semicircular canal

Figure 12.2 • The peripheral vestibular apparatus.

Clinical syndromes

A syndromic approach to the diagnosis of vertigo is a useful aid. There are four basic clinical presentations: acute vestibulopathy, recurrent vestibulopathy, motion-induced dizziness, and disequilibrium.

Acute vestibulopathy

The most common cause is vestibular neuronitis (also known as acute peripheral vestibulopathy, vestibular neuritis). This classically causes acute severe vertigo accompanied by ataxia, nausea, and vomiting. Auditory symptoms and signs are usually absent. Vertigo is aggravated by head movement and usually persists for longer than a day with recovery often occurring over days to weeks. The etiology is assumed to be viral in the majority of cases, but ischemia involving the internal auditory artery may also cause a similar syndrome, particularly in older age groups with vascular risk factors (Kim et al 1999). Recovery of the acute vertigo occurs over hours to days but may be followed by persistent chronic motion-induced symptoms (see motion-induced dizziness, below).

Other causes of acute vertigo include head trauma and stroke. Brainstem and cerebellar strokes can sometimes present with acute vertigo. Demyelinating diseases such as multiple sclerosis may occasionally cause acute vertigo that may resemble the presentation of vestibular neuronitis. A careful history and examination will usually detect other neurological features.

Recurrent vestibulopathy

Patients with this syndrome present with recurrent attacks of vertigo, often lasting several hours, and are usually symptom-free between attacks. Meniere's disease and migraine are the most common causes.

Meniere's disease, or endolymphatic hydrops, classically presents with a history of recurrent spontaneous vertigo accompanied by fluctuating auditory symptoms (tinnitus, hearing loss, and aural fullness). The hearing can recover between attacks but there is often a stepwise or gradual loss of hearing.

Migraine is a common cause of recurrent vertigo and should be suspected if there are no conspicuous auditory features. It can occur as an aura preceding or accompanying a migraine headache, or even as an isolated phenomenon (Kayan et al 1984). Rarely, patients present with chronic fluctuating spontaneous and motion-induced vertigo, punctuated by intermittent headaches (Waterston 2004). A history of headache should be sought as this may not be volunteered by the patient if the headaches are mild. Other features such as visual phenomena and photophobia may aid the diagnosis.

Other causes of recurrent vertigo are uncommon. Vertebrobasilar ischemia does not usually cause isolated vertigo. Occasionally patients present with intermittent vertigo of short duration (often up to a minute), which is postulated to be due to ischemia of the vestibular labyrinth, however these episodes rarely persist in isolation for more than a few months (Grad et al 1989). Generally, there are other associated symptoms such as diplopia, dysphagia, visual field defects, and focal motor and sensory features.

Motion-induced dizziness

Patients in this category present with short-lived bouts of motion-induced vertigo without spontaneous symptoms. The two most common causes are an uncompensated peripheral vestibular lesion (e.g. incomplete recovery following a bout of vestibular neuronitis) and BPPV.

BPPV is one of the most common vestibular conditions, accounting for 25% of presentations in patients with vestibular disorders (Herdman 1997). The presentation is usually distinctive with a history of short-lived bouts of vertigo triggered by head extension, bending forwards, lying down and rolling over in bed. Otoconial deposits or crystals, which are thought to arise from the utricular matrix, form a heavy mass most commonly in the posterior semicircular canal and, in response to provocative head movements, result in excessive displacement of the sensory organ, or cupula, via a plunger effect. This condition should be regarded as a syndrome which can occur either without any obvious cause, or as a secondary feature of other conditions, particularly head trauma, vestibular neuronitis, and Meniere's disease. In many cases the condition is self-limiting, but it can persist chronically or recur periodically over several years in the absence of treatment. BPPV can co-exist with headaches and neck pain and these conditions need to be considered in patient assessment.

Vertebrobasilar insufficiency due to cervical spondylosis has been promoted as a common cause of motion-induced vertigo due to osteophytic encroachment on vertebral artery flow in the neck during head rotation; however, early case descriptions had poor clinicopathological correlation (Sheehan et al 1960). While physiological obstruction of one vertebral artery has been demonstrated during angiographic studies, symptomatic cerebral ischemia is rare because of the anastomotic supply from the contralateral vertebral artery. Symptoms may occur in the presence of atypical anatomy where there is no anastomotic circulation because one vertebral artery terminates in the posterior inferior cerebellar artery (Strupp et al 2000).

Disequilibrium

There are many causes of this presentation that typically manifests with balance problems and falls (Box 12.1). The patient may still use the

---

Box 12.1

Major causes of disequilibrium.

CNS
- Cerebellar disease
- Parkinson's disease
- Vascular disease
- Multiple sclerosis
- Normal pressure hydrocephalus

Proprioceptive loss
- Spinal cord disease
- Peripheral neuropathy

Other
- Bilateral vestibular hypofunction
- Aging
- Hypothyroidism
- Multi-sensory dizziness/disequilibrium

---

term 'dizziness'. However, it is apparent that the symptoms are only present during standing and walking. Multisensory dizziness or disequilibrium is a term used to describe a syndrome occurring in older subjects manifest by disequilibrium and vague, non-specific dizziness when walking. It is caused by multiple sensory deficits that may include visual impairment, peripheral neuropathy, vestibular dysfunction and cervical spondylosis. A neurological examination may reveal signs indicative of specific pathology in the brain, spinal cord, or peripheral nerves. These patients often have lower limb orthopedic impairments that will accentuate the disability. Importantly, sedative and vestibular suppressant drugs have the potential to exacerbate the problem.

Ataxia, disequilibrium and motion-induced oscillopsia (oscillation of the visual scene due to failure of the vestibuloocular reflex) are the usual presenting symptoms of bilateral vestibular failure. The most common cause is gentamicin toxicity. Vertigo is not usually a feature because the vestibular loss is almost always bilateral and symmetrical.

Other conditions

Cervicogenic dizziness can be difficult to diagnose and usually requires exclusion of other vestibular disorders. Patients tend not to have rotatory vertigo; they usually present with non-specific dizziness, and/or disequilibrium, that may be associated with neck movement. Neck pain and stiffness may also be present. The symptoms may be associated with neck movement. Dizziness of cervical origin is thought to be due to abnormal afferent input to the vestibular nuclei from receptors in the upper cervical spine (Furman et al 2000). Diagnostic confusion may arise when there is a combined vestibular and cervical spine problem, a common occurrence where there is a history of head and neck trauma or secondary cervicogenic dysfunction complicating a primary vestibulopathy.

Tinnitus and vertigo are also reportedly common in patients with bruxism, but the mechanism of this association is unknown.

Clinical assessment

Vertigo can be simply defined as an illusion of movement. Spinning sensations are most commonly described and occur as a result of semicircular canal involvement. Linear sensations of rocking, tilting, and sudden dropping also occur and probably reflect involvement of the otolith organs (utricle and saccule) which sense linear motion (Krebs et al 1991).

The major differential diagnosis is lightheadedness or presyncope, for which there are numerous causes. Many patients have difficulty describing their symptoms, in particular 'dizziness' and it may not be clear whether the patient is describing a vestibular sensation. A history of non-specific dizziness that is aggravated by or associated with head movements suggests a vestibular etiology.

History

It is important to note the characteristics of the vertigo and any associated features, such as auditory symptoms, cervical spine dysfunction and headache. Self report scales such as the Vestibular Symptom Index can quantify the intensity of vestibular symptoms (Black et al 2000).

Visual vertigo, the induction of dizziness by visual stimuli, such as motion on cinema screens and walking down supermarket aisles, is commonly reported by patients with vestibular disorders and may be so severe that some patients develop frank agoraphobic symptoms.

Most cases of vertigo result from peripheral vestibular disorders or benign CNS conditions such as migraine. However it is important to exclude serious CNS causes such as vertebrobasilar ischemia, space occupying lesions, and demyelination. The diagnosis is made easier when there are associated auditory or focal neurological symptoms. Unilateral auditory symptoms are rarely seen with brain stem lesions. However isolated vertigo can sometimes be a presenting feature.

Examination

A neurological examination is important to identify focal signs that may indicate central pathology. Particular emphasis is placed on assessment of standing and walking balance, and examination of eye movements to look for nystagmus and other eye movement abnormalities. Acute peripheral vestibular disorders typically cause a mixed torsional and horizontal nystagmus that beats away from the side of the lesion and abates quickly as the acute vertigo settles. Features of nystagmus due to central lesions are listed in Box 12.2.

The Dix-Hallpike maneuver (Fig. 12.3) is an assessment procedure to identify BPPV. It is an essential part of the examination of most

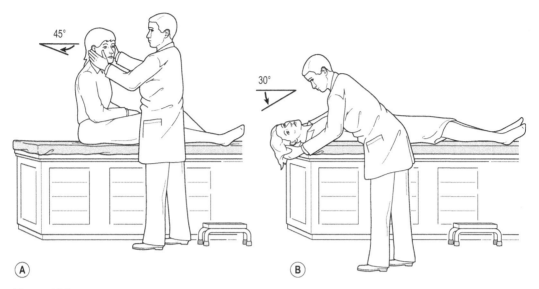

Figure 12.3 • The Dix-Hallpike maneuver. A. Starting position, head rotated 45°. B. Finishing position, 30° neck extension and 45° rotation maintained.

patients presenting with vertigo (Herdman 1997). A positive test comprises:

- a mixed torsional and upbeating nystagmus which begins after a short latent period
- presence of moderately severe vertigo, which lasts up to 60 seconds, and
- less marked response with repeated maneuvers (habituation).

Nystagmus that does not have all of these characteristics may be seen in unusual variants of BPPV involving other semicircular canals but can also be a rare presenting feature of brain stem or cerebellar lesions.

Another useful test for identifying unilateral vestibular hypofunction is the Head Thrust Test (Halmagyi and Curthoys 1988). The patient's head is gently held by the practitioner, they are asked to focus on a target straight ahead, and without warning their head is given a small (5–10°) fast turn to one side, and the eye response is observed. In a normal response the eyes remain fixed on the target, whereas a positive test involves a corrective eye motion (saccade) back towards the target when the head movement stops. The presence of a corrective saccade is suggestive of unilateral vestibular hypofunction on the side the head was being turned towards. Performing this test in 30° flexion of the cervical spine can increase the diagnostic accuracy of the test (Schubert et al 2004).

'Red flags' signifying possible CNS disease are listed in Box 12.2. Vertigo due to central

Box 12.2

Red flags indicating possible CNS disease.

- Focal neurological signs
- Ataxia and nystagmus out of proportion to vertigo
- Direction changing nystagmus on lateral gaze to both sides, or gaze-evoked nystagmus
- Pure vertical (upbeating or downbeating) nystagmus
- Other eye movement abnormalities, e.g. gaze palsy, skew deviation (vertical misalignment of the eyes)

lesions may occasionally be severe, as in brainstem strokes. However, when there appears to be a degree of ataxia that is out of proportion to the vertigo, central pathology should be suspected. The exception to this rule is bilateral vestibular failure.

Balance and mobility assessment

Whilst dizziness is often the most common symptom of vestibular dysfunction, balance and mobility are often also impaired. These problems also increase the risk of falling (Tinetti et al 2000), with up to 64% of patients with bilateral vestibular dysfunction over the age of 65 years reporting at least one fall in a 12 month period (Herdman et al 2000). A detailed assessment of the patient with suspected vestibular dysfunction should include a series of tests that challenge balance and focus on the vestibular system. Examples of appropriate tests, issues relating to their use in vestibular patients, and typical scores for vestibular patients and healthy older people are described in Table 12.1.

Function, handicap and psychological assessment

Vestibular dysfunction can have a primary or secondary effect on functional status and level of handicap. The Dizziness Handicap Inventory (DHI) is a validated 25-item questionnaire evaluating the individual's self-perceived physical, emotional and functional handicap in relation to vestibular disorders (Jacobson et al 1990). Psychological problems are common in patients with vestibular dysfunction, particularly those with chronic symptoms (Yardley et al 2001). Of a sample of chronic dizzy patients, 38% had a primary psychological diagnosis causing, or a secondary psychological diagnosis contributing to,

their dizziness (Sloane et al 1994). As well as the emotional component of the DHI, the Hospital Anxiety and Depression Scale (HADS) has been used in identifying psychological issues in people with vestibular dysfunction (Zigmond et al 1983).

Cervical spine assessment

Cervical spine dysfunction is a less commonly identified cause of dizziness, but should be considered in the differential diagnosis, particularly if vestibular symptoms exist in the presence of neck pain, reduced cervical range of motion, and/or headache (Wrisley et al 2000). Examination includes active and passive range of cervical motion and manual posteroanterior pressure over the upper cervical facet joints. Significant findings include the reproduction of vestibular symptoms with manual examination at one or more spinal levels.

Investigations to aid diagnosis

Neuroimaging in the form of a computerized tomographic (CT) brain scan or magnetic resonance imaging (MRI) should be performed if central pathology is suspected. Some pathology, such as demyelination and posterior circulation ischemia, may only be visible on MRI.

Audiometry is used to document the presence and patterns of associated hearing loss (e.g., in Meniere's disease). Brainstem auditory evoked potentials have traditionally been used to exclude eighth nerve and brainstem pathology; however MRI is now the gold standard. Results of other vestibular investigations, such as caloric and rotational chair testing, Vestibular Evoked Myogenic Potential (VEMP), and Subjective Visual Vertical (SVV) testing may be helpful in documenting peripheral vestibular dysfunction.

Table 12.1 Selected clinical balance and mobility assessment tools with scores reported for healthy older people and people with vestibular dysfunction.

Assessment tool	Description of task	Usefulness for vestibular patients	Scores reported for vestibular samples	Scores reported for healthy older subjects
Clinical Test of Sensory Integration of Balance (Shumway-Cook et al 1986)	Performance timed up to 30 seconds on 6 sensory tasks: –EO, Firm –EC, Firm –VC, Firm –EO, Foam –EC, Foam –VC, Foam	– Need to select most appropriate foot position, and standardize for repeated testing – The EC and VC tasks on foam require an intact vestibular system to provide a frame of reference – vestibular patients often have difficulty with these tasks.	Mean age 59.8 years (Cohen et al 1993) Feet *together* (trial 3 of 3) EO, Firm 30s EC, Firm 30s VC, Firm 30s EO, Foam 26s EC, Foam 16s VC, Foam 12s	Asymptomatic subjects aged 65–84 years (Cohen et al 1993) Feet together** EO, Firm 30s EC, Firm 30s VC, Firm 30s EO, Foam 29s EC, Foam 17s VC, Foam 19s
Timed Up and Go Test (Podsiadlo et al 1991)	Timed task, standing up from a chair, walking 3 meters, turning, returning to chair and sitting down (sec)	Using a dual task such as carrying a tray of glasses, or head turning during the task can improve sensitivity in detecting mild balance problems, and identifying visual fixation.	14.0 (5.0) (Whitney et al 2004)	Females $\geq$ 70 years 9.1 sec (Hill et al 1999)
Step Test (Hill et al 1996)	Number of completed steps stepping one foot on then off a 7.5 cm block in 15 sec	This is a higher level dynamic balance task, sensitive to mild balance dysfunction (a number of other commonly used balance tests have ceiling effects).	Mean age 53.2 years, patients with canal and otolith dysfunction (Murray 2005) 12.9 (6.2)	Subjects $\geq$ 60 years (Hill et al 1996) 16 steps/15s
Sharpened Romberg	Timed task, standing one foot directly in front of the other, up to a maximum of 30 ooo. Can be assessed with dominant leg behind, or non-dominant leg behind	Challenging static balance task. Has been used more often with eyes closed in vestibular patients.	Ceiling effect with EO, with 68% of sample with chronic vestibular dysfunction able to balance 30 sec with EO. 34% unable to complete with EC (Murray et al 2007)	Healthy older women able to do EO > 30 sec; and EC for mean score > 14 ooo (Briggs et al 1989)
Functional Gait Assessment (Wrisley et al 2004)	Ten item assessment tool, based on the Dynamic Gait Index, (Wrisley et al 2003) that evaluates a range of tasks relevant to vestibular patients		Mean age 58.7 years (Wrisley et al 2004) 20 (6.6)	Normal performance on each item rated as 3, maximum overall score for 10 items is 30

EO = eyes open, EC = eyes closed, VC = visual conflict (visual sensory cues in conflict with other sensory cues measured using a visual conflict dome), Firm = firm surface, Foam = foam surface.
** Samples not comprehensively screened, so may under-estimate scores for healthy older adults.

Medical management

The nature of vestibular dysfunction, and its impact on physical, functional, and emotional wellbeing often necessitate that medical management occur within a multidisciplinary team management program. Medical components of the management program may include medication prescription or withdrawal, dietary advice, support, and/or surgery. These are discussed briefly.

Vestibular suppressant drugs are indicated only for the treatment of acute vertigo. Long term use of these drugs carries the risk of neurological complications such as drug-induced Parkinsonism and tardive dyskinesia. There is also some anecdotal evidence that prolonged drug therapy may retard the process of central compensation.

Specific medical treatments are indicated in the treatment of conditions such as migraine or Meniere's disease. Medications used for migraine prophylaxis include pizotifen, propanolol and verapamil. Salt restriction and diuretic therapy are the major medical treatment modalities in Meniere's disease. Betahistine, a vasodilator, can also be helpful in these patients. It has been proposed that this medication improves blood flow to the inner ear although the exact mechanism of its action remains unclear.

Surgery may be indicated for management of Meniere's disease when medical therapy fails. Endolymphatic sac surgery is designed to reduce the pressure in the endolymph compartment. Labyrinthectomy or vestibular nerve section may be performed when sac surgery fails. However, this procedure is reserved for unilateral cases. Chemical vestibular ablation, via one or more gentamicin injections into the middle ear cavity, has proved to be a useful and less invasive management option in some cases (Monsell et al 1993).

When physical therapies for BPPV (see below) are unsuccessful, a surgical procedure to plug, and effectively paralyze, the offending canal may be considered.

Physical management

Management of BPPV

A simple treatment procedure called particle repositioning has been found to result in complete resolution of symptoms in up to 90% of patients with BPPV within 1–2 treatment sessions (Epley 1992, Lynn et al 1995). The treatment maneuver involves the practitioner moving the patient's upper body, neck and head through a series of positions (Epley 1992),which are thought to result in movement of the otoconial deposits out of the offending semicircular canal into the utricular cavity. Home exercise therapy, namely the Brandt-Daroff exercises, is also effective in the treatment of BPPV (Brandt et al 1980).

Management of cervicogenic dizziness

Treatment for cervicogenic dizziness may include mobilization of the symptomatic unilateral facet joint/s and surrounding soft tissues (Wrisley et al 2000), stabilization exercises for the cervical spine and trunk, and implementing minor ergonomic changes. This approach has been shown to reduce neck pain, reduce the frequency of dizziness, and improve balance performance (Karlberg et al 1996).

Vestibular rehabilitation

Vestibular rehabilitation (VR) is an approach based around exercise for the treatment of vestibular dysfunction, primarily incorporating exercises designed to encourage the process of central compensation. It was first reported in the 1940s with the work of Cawthorne and Cooksey (Cawthorne 1944). These pioneers in the area stressed that patients should be encouraged to move into the positions that provoked their symptoms.

Commonly, patients with acute or chronic vestibular pathology avoid activities that trigger their dizziness. However, in most cases, this approach can actually slow down or impede recovery. Approaches to VR have been shown to result in significantly improved symptoms and balance even in acute conditions such as vestibular neuronitis (Strupp et al 1998).

VR is an evolving area and results of ongoing clinical research in this field will further refine treatment paradigms.

Who is appropriate for vestibular rehabilitation?

Vestibular rehabilitation is considered an appropriate treatment strategy for individuals with a stable uncompensated vestibular lesion. Patient selection for this type of intervention can be determined from the clinical assessment and specific goals for rehabilitation are set at this time (Whitney et al 2000a).

Patients with spontaneous attacks of vertigo generally do not respond well to physical treatment programs because of the unstable nature of their vestibular pathology. Criteria for inclusion in a program of VR include:

- A history of positional or motion-provoked symptoms of dizziness/vertigo;
- Evidence of impaired balance performance;
- Substantial limitations in activities of daily living (Shepard et al 1993).

What exercises should be included?

Exercise prescription is largely based on findings from the subjective and objective assessment. The exercise program may be delivered as a therapist supervised program, an independent home exercise program, or a combination of the two. Home exercise programs are often prescribed to be done at least once a day, with a written and/or graphic description of the exercise and dosage provided to the patient. Examples of exercise types that can be used in a home exercise program or supervised by a physiotherapist include:

- vestibular adaptation (gaze stability) exercises (Herdman 1998), involving visual fixation on a target while the head is moving. Often recommended to be undertaken for short periods several times daily;
- habituation exercises (Norre et al 1980), involving repeated exposure to positions and movements that provoke or exacerbate symptoms. May include the Brandt-Daroff exercises for BPPV;
- balance and gait training (Clendaniel et al 1997). Exercises are selected to target identified balance problems, in a safe manner;
- general fitness training (Shepard et al 1990); and
- functional retraining (Cohen 1994).

The structure and length of the programs described in the literature varies considerably, making comparison between studies difficult. Traditionally, a generic approach such as Cawthorne and Cooksey exercises has been used. These exercises were often provided as a handout with no direct supervision or review of performance. A customized approach is now advocated, where specific exercises are chosen and reviewed by the therapist to meet individual needs and functional deficits (Black et al 2003). Further research is required to assess the effectiveness of customized versus generic exercise program of vestibular rehabilitation.

Further research is also required to evaluate the relative benefits of a supervised program of exercises compared to an unsupervised home program. Using both types of approach, studies have reported significant improvements in vestibular handicap and balance performance following 4–10 weeks of the program (Black et al 2000, Cass et al 1996, Krebs et al 2003, Murray et al 2001). Although the type of approach adopted may vary, a recent randomized controlled study determined that there were no significant differences in outcome between individuals receiving a home program of VR with or without additional supervised sessions (Kammerlind et al 2005).

Additional potential components of a vestibular rehabilitation program include:

- education (Whitney et al 2000b) including information about the condition, likely prognosis, strategies to maximize recovery and minimize development of secondary problems;
- psychological counseling (Yardley et al 1994);
- fall prevention strategies (Macias et al 2005);
- interventions for secondary limitations, such as neck and back pain, muscle weakness, limited joint range of movement and headaches (Cass et al 1996).

Other methods have recently been described which may enhance the response to vestibular rehabilitation of individuals with chronic vestibular dysfunction. Included is a simulator-based desensitization program (incorporating controlled exposure to visual motion and visual-motor conflict environments) (Pavlou et al 2004).

How effective is vestibular rehabilitation?

Several studies have provided evidence regarding the effectiveness of VR in successfully treating individuals with a range of acute and chronic vestibular disorders (Cass et al 1996, Murray et al 2001, Shepard et al 1993). Significant improvements in symptom severity, self-reported handicap, levels of disability and balance performance have been described. Recent research has also identified a reduction in falls risk following VR (Macias et al 2005).

Predictors of outcome following vestibular rehabilitation

Late presentation for an assessment of vestibular function, late initiation of VR, and non-compliance with the therapy program have been identified as factors most predictive of unsuccessful outcome (Bamiou et al 2000). Work done by Yardley and co-workers (Yardley et al 2004) found that compliance with the exercise program and levels of commitment and as well as motivation influence outcomes.

Damage to central nervous system links from the vestibular apparatus may also influence recovery. Although individuals with central vestibular dysfunction can respond to vestibular rehabilitation (Suarez et al 2003), they appear to improve more slowly than those with peripheral disorders (Shepard et al 1993).

Age does not appear to be a significant factor in predicting the outcome of VR (Whitney et al 2002). However, Hall and colleagues (2004) reported that a significantly greater proportion of older adults (45%) remained at risk for future falls at the completion of VR compared to younger individuals (11%).

Conclusion

Vestibular dysfunction is a relatively common, though often unrecognized health problem that can have substantial impact on an individual's function, psychological status, and well being. Symptoms associated with vestibular dysfunction may include dizziness, nausea, headache, and neck pain. The ability to recognize that symptoms common to many possible diagnoses may be due to vestibular dysfunction is an important clinical skill. A comprehensive assessment, often including formal vestibular function testing, and an individualized program of vestibular rehabilitation can improve outcomes.

References

Bamiou D, Davies R, McKee M et al 2000 Symptoms disability and handicap in unilateral peripheral vestibular disorders. Scandinavian Audiology 29:238-244.

Black F, Pesznecker S 2003 Vestibular adaptation and rehabilitation. Current Opinion Otolaryngology Head and Neck Surgery 11:355-360.

Black F, Angel C, Pesznecker S et al 2000 Outcome analysis of individualised vestibular rehabilitation protocols. American Journal of Otology 21:543-551.

Brandt T, Daroff R 1980 Physical therapy for benign paroxysmal positional vertigo. Archives of Otolaryngology 106:484-485.

Briggs R, Gossman M, Birch R et al 1989 Balance performance among non-institutionalised elderly women. Physical Therapy 69:748-756.

Cass S, Borello-France D, Furman J 1996 Functional outcome of vestibular rehabilitation in patients with abnormal sensory organisation testing. American Journal of Otology 17:581-594.

Cawthorne T 1944 The physiological basis for head exercises. Journal of the Chartered Society of Physiotherapists 30:106-107.

Clendaniel R, Tucci D 1997 Vestibular rehabilitation strategies in Menieres Disease. Otolaryngologic Clinics of North America 30:1145-1158.

Cohen H 1994 Vestibular rehabilitation improves daily life function. 48:919-925.

Cohen H, Blatchly C, Gombash L 1993 A study of the clinical test of sensory interaction and balance. Physical Therapy 73:346-351.

Colledge N, Wilson J, MacIntyre C et al 1994 The prevalence and characteristics of dizziness in an elderly community. Age and Ageing 23:117-120.

Curthoys I, Halmagyi G 1995 Vestibular compensation: a review of the oculomotor neural and clinical consequences of unilateral vestibular loss. Journal of Vestibular Research 5:67-107.

Epley J 1992 The canalith repositioning procedure: For treatment of benign paroxysmal positional vertigo. Otolaryngology Head and Neck Surgery 107:399-404.

Furman J, Whitney S 2000 Central causes of dizziness. Physical Therapy 80:179-187.

Grad A, Baloh R 1989 Vertigo of vascular origin: clinical and electronystagmographic features in 89 cases. Archives of Neurology 46:281-284.

Hall C, Schubert M, Herdman S 2004 Prediction of falls risk reduction as measured by dynamic gait index in individuals with unilateral vestibular hypofunction. Otology and Neurotology 25:746-751.

Halmagyi M, Curthoys I. 1988. A clinical sign of canal paresis. Arch Neurol 45(7):737-739.

Herdman S 1997 Advances in the treatment of vestibular disorders. Physical Therapy 77:602-618.

Herdman S 1998 Role of vestibular adaptation in vestibular rehabilitation. Otolaryngology Head and Neck Surgery 119:49-54.

Herdman SJ, Blatt P, Schubert MC et al 2000 Falls in patients with vestibular deficits. Am J Otol 21:847-851.

Hill K, Bernhardt J, McGann A et al 1996 A new test of dynamic standing balance for stroke patients: Reliability validity and comparison with healthy elderly. Physiotherapy Canada 48:257-262.

Hill K, Schwarz J, Flicker L et al 1999 Falls among healthy community dwelling older women: A prospective study of frequency circumstances consequences and prediction accuracy. Australian and New Zealand Journal of Public Health 23:41-48.

Honrubia V, Hoffman L 1993 In: Jacobson G, Newman C, Kartush J (eds) Handbook of balance function testing. Mosby Year Book, St Louis.

Jacobson G, Newman C 1990 The development of the Dizziness Handicap Inventory. Archives of Otolaryngology and Head and Neck Surgery 116:424-427.

Kammerlind A, Ledin T, Skargren E et al 2005 Long-term follow-up after acute unilateral vestibular loss and comparison between subjects with and without remaining symptoms. Acta Otolaryngology 125:946-953.

Karlberg M, Magnusson M, Malmstrom E et al 1996 Postural and symptomatic improvement after physiotherapy in patients with dizziness of suspected cervical origin. Archives of Physical Medicine and Rehabilitation 77:874-882.

Kayan A, Hood J 1984 Neuro-otological manifestations of migraine. Brain 107:1123-1142.

Kim J, Lopez I, Di Patre P et al 1999 Internal auditory artery infarction: Clinicopathologic correlation. Neurology 52:40-44.

Krebs D, Lockert J 1991 In: Spivack B (ed) Evaluation and management of gait disorders. Marcel Dekker Inc., New York.

Krebs D, Gill-Body K, Parker S et al 2003 Vestibular rehabilitation: useful but not universally so. Otolaryngology Head and Neck Surgery 128:240-250.

Lynn S, Pool A, Rose D et al 1995 Randomized trial of the canalith repositioning procedure. Otolaryngology and Head and Neck Surgery 113:712-720.

Macias J, Massingale S, Gerkin R 2005 Efficacy of vestibular rehabilitation therapy in reducing falls. Acta Otolaryngology Head Neck Surgery 133:323-325.

Monsell E, Cass S, Rybak L 1993 Therapeutic use of aminoglycosides in Menierres disease. Otolaryngolic Clinics of North America 26:737-746.

Murray KJ, Hill K, Phillips B et al 2005 A pilot study of falls risk and vestibular dysfunction in older fallers presenting to hospital Emergency Departments. Disability and Rehabilitation. 27(9):499-506.

Murray K, Hill K, Carroll S 2001 Relationship between change in balance and self-reported handicap following a course of vestibular rehabilitation therapy. Physiotherapy Research International 6:251-263.

Murray K, Hill K, Phillips B et al 2007 The influence of otolith dysfunction on the clinical presentation of people with a peripheral vestibular disorder. Physical Therapy 87:143-152.

Norre M, De Weerdt W 1980 Treatment of vertigo based on habituation. Journal of Laryngology and Otology 94:689-696.

Oghalai J, Manolidis S, Barth J et al 2000 Unrecognised benign paroxysmal positional vertigo in elder patients. Otolaryngology and Head and Neck Surgery 122:630-634.

Pavlou M, Lingeswaran A, Davies R et al 2004 Simulator based rehabilitation in refractory dizziness. Journal of Neurology 251:983-985.

Podsiadlo D, Richardson S 1991 The timed Up & Go: A test of basic functional mobility for frail elderly persons. Journal of the American Geriatrics Society 39:142-148.

Schubert M, Tusa R, Grine L et al. 2004 Optimising the sensitivity of the head thrust test for identifying vestibular hypofunction. Physical Therapy 84:151-158.

Sheehan S, Bauer R, Meyer J 1960 Vertebral artery compression in cervical spondylosis. Neurology 10:968-986.

Shepard N, Telian S, Smith-Wheelock M 1990 Habituation and balance retraining therapy. Diagnostic Neurotology 8:459-475.

Shepard N, Telian S, Smith-Wheelock M et al 1993 Vestibular and balance rehabilitation therapy. Annals of Otology Rhinology Laryngology 102:198-205.

Shumway-Cook A, Horak F 1986 Assessing the influence of Sensory Interaction on Balance: suggestion from the field. Physical Therapy 66:1548-1550.

Sloane P, Baloh R 1989 Persistent dizziness in geriatric patients. Journal of the American Geriatrics Society 37:1031-1038.

Sloane PD, Hartman M, Mitchell CM 1994 Psychological factors associated with chronic dizziness in patients aged 60 and older. Journal of the American Geriatrics Society 42:847-852.

Strupp M, Arbusow V, Maag K et al 1998 Vestibular exercises improve central vestibulospinal compensation after vestibular neuritis. Neurology 51:838-844.

Strupp M, Planck J, Arbusow V et al 2000 Rotational vertebral artery occlusion syndrome with vertigo due to labyrinthine excitation. Neurology 54:1376-1379.

Suarez H, Arocena M Suarez A et al 2003 Changes in postural control parameters after vestibular rehabilitation in patients with central vestibular disorders. Acta Otolaryngology 123:143-147.

Tinetti ME, Williams CS, Gill TM 2000 Health functional and psychological outcomes among older persons with chronic dizziness. Journal of the American Geriatrics Society 48:417-421.

Waterston J 2004 Chronic migrainous vertigo. Journal of Clinical Neuroscience 11:384-386.

Whitney S, Herdman S 2000a In: Herdman S (ed) Vestibular rehabilitation. F.A. Davis Company, Philadelphia.

Whitney S, Rossi M 2000b Efficacy of vestibular rehabilitation. Otolaryngology Clinics of North America 33:659-673.

Whitney S, Wrisley D, Marchetti G et al 2002 The effect of age on vestibular rehabilitation outcomes. Laryngoscope 112:1785-1790.

Whitney S, Wrisley D, Brown K et al 2004 Is perception of handicap related to functional performance in persons with vestibular dysfunction?. Otology and Neurotology 25: 139-143.

Wrisley D, Sparto P, Whitney S et al 2000 Cervicogenic dizziness: a review of diagnosis and treatment. Journal of Orthopaedic and Sports Physical Therapy 30:755-766.

Wrisley D, Walker M, Echternach J et al 2003 Reliability of the Dynamic Gait Index in people with vestibular disorders. Archives of Physical Medicine & Rehabilitation 84: 1528-1533.

Wrisley D, Marchetti G, Kuharsky K et al 2004 Reliability internal consistency and validity of data obtained with the Functional Gait Assessment. Physical Therapy 84:906-918.

Yardley L, Luxon L 1994 Treating dizziness with vestibular rehabilitation. British Medical Journal 308:1252-1253.

Yardley L, Redfern M 2001 Psychological factors influencing recovery from balance disorders. Anxiety Disorders 15:107-119.

Yardley L, Donovan-Hall M, Smith H et al 2004 Effectiveness of primary care-based vestibular rehabilitation for chronic dizziness. Annals of Internal Medicine 141:598-605.

Zigmond A, Snaith R 1983 The Hospital Anxiety and Depression Scale. Acta Psychiatry Scandinavia 67:361-370.

Measurement of headache

Ken Niere

Many practitioners treat headache but the question arises of how to verify whether patients have benefited from treatment. In this chapter the author, a musculoskeletal physiotherapist and clinical researcher, reviews the methods and tools used to measure headache and related impairments (including direct behavioral effects) in clinical and research settings.

Researchers are currently evaluating headache-specific questionnaires and outcome measures to assess their reliability and specificity. The outcome measures will help clinicians and researchers to evaluate current therapeutics. Headaches are subjective experiences of pain located somewhere in the head. A substantial number of conditions can give rise to headaches. This is reflected in the most recent International Headache Society (2004) headache classification document where 14 broad categories and numerous subcategories are listed and described in an exhaustive 114 page document (see Ch. 1). Similarly, there are numerous proposed treatments and management strategies for headache. No matter what the treatment, whether in a clinical or experimental context, it is essential to monitor the response to treatment. To do this we must be able to measure the headache at specific points in the management process.

Issues surrounding measurement of headache are similar to those involving measurement of pain. Pain and headache-related symptoms are subjective in nature and clinicians are reliant on patient descriptions. Pain is understood to be a complex, multidimensional experience encompassing sensory, affective, and motivational domains. Hence, accurate and complete measurement of headache symptoms will need to reflect these domains. Parameters that can be used to measure headaches include the intensity and nature of the symptoms as well as temporal features such as frequency and duration. The consequences of the headache, such as medication usage and behavioral and lifestyle impact, can also be measured.

Clinical measurement of headache

What is important for the patient with headache? This will vary among individuals according to the nature and characteristics of their headaches, their work and social situation, and their attitudes and beliefs towards their problem. Symptom relief may not be the main expectation of patients with headache presenting to a health practitioner. For example, in a survey of 100 outpatients with headache and 50 treating physicians by Packard (1979), 66% of physicians indicated that they believed pain relief was the patient's primary objective while only 31% of patients indicated that pain relief was their main expectation. This study found that 46% of patients primarily wanted an explanation of what was causing their headache. If the clinician lacks awareness of these expectations an unsatisfactory treatment outcome may occur, despite accurate headache measurement. Patient expectations may also influence the choice of outcome measures. In 1997 we surveyed 154 patients presenting for physiotherapy treatment of their headaches (Niere & Robinson 1997) and found that 66% chose reduction in headache frequency as the most important indicator of treatment success, compared to 21% who chose reduced intensity, and 5% who felt that decreased duration was the most important indicator. Interestingly, improvement in activities of daily living (ADL) was indicated as most important by only 8%. When asked to indicate the minimum acceptable level of improvement two months after commencing physiotherapy treatment, 29% expected to be completely better while the average level of minimum expected improvement was 78%. In general, subjects with a longer history of headache had lower expectations of treatment while those with shorter histories had higher expectations.

Headaches are often of finite duration, or may be episodes of increased pain superimposed upon a background of ongoing pain. Abolition of the headache (that is, frequency and other measures revert to zero) could be considered the ultimate aim of any therapy. However, this may not be realistic or possible. When considering outcome measures for physical treatment of headache in clinical trials and practice, the parameters of headache frequency, duration, and intensity are commonly

used (Jull et al 2002, Niere & Robinson 1997, Vernon 1982, Whittingham et al 1994).

Headache measurement in the clinical situation is usually by patient retrospective report, either via interview or questionnaire (Niere & Robinson 1997) although headache diaries are recommended for data collection in clinical trials and appear to be regarded as the 'gold standard' (International Headache Society 1995). The content of a headache diary may vary depending on the population being studied. Typically a patient would be asked to record the number of hours during the day that they had a headache, the intensity on a visual analogue scale (VAS), and the amount and type of medication taken (Fig. 13.1). Other items such as diet and activities may also be included if an aim is to identify possible precipitating factors. Patients may be required to complete the diary at regular points during the day or simply at the end of the day before retiring. A potential problem with headache diaries is a lack of compliance, in that patients may omit recordings and simply complete their entries at a later date or time (Collins & Thompson 1979). Another limitation is they need to be completed over a set period of time before the data is interpretable and clinically useful. Depending on the frequency and type of headaches measured, this baseline period may vary from one week to four or more weeks, with the longer time frames likely to increase the risk of non-compliance.

If patient estimates of headache parameters are used it is useful to know how accurate these estimates are in relation to headache diaries. In a headache population from a general community Blizaard et al (2000) compared diary and questionnaire reports for headache frequency over a one month period and found only moderate agreement. Niere and Jerak (2004) examined the accuracy of retrospective patient reports with respect to daily headache

Please complete this form every evening before going to bed

Name ....

Day ....   Date ..../........./.........

1. Have you taken any medication today for your headache?   Yes ☐   No ☐
If yes, name and strength (mg) and number taken of medication(s)

....

....

2. ☐ I have not had a headache today (Thank you, there is no need to answer the other questions)
or ☐ I have had a headache today (please complete the other questions)

3. Please shade the area where you felt your headache and any associated neck pain.

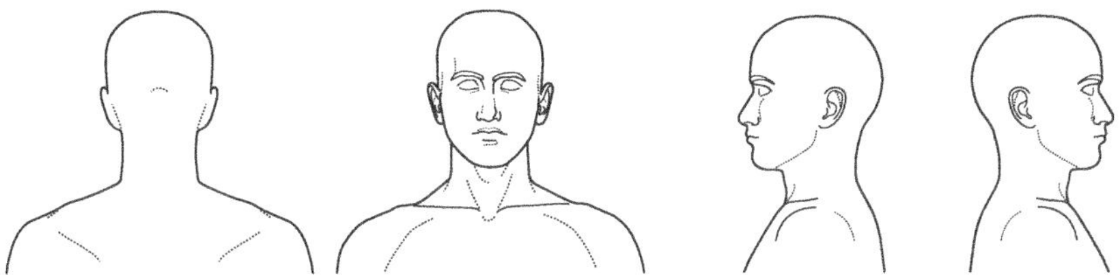

| Back | Front | Left | Right |

4. Please mark on the scale below your estimate of the intensity of today's headache.

No headache _____ Worst possible headache

5. How many hours did you have a headache today? .... hours

6. Can you nominate what provoked today's headache?

....

Figure 13.1 ● Example of a headache diary.

diaries for the measurement of frequency, duration and intensity of headaches in a sample of 40 participants. We found that correlation coefficients (Spearman's rho) for questionnaire and diary data for headache frequency and duration were 0.80 and 0.72 respectively, while that for intensity was only 0.51 (range: 0 indicating no correlation to 1.0 indicating perfect correlation). We also found that, when compared to diary data, subjects tended to under estimate headache frequency, but over estimate duration and intensity. Andrasik and Holroyd (1980) investigated the relationship between diary data for headache frequency, intensity, and duration collected hourly over a two-week period with that obtained from a questionnaire completed at the end of the two weeks. They found that subjects reported fewer headaches per week and significantly greater headache intensities in questionnaires compared to the diary data. Intensity and duration correlated poorly between the two methods (r = 0.23 and 0.29 respectively) while the strongest correlation was found between data for frequency (r = 0.71). However, the study tested only subjects with tension type headache and the instrument for measuring subject report was not detailed. A more recent study (Stewart et al 1999b) of 132 subjects with migraine, compared diary reports and data collected with the Headache Impact Questionnaire (Stewart et al 1998) over a three month period. Correlation coefficients for migraine frequency and intensity were 0.67 and 0.74 respectively, suggesting that when the headache is severe, as in migraine, recall of intensity is likely to be more accurate.

Accuracy of memory for headache pain

It is likely that severe pain is more easily remembered and reported by the patient (Rasmussen et al 1991). Hunter et al (1979) reported accurate five-day recall of acute head pain following neurosurgical procedure as measured by the McGill Pain Questionnaire (MPQ) (Melzack 1975). They also found that recall of sensory descriptors on the MPQ was more reliable than for the affective descriptors. In a general headache population Niere and Robinson (1997) found that memory for headache intensity was less reliable than for frequency and duration. Using intraclass correlation coefficients (ICC) they found relatively low 24 hour test-retest reliability (ICC = 0.64) when headache intensity was measured on a VAS. Although recall of headache intensity is relatively accurate in migraine it appears that

the severity of the less severe headaches in this general headache population was more difficult to remember. Test-retest scores (ICC) for headache frequency and duration in the same study were 0.95 and 0.98 respectively. It has been suggested that when documenting usual pain, there is a tendency to use present pain as a reference point (Eich et al 1985, Feine et al 1998, Turk & Okifuji 1999). This is supported by studies of headache (Rachman & Eyrl 1989) and chronic pain (Feine et al 1998, Jamieson et al 1989, Linton & Melin 1982). Therefore, clinicians should be aware that pain may be over estimated if the patient has a severe headache when asked to remember usual pain levels. Similarly, if the patient is pain free or has a mild headache, the usual intensity may be underestimated. Reporting of acute pain is also likely to be increased by negative affect (Gedney & Logan 2004, Tasmuth et al 1996). Other factors that can influence pain memory include emotional distress, domestic conflicts, decreased activity levels, reliance on medication (Jamieson et al 1989) or level of catastrophizing (Lefebvre & Keefe 2002). It has been suggested that averages of current, usual, and worst pain levels may be more reliable than single ratings for chronic pain (Dworkin et al 1990) although it is not known whether this would be generalizable to patients with headache.

Another factor influencing patient assessment of pain intensity may be that commonly used tools to measure pain, such as the VAS or numerical rating scale (NRS) do not adequately reflect the whole pain experience. It is generally understood that pain has affective and cognitive elements as well as sensory components. The influence of affective and cognitive factors may make pain intensity harder to recall. The use of pain measures that incorporate both sensory and affective dimensions of pain, such as the MPQ or the Short-Form MPQ, may give more accurate results than unidimensional measures.

Measurement of headache pain

There are many different ways to measure pain and hence headache intensity. The methods that are most commonly used or applicable to clinical practice will be reviewed here.

Descriptive rating scales

A descriptive rating scale (DRS) usually consists of a series of pain descriptors from which patients choose the most accurate descriptor for their pain. A numerical value may be assigned to each descriptor. Examples of DRS (often referred to as verbal rating scales) for pain intensity and pain affect are given in Figure 13.2. For these the descriptors 'none' and 'bearable' would be scored as zero, 'mild' and 'uncomfortable' would be scored as one, 'moderate' and 'awful' would be scored as two, and so on.

A DRS is usually easy to understand and use. However, they may be relatively insensitive, which would necessitate large changes in order to reliably detect differences between testing. It cannot be assumed that there are equal spacings between ratings. For example, moderate (which would be given a value of two) is not necessarily twice as painful as mild (which would be given a value of one). Hence, they do not necessarily provide interval or ratio data so analysis of group data should be performed using non-parametric methods.

Numerical rating scales

A numerical rating scale (NRS) requires the patient to rate their pain on a defined scale. For example, 0–10 where 0 is no pain and 10 is the worst pain imaginable (Fig. 13.3). Commonly used NRS are 11 point (0–10), 21 point

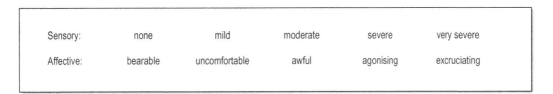

Figure 13.2 • Examples of descriptive rating scales for sensory and affective domains of pain.

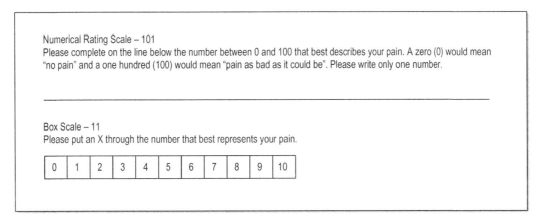

Figure 13.3 • Examples of numerical rating scales. A 101 numerical rating scale (above) and an 11 point box scale below.

(0–20) and 101 point (0–100) (Jensen & Karoly 2001). Jensen et al (1996) used a 101-point scale on 124 chronic pain patients and found that 90–98% of patients used the scale in multiples of five (equivalent to a 21-point scale). Over 50% of subjects rated their pain in multiples of 10 (equivalent to an 11-point scale). They concluded that 11- and 21-point scales were sensitive enough to measure chronic pain. Kwong & Pathak (2007) found that an 11-point scale for measuring intensity of migraine was 55% more sensitive than a 4-point scale (none, mild, moderate, severe) in detecting clinically important differences. Numerical rating scales may be administered verbally, where patients are asked to rate their pain and the therapist records the value. They may also be applied in written form, completed independently by the patient, either as a single rating or where the numbers are written in

ascending order and the patient is asked to circle or select the number corresponding to their pain. Advantages of NRS are that they are easily understood and quickly administered. They have been reported to be sensitive to change and correlate well with other pain intensity measures (Jensen & Karoly 2001). They do not appear to have ratio properties, meaning that a rating of 10, for example, does not necessarily indicate twice as much pain as a rating of five.

Visual analogue scales

A visual analogue scale (VAS) usually consists of a 100 mm line anchored at each end by descriptors (Fig. 13.4). Patients place a mark on the scale that corresponds to their pain. The distance (usually in mm) from the lower end of the scale is then measured and recorded. Visual analogue scales are generally easy to understand

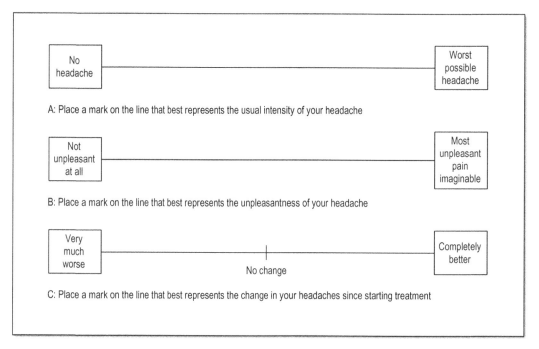

Figure 13.4 • Examples of visual analogue scales for measurement of: A = usual headache intensity, B = unpleasantness of headache pain, and C = change in headaches.

and complete although 3–11% of patients may not be able to complete them (Ogon et al 1996). Patients have been shown to use all parts of the scale and no single point seems to be favored (Huskisson 1974). It is likely that the VAS is more sensitive than the DRS in detecting treatment changes (Jensen & Karoly 2001). The VAS can also be used to measure pain relief, treatment effect or change in condition, depending on the anchor descriptors (Fig. 13.4). The VAS correlates highly with descriptive and numerical rating scales and is thought to produce ratio data, at least for group measurements (Price et al 1983, Jensen & Karoly, 2001). The VAS appears to be more reliable for current pain than remembered pains. In a series of 65 chronic low back pain patients. Love et al (1989) calculated reliability of present pain: r = 0.77, worst pain: r = 0.49, and best pain: r = 0.57. Although not demonstrated on patients with headache, this point should be considered when asking patients to remember their headache intensity. A disadvantage of the VAS is that it is unidimensional. Other dimensions have to be measured separately. Also, patients may not understand the requirements for completion, particularly if they have impaired cognitive function.

McGill Pain Questionnaire

The McGill Pain Questionnaire (MPQ) (Melzack 1975) was designed to reflect the sensory, affective, and evaluative dimensions of pain. The MPQ contains 78 pain descriptors assigned to 20 categories within sensory, affective, evaluative and miscellaneous subclasses, a body chart, nine temporal adjectives and a 'present pain index' that is rated out of five. The descriptors are assigned an intensity value in each of 20 sections, starting at one for the word with the least pain value. Scoring is via a Pain Rating Index (PRI) for each subclass and a total PRI. The number of words chosen and the score on the PPI can also be used. The MPQ takes approximately 5–10 minutes to complete once a patient has had some experience with it, but may take 15–20 minutes if they are unfamiliar with it (Melzack 1975). The MPQ may be read to the patient by the researcher/clinician or completed by patients themselves, although scores may be higher when the patient has the MPQ read to them (Klepac et al 1981). The construct validity of the MPQ has been reinforced by studies that confirm the three-factor (sensory, evaluative and affective) structure (Lowe et al 1991, Turk et al 1985). The test-retest reliability or reproducibility of the MPQ has been calculated at 0.83 over 'several days' in 65 chronic low back pain patients (Love et al 1989). In a study of 16 patients with acute head pain after neurosurgical procedure Hunter et al (1979) reported reproducibility over a five day period of greater than 0.89. It has been reported that the MPQ is sensitive to changes in pain related to various clinical syndromes (Melzack & Katz, 2001) although it does not appear to have been tested on benign, recurrent headache. The MPQ has been used widely for research but is clinically less practical due to the time taken to complete than other less complex scoring systems.

Short-form McGill Pain Questionnaire

The Short-form McGill Pain Questionnaire (SFMPQ) was developed to provide an instrument that could be completed in less time than the MPQ but would still reflect both the sensory and affective dimensions of pain (Melzack 1987). The SFMPQ consists of 15 descriptors from the MPQ that were chosen by greater than 33% of patients with nine different pain syndromes including headache, low back pain, arthritis and dental pain. Of the 15 descriptors, 11 are from the sensory section of the MPQ and 4 are from the affective section. Each descriptor is ranked on an intensity scale of

0 = none, 1 = mild, 2 = moderate and 3 = severe. A VAS and a 0–5 numerical rating scale are also included. Scoring is by adding the rankings for the descriptors although sensory and affective descriptors may be scored separately (Melzack 1987). The VAS and numerical rating scale scores are not usually incorporated with the descriptor scores. The SFMPQ takes approximately five minutes to complete and score.

The SFMPQ was tested against the MPQ on 40 post-surgical, 20 obstetric, and 10 musculoskeletal pain patients (Melzack 1987). The procedure was repeated for dental patients. The results showed significant correlations (r = 0.65 to 0.93) between sensory, affective, and total scores for pre-and post-intervention scores. These results indicate that the SFMPQ may provide similar data to the MPQ on the different dimensions of the pain experience, but in a more practical and timely manner than the longer version of the questionnaire.

Measurement of musculoskeletal impairment

Where treatment of spinal and/or TMD aims to improve a patient's headaches, parameters such as range of motion and tests of muscle function may be necessary to determine the extent of musculoskeletal impairment in a particular presentation. The pattern and magnitude of musculoskeletal impairment should be consistent with the pattern of headache intensity, frequency, and duration. The degree of change in the musculoskeletal impairments with treatment should be proportional to the improvement in the headache parameters to justify continued treatment. The role that the physical impairment plays in the headache can be clarified by careful monitoring of physical and headache parameters (Jull & Niere 2004). For example, if the physical measures improve but the headache parameters stay the same it is

unlikely that the musculoskeletal impairment is responsible for the headaches. Where physical parameters improve but are not sustained and the headaches do not improve substantially, the physical impairments are probably secondary to the headache that is likely to have another etiology (Jull & Niere 2004).

Measurement of headache-related disability

It is now widely accepted that best clinical practice incorporates a patient-centered approach to management of headache (Andrasik et al 2005). Hence, it is important for the clinician to appreciate and be able to measure the impact of headache on a patient's quality of life, both during and between headache attacks. Cavallini et al (1995) found that patients with headache often suffer from diminished ability to perform activities of daily living (ADL) during headache attacks. They also found that patients with headaches suffered from reduced motor performance, disturbed interpersonal relationships and feelings of inadequacy. Subjects also reported distress caused by imminence of attacks and that their headaches negatively affected relationships with family, friends and colleagues, often disturbing the planning of their social lives. Other research has also shown decreased quality of life in headache sufferers, including those with cervicogenic headache (Diener 2001, Kryst & Scherl 1994, Marcus 2003). Over the past two decades a number of questionnaires have been developed to gauge headache-related disability. These have generally been related to specific headache types, most notably migraine, or were developed within secondary referral headache clinics. One of these, the Headache Disability Inventory (HDI) (Jacobsen et al 1994) comprises 25 statements (items) derived from case history responses of patients with headache, each measured on a scale or 4 (yes), 2 (sometimes) or 0 (no). Measured psychometric properties of the HDI include internal consistency ($\alpha = .89$) and two-month reproducibility ($r = 0.83$) (Jacobsen et al 1994). However, it has been estimated that a change score of at least 30 points is necessary to be 95% sure of a real change in patient condition (Jacobsen et al 1994), a factor that may limit the clinical utility of the questionnaire. Descriptions of three of the more recently developed questionnaires follow.

Migraine Disability Assessment Scale

In 1998 an international, expert working group proposed a 16 item Headache Impact Questionnaire (HImQ) to measure the effects of migraine on quality of life (Stewart et al 1998). From the HImQ Stewart et al (1998) developed an 8-item, migraine-specific quality of life (QoL) questionnaire that was subsequently reduced to the five question Migraine-specific Disability Assessment Scale (MIDAS)(Stewart et al 1999a) based on a three month time frame. The MIDAS items are:

1. On how many days in the last 3 months did you miss work or school because of your headaches?

2. How many days in the last 3 months was your productivity at work or school reduced by half or more because of your headaches? *(Do not include days you counted in question 1 where you missed work or school.)*

3. On how many days in the last 3 months did you not do household work because of your headaches?

4. How many days in the last 3 months was your productivity in household work reduced by half or more because of your headaches? *(Do not include days you counted in question 3 where you did not do household work.)*

5. On how many days in the last 3 months did you miss family, social or leisure activities because of your headaches?

The MIDAS also includes one question on headache frequency and one question on headache intensity, although these are not included in the total score. Stewart et al (2001) tested the psychometric properties of the MIDAS and found internal consistency of at least 0.73 (Cronbach's α) and reproducibility of 0.80 (Pearson's r). The MIDAS has been translated into a number of languages. To date, there do not appear to be published data related to minimum detectable change, so clinicians using the MIDAS with individuals cannot be sure what proportion of change score is likely to be due to measurement error.

Potential weaknesses of the MIDAS are that days where productivity is reduced by less than 50% are not included in the score and days where productivity is reduced by more than 50% are given the same weighting as days that were completely missed. For individuals where migraines inhibit rather than prohibit activity the MIDAS may be less sensitive. Also, the MIDAS relies on the accuracy of the patient's memory over a 3-month period for estimating days lost or productivity reduced by more than 50%. Stewart et al (2000) compared MIDAS scores to a 90-day daily diary in 144 migraine sufferers. They found that responses to MIDAS questions about number of days where productivity in work or household work was reduced by greater than 50%, was significantly overestimated compared to diary data. Responses to other items were similar between the two measures while the correlation between diary and total MIDAS scores for the population was fair at only 0.63. Although the MIDAS appears a suitable instrument for measuring migraine-related disability, it is not known if it would be suitable for measuring disability in patients with other headache types. Studies by Solomon et al (1994) and Solomon (1997) used the medical outcomes study instrument to establish whether quality of life differs among headache diagnoses. They found that quality of life profiles for each of the common benign headache disorders (migraine, tension-type, mixed, and cluster) appear to be unique for the specific headache diagnosis. The MIDAS does not appear to have been tested on other headache types.

Headache Disability Questionnaire

With the aim of measuring headache-related activity restriction in patients presenting for physiotherapy, Niere and Quin (2009) reduced the 16-item Headache Impact Questionnaire into a 9-item questionnaire based on responses made by 111 patients receiving physiotherapy treatment for their headaches. Items were included or rejected based on floor or ceiling effects, item-total correlations and factor analysis. Of the 111 patients, 36% were diagnosed with cervicogenic headache, 30% with tension-type headache, 14% with migraine without aura, and 7% had migraine with aura. A diagnosis of 'other' was made in 14%. The HDQ consists of nine items measuring pain intensity, number of days over a one-month period where activity was prevented for a day or more, and the degree to which activities were curtailed due to headaches (Fig. 13.5). Although the HDQ and MIDAS were both developed from the HImQ, the HDQ differs from the MIDAS in that it encompasses decreased efficiency of tasks rather than days where tasks are missed or productivity is decreased by at least half due to the headache. Each item is graded on 11 point scale (0–10). The item scores are then added to give a total out of 90. It takes 5–10 minutes to complete and score. The HDQ has been found to have a three-factor structure encompassing activity limitation, activity prevention and pain intensity, with internal consistency reflected by Cronbach's α of 0.80, indicating that each item contributes evenly to the overall score (Niere & Quin 2009).

A further study of the HDQ by Muller (2007) reported 24 hour reproducibility of $r = .91$ and one month reproducibility of $r = .89$. The minimal detectable change (MDC_{90}) was calculated as 11.2 points, meaning that if a score changed by this magnitude, the researcher or clinician could be 90% confident that the change was not due to error. The HDQ would appear to be an appropriate instrument for measuring headache related disability in a general population of headache patients.

Headache Impact Test

The Headache Impact Test (HIT-6) is a standardized 6-item questionnaire that was developed by reducing a pool of 54 items used for computerized adaptive testing (CAT) of headache impact (Bjorner et al 2003) and 35 further items suggested by clinicians. Item selection was achieved by evaluations of content validity, internal consistency, score distributions, linguistic analyses, and item response theory (Kosinski et al 2003). The HIT-6 items are:

1. When you have headaches, how often is the pain severe?

2. How often do headaches limit your ability to do usual daily activities, including household work, work, school, or social activities?

3. When you have a headache, how often do you wish you could lie down?

4. In the past 4 weeks, how often have you felt too tired to do work or daily activities because of your headaches?

5. In the past 4 weeks, how often have you felt tired or fed up or irritated because of your headaches?

6. In the past 4 weeks, how often did headaches limit your ability to concentrate on work or daily activities?

Name: ....   Date: ..../.........../...........   Score   / 90

Please read each question and circle the response that best applies to you

1. How would you rate the usual pain of your headache on a scale from 0 to 10?

0	1	2	3	4	5	6	7	8	9	10	WORST
NO											PAIN
PAIN											

2. When you have headaches, how often is the pain severe?

Never	1-9%	10-19%	20-29%	30-39%	40-49%	50-59%	60-69%	70-79%	80-89%	90-100%	ALWAYS
0	1	2	3	4	5	6	7	8	9	10	

3. On how many days in the last month did you actually lie down for an hour or more because of your headaches?

None	1-3	4-6	7-9	10-12	13-15	16-18	19-21	22-24	25-27	28-31	EVERY DAY
0	1	2	3	4	5	6	7	8	9	10	

4. When you have a headache, how often do you miss work or school for all or part of the day?

None	1-9%	10-19%	20-29%	30-39%	40-49%	50-59%	60-69%	70-79%	80-89%	90-100%	EVERY DAY
0	1	2	3	4	5	6	7	8	9	10	

5. When you have a headache while you work (or school), how much is your ability to work reduced?

NOT	1-9%	10-19%	20-29%	30-39%	40-49%	50-59%	60-69%	70-79%	80-89%	90-100%	UNABLE
0	1	2	3	4	5	6	7	8	9	10	TO WORK
REDUCED											

6. How many days in the last month have you been kept from performing housework or chores for at least half of the day because of your headache?

None	1-3	4-6	7-9	10-12	13-15	16-18	19-21	22-24	25-27	28-31	EVERY DAY
0	1	2	3	4	5	6	7	8	9	10	

7. When you have a headache, how much is your ability to perform housework or chores reduced?

NOT	1-9%	10-19%	20-29%	30-39%	40-49%	50-59%	60-69%	70-79%	80-89%	90-100%	UNABLE
0	1	2	3	4	5	6	7	8	9	10	TO PERFORM
REDUCED											

8. How many days in the last month have you been kept from non-work activities (family, social or recreational) because of your headaches?

None	1-3	4-6	7-9	10-12	13-15	16-18	19-21	22-24	25-27	28-31	EVERY DAY
0	1	2	3	4	5	6	7	8	9	10	

9. When you have a headache, how much is your ability to engage in non-work activities (family, social or recreational) reduced?

NOT	1-9%	10-19%	20-29%	30-39%	40-49%	50-59%	60-69%	70-79%	80-89%	90-100%	UNABLE
0	1	2	3	4	5	6	7	8	9	10	TO PERFORM
REDUCED											

Figure 13.5 • The headache disability questionnaire.

The response choices for each item are: never (scored as 6), rarely (8), sometimes (10), very often (11), and always (13). The possible scores therefore range from 36 to 78. In an internet survey of 1103 participants with headache the HIT-6 has demonstrated internal consistency of Cronbach's $\alpha = 0.89$ and 14 day reproducibility of 0.80 (540 participants at follow up) (Kosinski et al 2003). The minimum important difference for the HIT-6 has been calculated as 2.3 units

(95% CI 0.3 to 4.3) in a population of 71 patients with chronic daily headache (Coeytaux et al 2006). Although the HIT-6 appears to be used widely, at least over the internet where scores are calculated automatically, a potential weakness is the difficulty in calculating scores for the pen and paper version. Also derived scores are not intuitively meaningful because of the relatively narrow scoring range and the minimum score of 36 representing no headache related disability.

Conclusion

There is a vast range of conditions that can cause headaches and a similarly large number of proposed treatments. To gauge treatment efficacy, it is essential to be able to measure patients' headaches or their direct behavioral effects. All headaches have at least one thing in common — pain felt in the head. This pain can be measured, as can its frequency and duration, although the clinician or researcher should be mindful of the strengths and weaknesses of any method they use to measure different aspects of headache pain. Given the multidimensional nature of any pain, and hence headache, it is recommended that a range of methods be used to judge treatment outcome accurately. As a general rule, it is recommended that outcomes should include headache frequency, at least one pain measure, and a valid and reliable tool to measure headache-related disability.

References

Andrasik F, Holroyd KA 1980 Reliability and concurrent validity of headache questionnaire data. Headache 20: 44-46.

Andrasik F, Mccrory DC, Wittrock DA 2005 Outcome measurement in behavioural headache research: headache parameters and psychosocial outcomes. Headache 45:429-437.

Bjorner JB, Kosinski M, Ware JE Jr 2003 Calibration of an item pool for assessing the burden of headaches: An application of item response theory to the Headache Impact Test (HIT™). Quality of Life Research 12 (8):913-933.

Blizzard L, Grimmer KA, Dwyer T 2000 Validity of a measure of the frequency of headaches with overt neck involvement, and reliability of measurement of cervical spine anthropometric and muscle performance factors. Archives of Physical Medicine and Rehabilitation 1204-1210.

Cavallini A, Micieli G, Bussone G et al 1995 Headache and quality of life. Headache 35:29-35.

Coeytaux RR, Kaufman JS, Chao R et al 2006 Four methods of estimating the minimal important difference score were compared to establish a clinically significant change in the headache impact test. Journal of Clinical Epidemiology 59:374-380.

Collins FL, Thompson JK 1979 Reliability and standardization in the assessment of self-reported headache pain. Journal of Behavioural Assessment 1:73-86.

Diener I 2001 The impact of cervicogenic headache on patients attending a private physiotherapy practice in cape town. South African Journal of Physiotherapy 57:35-39.

Dworkin SF, Von Korff M, Whitney CW et al 1990 Measurement of characteristic pain intensity in field research. Pain Supplement 5:S290.

Eich E, Reeves JL, Jaeger B, Graff-Radford SB 1985 Memory of pain: relation between past and present pain intensity. Pain 23:375-379.

Feine JS, Lavigne GJ, Dao TT et al 1998 Memories of chronic pain and perceptions of relief. Pain 77.

Gedney JJ, Logan H 2004 Memory For stress-associated acute pain. Journal of Pain 5:83-91.

Hunter M, Philips C, Rachman S 1979 Memory for pain. Pain 6:35-46.

Huskisson S 1974 Measurement of pain. Lancet 2:1127-1131.

International Headache Society, Headache Committee On Clinical Trials 1995 Guidelines for trials of drug treatments in tension-type headache. Cephalalgia 15:165-179.

International Headache Society 2004 The international classification of headache disorders, 2nd edn. Cephalalgia 24(Supplement 1).

Jacobsen G, Ramadan N, Aggarwal S, Newman C 1994 The Henry Ford Hospital headache disability inventory (HDI). Neurology 44:837-842.

Jamieson R, Sbrocco T, Parris W 1989 The influence of physical and psychosocial factors on accuracy of memory for pain in chronic pain patients. Pain 37:289-294.

Jensen MP, Turner LR, Turne RJA, Romano JM 1996 The use of multiple-item scales for pain intensity measure in chronic pain patients. Pain 67:35-40.

Jensen MP, Karoly P 2001 Self-report scales and procedures for assessing pain in adults. In: Turk DC, Melzack R (eds) Handbook of pain assessment, 2nd edn. Guilford Press, New York.

Jull G, Trott P, Potter H et al 2002 A randomized controlled trial of exercise and manipulative therapy for cervicogenic headache. Spine 27:1835-1843.

Jull GA, Niere KR 2004 The cervical spine and headache. In: Boyling JD, Jull G (eds) Grieve's modern manual therapy of the vertebral column, 3rd edn. Churchill Livingstone, Edinburgh.

Klepac RK, Dowling J, Rokke P et al 1981 Interview vs paper-and-pencil administration of the McGill pain questionnaire. Pain 11:241-246.

Kosinski M, Bayliss MS, Bjorner JB et al 2003 A six-item short-form survey for measuring headache impact: The HIT-6™. Quality Of Life Research 12:963-974.

Kryst S, Scherl E 1994 A population-based survey of the social and personal impact of headache. Headache 34:344-350.

Kwong Wj, Pathak DS 2007 Validation of the eleven-point pain scale in the measurement of migraine headache pain. Cephalalgia 27:336-342.

Lefebvre JC, Keefe FJ 2002 Memory for pain: the relationship of pain catastrophising to the recall of daily rheumatoid arthritis pain. Pain 18:56-63.

Linton SJ, Melin L 1982 The accuracy of remembering chronic pain. Pain 13.

Love A, Leboef C, Crisp TC 1989 Chiropractic chronic low back pain sufferers and self-report assessment methods. part 1 a reliability study of the visual analogue scale, the pain drawing and the McGill pain questionnaire. Journal of Manipulative and Physiological Therapeutics 12:21-25.

Lowe NK, Walker SN, Mccallum RC 1991 Confirming the theoretical structure of the McGill pain questionnaire in acute clinical pain. Pain 46:53-60.

Marcus D 2003 Disability and chronic posttraumatic headache. Headache 43:117-121.

Melzack R 1975 The McGill pain questionnaire: major properties and scoring methods. Pain 1:277-299.

Melzack R 1987 The short-form McGill pain questionnaire. Pain 30:191-197.

Melzack R, Katz J 2001 The McGill pain questionnaire: appraisal and current status. In: Turk DC, Melzack R (eds)

Handbook of Pain Assessment, 2nd edn. Guilford Press, New York.

Muller P 2007 Reproducibility and responsiveness of the headache disability questionnaire. Honorsthesis, La Trobe University, Melbourne.

Niere K 1997 Expectations of physiotherapy treatment in headache patients. In: Gerrard B (ed) Tenth Biennial Conference of the Manipulative Physiotherapists' Association of Australia. APA, Melbourne.

Niere K, Jerak A 2004 Comparison of patient report by questionnaire and headache diary for measurement of headache frequency, intensity and duration. Physiotherapy Research International.

Niere K, Quin A 2009 Development of a headache-specific disability measure for patients attending physiotherapy. Manual Therapy 14:45-51.

Niere KR, Robinson PM 1997 Determination of manipulative physiotherapy treatment outcome in headache patients. Manual Therapy 2:199-205.

Ogon M, Krismer M, Sollner W et al 1996 Chronic low back pain measurement with visual analogue scales in different settings. Pain 64:425-428.

Packard RC 1979 What does the headache patient want? Headache 19:370-374.

Price D, Mcgrath P, Rafii A, Buckingham B 1983 The validation of visual analogue scales as ratio measures for chronic and experimental pain. Pain 17:45-56.

Rachman S, Eyrl K 1989 Predicting and remembering chronic pain. Behavioural Research and Therapy 27:621-635.

Rasmussen BK, Jensen R, Olesen J 1991 Questionnaire versus clinical interview in the diagnosis of headache. Headache 31:290-295.

Solomon G 1997 Evolution of the measurement of quality of life in migraine. Neurology 48(suppl 3): S10-S15.

Solomon G, Skobieranda F, Gragg L 1994 Does quality of life differ among headache diagnoses? Analysis

using the medical outcomes study instrument. Headache 34:143-147.

Stewart WF, Lipton RB, Simon D et al 1998 Reliability of an illness severity measure for headache in a population sample of migraine sufferers. Cephalalgia 18:44-51.

Stewart WF, Lipton RB, Kolodner K et al 1999a Reliability of the migraine disability assessment score in a population-based sample of headache sufferers. Cephalalgia 19:107-114.

Stewart WF, Lipton RB, Simon DEA 1999b Validity of an illness severity measure for headache in a population sample of migraine sufferers. Pain 79:291-301.

Stewart WF, Lipton RB, Kolodner KB et al 2000 Validity of the migraine disability assessment (midas) score in comparison to a diary-based measure in a population sample of migraine sufferers. Pain 88:41-52.

Stewart WF, Lipton RB, Dowson AJ, Sawyer J 2001 Development and testing of the migraine disability assessment (Midas) questionnaire to assess headache-related disability. Neurology 56:S20-S28.

Tasmuth T, Estlanderb AM, Kalso E 1996 Effect of present pain and mood on the memory of past postoperative pain in women treated surgically for breast cancer. Pain 68:343-347.

Turk DC, Okifuji A 1999 Assessment of patients' reporting of pain: an integrated perspective. Lancet 353:1784-1788.

Turk DC, Rudy TE, Salovey P 1985 The McGill pain questionnaire reconsidered: confirming the factor structure and examining appropriate uses. Pain 6:385-397.

Vernon HT 1982 Chiropractic manipulative therapy in the treatment of headaches: a retrospective and prospective study. Journal of Manipulative and Physiological Therapeutics 5:109-112.

Whittingham W, Ellis WB, Molyneux TP 1994 The effect of manipulation (toggle recoil technique) for headaches with upper cervical joint dysfunction: a pilot study. Journal of Manipulative and Physiological Therapeutics 17:369-375.

Section Two

Approaches

14

Physiotherapy management of cervicogenic headache: Part 1

Gwendolen Jull

Frequent intermittent headaches, including cervicogenic headache, are common and patients often present to physiotherapists for management. In this chapter the author, a musculoskeletal physiotherapist, evaluates the literature associated with the identification of cervicogenic headache. Differential diagnosis and the role of musculoskeletal and sensorimotor impairments are discussed.

The most common types of frequent intermittent headache are the primary headaches of migraine with and without aura and tension-type headache, and the secondary headache form, cervicogenic headache. Cervicogenic headaches are reported by both genders although, like most headache types, the prevalence is higher in females (Nilsson 1995). Cervicogenic headaches are not restricted to any age group and can be reported by the young to the aged (Fredriksen et al 1987).

The cervical spine and headache

The term 'cervicogenic' is both a generic term to describe headaches arising from cervical musculoskeletal disorders as well as a term for a specific type of headache. The headache type *cervicogenic headache* was defined by Sjaastad et al (1983) on the presence of a set of clinical features. The criteria have been updated with further research in the field (Sjaastad et al 1998). Cervicogenic headache as a distinct headache classification is recognized by the International Headache Society (IHS) (Headache Classification Committee of the International Headache Society 2004).

Cervicogenic headache can be described as a referred pain. The neurophysiological mechanism for cervical spine referral of pain into the head is convergence between cervical afferents from the upper three cervical nerves and afferents from the trigeminal nerve in the trigeminocervical nucleus (Bartsch & Goadsby 2003a, Bogduk 2004). Thus nociceptor afferents from any structure supplied by the upper three nerves are capable of causing headache. This is inclusive of osseous, articular, muscular, neural, and vascular structures, with the upper cervical joints being the most likely primary cause in most cases (Bogduk 2004, 2005). A number of experimental studies have confirmed this referral of pain by either producing head pain through noxious stimulation of upper cervical structures (Dreyfuss et al 1994, Dwyer et al 1990, Feinstein et al 1954) or relieving head pain by anesthetic blocks (Bogduk & Marsland

1988, Lord et al 1994). It is more difficult to explain a direct link between disorders in lower cervical segments/structures and headache. Impairments in other regions of the cervical or thoracic spines have been reported to accompany the upper cervical dysfunction (Bovim et al 1992, Jensen et al 1990, Jull 2002). More directly, there are reported cases where surgical interventions to lower cervical segments have alleviated headache (Fredriksen et al 2003, Persson & Carlsson 1999). It is possible that in such cases, co-existing upper cervical dysfunction was present and/or muscle spasm from the cervicobrachial syndrome simultaneously irritated upper cervical structures (Peterson et al 1975).

The generic term *cervicogenic headache* also implies that despite a certain pattern of clinical features for the headache, there is no unique patho-anatomical lesion, nociceptive cause, or segmental source for cervicogenic headache. Several pathological entities have been aligned with this headache type, including facet joint arthropathies and disc disease (Ahn et al 2005, Trevor-Jones 1964), trauma (Drottning et al 2002, Radanov et al 2001) or postural strain. The pathological debate becomes somewhat academic in any individual case of cervicogenic headache because, as reflects the situation in low back pain, neither plain X-rays nor magnetic resonance imaging (MRI) have been shown to be sensitive to detect relevant pathological change (Coskun et al 2003, Fredriksen et al 1989, Hinderaker et al 1995). Accordingly, the IHS diagnostic criteria explicitly reject radiological evidence of cervical spondylosis or osteochondrosis as valid evidence for a diagnosis of cervicogenic headache (Headache Classification Committee of the International Headache Society 2004).

There is now little dispute about the existence of cervicogenic headache. However, there is debate over its differential diagnosis from other common frequent intermittent headache types, notably migraine without aura and tension-type headache. There is symptomatic overlap between these headache types. In response, the IHS classification of headache disorders (Headache Classification Committee of the International Headache Society 2004) states that it is insufficient to list manifestations of headaches for diagnosis. Other criteria are required to diagnose cervicogenic headache. The IHS (Headache Classification Committee of the International Headache Society 2004) has indicated that to diagnose a cervicogenic headache, there must be evidence that the headache can be attributed to a neck disorder either by: *(a) demonstration of clinical signs that implicate a source of pain in the neck, or (b) abolition of headache following diagnostic blockade of a cervical structure or its nerve supply using placebo or other adequate controls* (p. 117).

Diagnosis of cervicogenic headache

The diagnostic criteria for cervicogenic headache as described by Sjaastad et al (1998) are presented in Box 14.1. Not all features will be present in every patient, but symptoms within Criteria 1 to 3 are mandatory while those in Criteria 4 to 6 are variably present and not obligatory to make the diagnosis of cervicogenic headache. None of the features, taken singularly, is unique to cervicogenic headache (Fishbain et al 2003, Leone et al 1995, 1998, Solomon & Lipton 1993). Vincent (1998) investigated the strength of a number of symptoms collectively to identify the headache types using the criteria for cervicogenic headache (Sjaastad et al 1990) and those of the IHS for tension-type and migraine headache. Although cervicogenic headache patients

Box 14.1

Diagnostic criteria for cervicogenic headache (adapted from Sjaastad et al 1998).

1. Symptoms and signs of neck involvement
   - (i) Precipitation of comparable head pain by:
     - – Neck movement or sustained awkward head postures, and/or
     - – External pressure over the upper cervical or occipital region on the symptomatic side
   - (ii) Restriction of range of motion in the neck
   - (iii) Ipsilateral neck, shoulder or arm pain

2. Response to diagnostic anesthetic blocks

3. Unilaterality of head pain, without sideshift

4. Head pain characteristics
   - (i) Moderate-severe, non-throbbing and non-lancinating pain, usually starting in the neck
   - (ii) Episodes of varying duration
   - (iii) Fluctuating continuous pain

5. (i) Lack of effect of idomethician
   - (ii) Lack of effect of ergotomine and sumatriptan
   - (iii) Female gender
   - (iv) Not infrequent history of head or indirect neck trauma

6. (i) Nausea
   - (ii) Phonophobia and photophobia
   - (iii) Dizziness
   - (iv) Ipsilateral blurred vision
   - (v) Difficulties on swallowing
   - (vi) Ipsilateral edema, mostly in the periocular area

reported myriad symptoms and aggravating features which overlapped with other headache types, Vincent (1998) found that the features which most distinguished cervicogenic headache were unilateral, side-locked headache, and headache association with neck postures or movements.

The pivotal symptom of neck pain is pertinent to a discussion of the differential diagnosis of cervicogenic headache. Patients and clinicians alike can be tempted to entertain the notion that neck pain accompanying headache suggests a cervical musculoskeletal cause or component. However, neck pain is not an uncommon accompaniment of migraine and tension-type headache (Bartsch & Goadsby 2003a, Leone et al 1998, Fishbain et al 2001, Solomon 1997) and can accompany temporomandibular joint dysfunction (Montgomery et al 1992). This is due to the bi-directional interactions between trigeminal afferents and afferents from the three upper cervical nerves in the trigeminocervical nucleus (Bartsch & Goadsby 2002, 2003b). In other words, as much as nociceptive activity in cervical afferents can result in referred pain to the head, nociceptive activity in the trigeminal afferents can refer pain into the neck. The pathogeneses of migraine and tension-type headache do not lie in cervical musculoskeletal dysfunction. There is no evidence of biological markers for the activation of the trigeminovascular system in cervicogenic headache as is found in migraine (Frese et al 2005). The question is whether a pain referred to the neck can, over time, set up secondary cervical musculoskeletal changes which could be assisted with physical therapies.

Another factor is a history of head or neck trauma associated with the onset of headache. It is also not illogical for either patients or clinicians to be tempted to accredit a cervicogenic origin of headache when the history of headache is related to a whiplash injury. However Radanov et al (2001), for example, investigated 112 patients with persistent headache following a whiplash injury and found that 37% of headaches were tension-type, 27% were migraine, 18% were cervicogenic, and 18% were unclassifiable. Thus the headache type is not necessarily cervicogenic even though related to a neck injury.

While some level of certainty can be gained from a collection of symptoms to diagnose cervicogenic headache (see Box 14.1), the long history of challenge in diagnosis continues today (Xiaobin et al 2005). It is evident that more evidence is necessary to define cervicogenic headache. It is suggested that this can be provided by a detailed examination of the cervical musculoskeletal system. The possible role of any cervical musculoskeletal dysfunction associated with neck pain in migraine and tension-type headache could also be determined from such an examination.

Cervical musculoskeletal impairment in headache

With the symptomatic overlap between frequent intermittent types and the frequent co-occurrence of neck pain, more evidence of a cervical origin of headache is required to make the diagnosis of cervicogenic headache. Both the IHS (Headache Classification Committee of the International Headache Society 2004) and the Cervicogenic Headache International Study Group classification criteria for cervicogenic headache (Sjaastad et al 1998) include the use of diagnostic anesthetic blocks (see Box 14.1, point 2). There are those who strongly advocate the use of diagnostic nerve or joint blocks as the only valid way to diagnose cervicogenic headache (Bogduk 2005). There is no in-principle objection to this stance. However for the blocks to be valid, they must be placebo-controlled and performed under fluoroscopic guidance (Lord et al 1995). The diagnostic techniques are not office procedures (Bogduk 2005). In view of the relative frequency of frequent intermittent headache in the

community, the resources, expertise and manpower requirements of this diagnostic procedure, it is unlikely to be able to serve in the diagnosis of the vast majority of potential cervicogenic patients. Cervicogenic headache patients are generally managed conservatively as a first line of treatment (Pollmann et al 1997). Diagnostic blocks should be considered, and are a necessary pre-treatment procedure, for those more severe and recalcitrant headaches (Drottning et al 2002, Lord & Bogduk 2002) to guide surgical techniques such as radiofrequency neurotomies (Govind et al 2003, McDonald et al 1999, van Suijlekom et al 1998).

The other evidence acceptable under the guidelines of the IHS to diagnose a cervicogenic headache is the demonstration of clinical signs that implicate a source of pain in the neck, using reliable and valid operational tests to establish causal relationships. The physical criteria for cervicogenic headache in the current classification criteria are sparse with only restricted neck motion and palpable tenderness over the upper cervical or occipital region on the symptomatic side listed (see Box 14.1). It is thus pertinent to review studies which have investigated cervical musculoskeletal impairment in cervicogenic headache patients and other neck disorders to determine the potential for tests of musculoskeletal features to distinguish this headache type from other frequent intermittent headache types.

Range of movement

Restriction of neck motion is one of the two published criteria for cervicogenic headache. Dumas et al (2001) measured range of motion in cervicogenic headache patients and compared ranges in those whose headaches were related to a motor vehicle crash to those whose headaches were of an insidious origin. They found that range of motion was significantly reduced in the whiplash group, but the insidious onset group was not different to the control group. However Zwart (1997) measured range of neck movement in subjects with cervicogenic headache, migraine, and tension-type headache and compared values to a non-headache control group. There was a significant reduction in range of movement (axial rotation and flexion/extension) in cervicogenic headache subjects compared to the other headache groups and asymptomatic controls. Notably, there were no differences in range of motion between the control subjects of similar mean age and the migraine and tension-type headache groups, despite a prolonged history of headache (migraine group, mean duration 13.4 years; tension-type headache, mean duration 10.4 years). This suggests that cervical musculoskeletal impairment may not accompany migraine and tension-type headache, despite headache chronicity, and would suggest that reduced range of movement might be a strong diagnostic characteristic of cervicogenic headache. Nevertheless, Bogduk (2005) highlights that there was some overlap in ranges of motion between the groups, thus preventing a diagnostic threshold of abnormality. Additionally the effects of age on range of motion must be considered when range of motion is taken as a singular feature (Chen et al 1999, Sjaastad et al 2003). Despite these issues, measurement of cervical range of movement could form part of a diagnostic battery of tests. This should be inclusive of a measure of head rotation with the neck positioned in full flexion to bias rotation to the C1–C2 segment (Hall & Robinson 2004) as this measure reliably detects cervicogenic headaches associated with dysfunction primarily at this segment (Ogince et al 2007).

Manual palpation of symptomatic joint dysfunction

Restricted movement is characteristic of cervicogenic headache yet radiological analysis has not proven to be successful in identifying symptomatic segments (Antonaci et al 2001, Fredriksen et al 1989, Pfaffenrath et al 1987). Manual palpation is an alternate clinical method of assessment to determine the presence of symptomatic segmental dysfunction. It is used by manual therapy practitioners of several health disciplines and relies on the provocation of pain and the perception of altered tissue compliance (often segmental muscle reaction) to gentle manual pressure applied rhythmically on each cervical segment.

It has been difficult to gain acceptable intra- and inter-rater reliability when the reliability of separate components of manual examination (magnitude of pain provocation and segmental mobility) are tested (Pool et al 2004). A recent study using one medical examiner (King et al 2007) demonstrated high sensitivity but low specificity of manual examination to detect the precise locations of symptomatic joints within a group of neck pain patients. However, in studies where the requirement of manual segmental examination is only to diagnose the presence or absence of symptomatic cervical joints in a patient's headache syndrome, results are indicating that it is a suitably reliable clinical test. This has been shown both directly and indirectly in various studies which have either tested the accuracy of manual examination or used manual examination to differentiate cervicogenic headache from other headache types or control subjects (Amiri et al 2007, Gijsberts et al 1999a & b, Jull et al 1988, 1997, 2007a, Zito et al 2006) to locate the segmental source of pain in cervicogenic headache (Hall & Robinson 2004, Jull et al 1988, Lord et al 1994, Ogince et al 2007).

Impairment in the muscle system

Impaired muscle function is a hallmark of musculoskeletal disorders. Recent research is beginning to unravel the complexity of the cervical and cervicobrachial muscle impairments associated with cervical spine disorders (Falla 2004). Impairment is present on a number of levels of function. These include the aberrant way in which muscles are used and coordinated in various tasks, as well as declines in fatigability, endurance capacity at both high and low loads, and muscle strength.

Changes in patterns of muscle activity

Several studies have documented changes in the patterns of usage of muscles in the cervicobrachial region in patients with neck pain disorders, using cognitive, functional and automatic tasks.

In the cognitive task of craniocervical flexion (craniocervical flexion test, CCFT), the pattern of activity between the deep (longus capitis and colli) and superficial cervical flexor muscles (sternocleidomastoid (SCM) and anterior scalene (AS) muscles) has been examined in a number of studies. The CCFT assesses the contractile capacity of the longus capitis and colli to perform, in five stages, progressively increasing inner range contractions in their primary anatomical action. These muscles have been shown to be important for the control of the cervical curve and segments (Mayoux-Benhamou et al 1994). A novel surface EMG electrode inbuilt into a nasopharyngeal catheter has recently allowed direct measurement of the longus capitis and colli in the CCFT in a laboratory setting (Falla et al 2003a, 2006). It has been shown that patients with neck pain demonstrate a reduced level of EMG activity in the longus capitis/colli across all stages of the CCFT test compared to control subjects and this is associated with higher measured activity in the SCM and AS in the neck pain patients (Falla et al 2004a). Several studies have shown this impairment in the deep cervical flexors as well as the altered muscle strategy in the superficial flexors in patients with cervical disorders, including cervicogenic headache, either using less invasive versions of the test by measuring the EMG activity in the superficial flexors only (Jull 2000, Jull et al 2004a, Sterling et al 2003, Zito et al 2006) (Fig. 14.1) or through clinical assessment of the stage of the test that neck pain patients

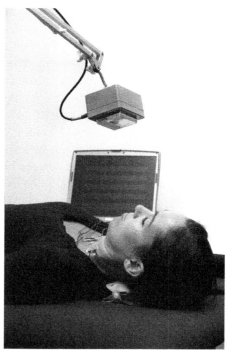

Figure 14.1 ● The craniocervical flexion test measuring activity in the sternocleidomastoid and anterior scalene muscles with surface EMG. A pressure sensor is positioned behind the neck to monitor the slight flattening of the cervical curve which accompanies the contraction of longus colli. The test is performed in five stages of increasingly inner range craniocervical flexion. Patients are guided to each stage with feedback from the pressure sensor.

and control subjects can achieve (Chiu et al 2005, Jull et al 1999, 2002, Petersen 2003).

Studies have also investigated the pattern of activity of cervicobrachial muscles in patients with neck pain of both insidious and traumatic onset during functional activities (Falla et al 2004b, Nederhand et al 2003). More specifically, activity in the upper trapezeii (Falla et al 2004b, Nederhand et al 2003) and SCM and AS muscles was measured (Falla et al 2004b) while subjects performed a repetitive unilateral task using their right hand, which involved marking three targets positioned on a desk in front of them. Collectively, these studies revealed that the neck pain subjects demonstrated higher co-activation of the contralateral upper trapezius, SCM and AS muscles compared to control subjects as well as a decreased ability to relax the muscles on completion of the task. This is analogous with the increased activity in the SCM and AS demonstrated in the CCFT. The ipsilateral upper trapezius demonstrated lesser activity, which could have been an adaptation to pain. Bansevicius and Sjaastad (1996) measured activity (EMG) of shoulder-neck and facial muscles as well as pain levels in cervicogenic headache subjects before, during, and after a stressful reaction time test. In the headache patients as compared to control subjects, pain values increased markedly for the shoulder region during the test, while pain values for the temple and neck increased in the post-test period. Upper trapezius activity increased significantly in the headache patients during the test while there was no significant increase in trapezius activity in control subjects. Thus altered patterns of muscle activity are present in patients with cervical musculoskeletal disorders in functional and stress related tasks.

The timing of cervical flexor muscle activation has also been measured in automatic function during postural perturbations in neck pain patients. Evidence indicates that there is a feed-forward response of the cervical muscles during postural perturbations, presumably to provide stability for the neck as well as the head for the visual and vestibular systems (Falla et al 2004c, Gurfinkel et al 1988). Falla et al (2004d) investigated temporal parameters of deep and superficial cervical flexor muscle activation in neck pain patients and controls using a rapid unilateral arm movement task to induce an internal postural perturbation. The neck pain subjects displayed delayed onsets of all muscles monitored in the task, the longus capitis/colli as well as the SCM and AS muscles, in comparison to the control subjects. The delays in the longus capitis/colli were the most substantial. These delays in neck muscle activity associated with arm movement indicate a deficit in the automatic feed-forward control of cervical spine stability in the neck pain patients. This change in the feed-forward response in persons already with neck pain, might leave the cervical spine further vulnerable to strain, a factor worth considering given the often recurrent and prolonged histories of pain commonly encountered in patients with neck pain and cervicogenic headache.

Muscle fatigability, endurance and strength

There is evidence that the neck muscles become more fatigable in patients with neck pain. Gogia and Sabbahi (1994) measured fatigue patterns of the neck flexors and extensors in neck pain patients. Muscle fatigue was evident in both flexors and extensors at 80% and 100% of maximum voluntary contraction (MVC) when compared to control subjects. However when measured at 50% MVC, fatigue was only evident in the neck flexors. Falla et al (2003b) examined fatigability of the sternocleidomastoid (SCM) and anterior scalene (AS) muscles during sustained cervical flexion contractions in patients with chronic neck pain and control subjects and investigated fatigue at lower levels of MVC (25% and 50%). Greater myoelectric manifestations of SCM and AS muscle fatigue were identified for the neck pain patient group. The results confirmed Gogia and Sabbahi's (1994) findings of greater fatigability of the cervical flexors in neck pain patients at moderate loads (50% MVC) but also established greater flexor muscle fatigability during low load sustained contractions (25% MVC). When functional requirements of every day activities are considered, this level of contraction is more commensurate with daily cervical muscle use than MVCs and has implications for the nature of rehabilitative exercise. Similarly, greater fatigability has been shown in the upper trapezius muscles in patients with neck pain with an active repetitive arm elevation task (Falla & Farina 2005).

In tandem with the findings of increased fatigability in the neck muscles, mechanical measures of muscle performance have revealed that reduced muscle endurance as well as decreased muscle strength is present in patients with neck disorders, including cervicogenic headache (Barton & Hayes 1996, Dumas et al 2001, Placzek et al 1999, Treleaven et al 1994, Watson & Trott 1993). Two researchers have specifically focused on the measure of craniocervical flexion, as distinct from cervical flexion, using specially designed dynamometers (O'Leary et al 2005, Watson & Trott 1993). Both studies determined that the craniocervical flexors had reduced strength and endurance compared to control subjects in line with the studies testing global cervical strength and endurance. Notably, O'Leary et al (2007) also found that neck pain patients had a significantly reduced capacity to sustain isometric craniocervical flexion muscle contractions at 20% of MVC and 50% of MVC, which not only

supports the findings of fatigability at these loads by Falla et al (2003b) but supports the need in rehabilitation to exercise the muscles over a range of contraction intensities.

Muscle length

Muscle stretching has been included in early multimodal management approaches for cervicogenic headache (Graff-Radford et al 1987, Jaeger 1989). Research into the prevalence of muscle tightness in cervicogenic headache is sparse, probably reflecting the difficulty in developing quantitative measures to represent the length of muscles in the cervicobrachial region. Three studies (Jull et al 1999, Treleaven et al 1994, Zito et al 2006) have used conventional clinical tests of muscle length to variously assess the upper trapezius, levator scapulae, scalene, suboccipital extensor and pectoral muscle groups in cervicogenic headache cohorts compared to control or other headache groups. The notable finding of these studies was that differences between headache and control groups were not remarkable. The overall incidence of clinically relevant muscle tightness was comparatively low albeit higher in the cervicogenic headache groups and distributed across the various muscles. Muscle tightness was not necessarily present in all headache subjects suggesting that assessment of the individual patient is necessary to guide prescription of any muscle lengthening exercises.

Sensorimotor system

There has been considerable interest in recent times in impairments in the sensorimotor system in patients with neck pain, particularly as symptoms of light-headedness or dizziness and unsteadiness are not infrequently reported. The deep muscles of the neck in particular have a vast density of muscle spindles (Bakker & Richmond 1982, Boyd-Clark et al 2002, Kulkarni et al 2001, Liu et al 2003), and there are complex functional and reflex interactions between the vestibular and visual systems and the cervical somatosensory system (Bolton & Tracey 1992, Corneil et al 2002, Gdowski & McCrea 2000, Hirai et al 1984, Isa & Sasaki 2002, Shinoda et al 1994, Xiong & Matsushita 2001) which are likely to provide the bases for these symptoms. The measures that have been made in patients with neck disorders include measures of joint position error, standing balance and eye movement control.

Joint position error

Joint position error (JPE) is commonly used as a measure of cervical kinesthetic sense. It is a measure of the ability to relocate the natural head posture whilst vision is occluded (Revel et al 1991). This test has been found to be the most repeatable and reliable of a group of similar tests (Kristjansson et al 2001, 2003). Greater cervical JPEs have been shown in persons with both idiopathic neck pain and neck pain associated with trauma (whiplash) (Heikkila & Astrom 1996, Heikkila & Wengren 1998, Kristjansson et al 2003, Revel et al 1991, Treleaven et al 2003). Dumas et al (2001) failed to find any difference in JPE in patients with cervicogenic headache of insidious or post-traumatic onset, but the authors had concerns with their methodology. It has also been shown that JPE is greatest in those subjects who report dizziness in association with their neck pain (Treleaven et al 2003).

Standing balance

Several studies have documented disturbances to standing balance in patients with neck pain using computerized dynamic posturography (Alund et al 1991, 1993, Karlberg et al 1995,1996, Kogler et al 2000, Sjostrom et al 2003, Treleaven et al 2005a). There are no known studies of balance, specific to cervicogenic headache. Nevertheless considering the frequency with which balance disturbances have been identified in patients with neck disorders, this is an area for future research. Clinical assessment of balance warrants consideration in the physical examination of cervicogenic headache patients.

The clinical test for sensory interaction in balance that was developed by Shumway-Cook and Horak (1986) is suitable for the clinical environment. It consists of six tests that gradually alter the degree of difficulty for balance in bilateral stance. Balance is tested with eyes open, eyes closed and under visual conflict on firm and soft surfaces. Comfortable stance is commonly used, although narrow, tandem and unilateral stance can be used to challenge the cervical sensorimotor system at higher levels, which may be in order for cervical musculoskeletal disorders.

Eye movement control

As with standing balance, there are no known studies that have specifically investigated eye movement control in a cervicogenic headache group. However a number of studies have been undertaken which have identified abnormalities in eye movement, using electro-oculography, in patients with both idiopathic neck pain and whiplash associated disorders (Gimse et al 1996, Heikkila et al 1998, Hildingsson et al 1989, 1993, Tjell & Rosenhall 1998, Treleaven et al 2005b).

Abnormalities of smooth pursuit eye movements may be present in disorders of the vestibular system, the central nervous system as well as cervical disorders. The smooth pursuit neck torsion test was developed by Tjell and

Rosenhall (1998) to attempt to differentiate a cervical origin from these other causes. In the test, the eye movement pursuit is measured in a neutral head position and measured again when the neck is rotated (torsioned) via the trunk with the head kept still. The rotated position stimulates the cervical receptors but not the vestibular receptors. Tjell and Rosenhall (1998) were able to demonstrate that there was no change in smooth pursuit when measured in a neutral compared to a neck-rotated position in normal subjects or in subjects with central nervous system or vestibular dysfunction, but there was a difference in subjects with neck disorders.

The results from several studies of neck pain patients indicate that impairments in eye movement control are greater in subjects with whiplash associated disorders than those with idiopathic neck pain and within these categories, disturbances are greater in those who report the symptom of dizziness or light-headedness and visual disturbances (Gimse et al 1997, Tjell & Rosenhall 1998, Treleaven et al 2005b). As with balance disturbances, there is sufficient evidence of this impairment in eye movement control in patients with cervical disorders to warrant specific research in a cervicogenic headache cohort. It could be suggested that there are also sufficient indications to warrant tests of eye movement control in the clinical setting, especially in cervicogenic headache patients presenting with symptoms of light-headedness or dizziness, or visual disturbances in association with their headache (Fig. 14.2).

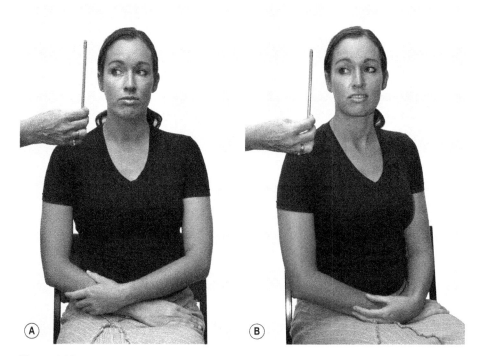

Figure 14.2 • Eye follow can be tested in the clinical setting by observing for saccades while the patient follows movement of a pen through an excursion of approximately 40° either side of the midline. Performance in a neutral position of the head is compared to that when the trunk is rotated beneath a stationary head (cervical torsion). An increase in the number of saccades in the neck torsion position suggests a cervical cause.

Neural system

Compression of neural structures is a rare cause of cervicogenic headache but cases of compression of the upper cervical nerve roots, the dorsal root ganglion or the greater occipital nerve have been recorded (Hildebrandt & Jansen 1984, Jansen 2000, Jansen et al 1989a, 1989b, Pikus & Phillips 1995). This usually results in a distinct neuropathic type pain and can be clearly identified (Bogduk 2004).

The dura mater of the upper cervical cord and the posterior cranial fossa receives innervation from branches of the upper three cervical nerves (Bogduk 2004) and as such, is capable of being one of the causes of cervicogenic headache. Anatomical studies have demonstrated fibrous connections between the rectus capitus posterior minor and the cervical dura mater (Hack et al 1995) and continuity has been observed between the ligamentum nuchae and the posterior spinal dura at the first and second cervical levels (Mitchell et al 1998). Neural tissues such as the dura could become a source of cervicogenic headache in association with, for example, inflammatory reactions from an upper cervical musculoskeletal disorder. Neural tissue may become sensitive to movement.

Little is known of the role of neural tissue mechanosensitivity in cervicogenic headache. In two studies which used the clinical structural differentiation test (passive upper cervical flexion, which is repeated with the neural tissues pre-tensioned by either straight leg raise or placement of the upper limb in the brachial plexus provocation test position) (Jull 1994), the incidence was low: 10% of 200 (Jull et al 2002) and 7.4% of 27 (Zito et al 2006) cervicogenic headache subjects. This suggests that although neural tissue mechanosensitivity may have a role in a few cervicogenic headache syndromes, in general it is not a strong characteristic sign.

Cervical posture

The forward head posture is believed to be a common poor postural position associated with cervicogenic headache. However studies in this area are divided in their findings and have not produced convincing evidence for a strong association between static measures of the forward head postural position and neck pain or neck pain and headache (Dumas et al 2001, Griegel-Morris et al 1992, Grimmer 1997, Lee et al 2003, Treleaven et al 1994, Watson & Trott 1993). Nevertheless, evidence is emerging that functional postures may have greater relevance. It has been shown that with sedentary work, for example at a computer, the head subtly drifts into a more forward position in persons with neck pain as opposed to those without neck pain (Falla et al 2007a, Szeto et al 2002) and this is associated with altered muscle recruitment patterns in the neck extensor and upper trapezius muscles in office workers with neck pain (Szeto et al 2003). This highlights the need for attention on training functional working postures in rehabilitation.

Patterns of impairment in cervicogenic headache

The attraction of anesthetic blocks is that they can definitively identify a pain source (joint blocks) or at least the segmental source of pain (nerve blocks) for the diagnosis of cervicogenic headache. It is a more challenging task to match this procedure with a single physical sign in the cervical musculoskeletal system due to the range of values that can be present in any single physical test (Bogduk 2005). Acknowledging this problem, a study was undertaken in which a battery of clinical measures was used to examine a community-based population with chronic frequent intermittent headache, inclusive of those with migraine, tension-type and cervicogenic headache (Amiri et al 2007, Jull et al 2007a). The range of cervical movement, the presence of painful cervical segmental dysfunction (manual examination), SCM activity in the CCFT, cervical flexor and extensor muscle strength, an ultrasound imaging measure of selected extensor muscles at the C2 level and cervical joint position error (JPE) were measured. Forty-five percent of the group reported one headache type and the remainder reported two or more concurrent headaches.

This study revealed that of subjects reporting one headache, the cervicogenic headache group had greater impairments in all cervical musculoskeletal measures with the exception of JPE. Interestingly, the musculoskeletal profile of those classified as tension-type or migraine was no different to the control group. It was further shown that a pattern of musculoskeletal impairment discriminated cervicogenic headache from migraine, tension-type, and control subjects with a high sensitivity and specificity. This pattern was inclusive of the presence of palpable symptomatic upper cervical joint dysfunction (C0–C3) in association with restricted range of motion (extension in this study) and impairment in the craniocervical flexion test. Furthermore when the subjects with two or more concurrent frequent intermittent headaches were grouped on these three factors, it was found that this pattern of musculoskeletal impairment was only present in those subjects who were classified with a

cervicogenic headache as one of their two or more headache types. Thus while a single physical measure in a headache patient, for example restricted range of movement, may not be unique to cervicogenic headache, if this restriction in range is accompanied by palpably painful upper cervical joint dysfunction and impairment in tests of cervical muscle function, then there is a high certainty for a diagnosis of cervicogenic headache.

Conclusion

Cervicogenic headache results in substantial quality of life burdens, comparable (albeit with differences) to that of migraine and tension-type headache (van Suijlekom et al 2003). The historical disputes about the existence of headaches related to cervical spine disorders have lost impetus. Nevertheless the challenge remains to accurately differentiate cervicogenic headache from other headache types so that the most appropriate treatment can be offered to the headache patient. Latest research suggests that this can be achieved with the presence of a pattern of symptoms characteristic of cervicogenic headache in combination with a pattern of cervical movement and muscle impairments. A better understanding of the precise nature of the impairments in the cervical musculoskeletal function associated with cervicogenic headache lays the basis for optimal programs of conservative management.

References

References appear at the end of Part 2 of this discussion (Chapter 15, p. 189).

Chapter Fifteen

15

Physiotherapy management of cervicogenic headache: Part 2

Gwendolen Jull

Physiotherapy management of cervicogenic headache is supported by high quality scientific research. In this chapter the author, a musculoskeletal physiotherapist, presents a multimodal management regimen addressing articular dysfunction, correction of muscle system impairments, and retraining of sensorimotor deficits. Patient education and promotion of healthy work and lifestyle practices are seen as integral to the program.

Conservative therapies are the first line approach to the management of cervicogenic headache (Pollmann et al 1997, Sjaastad et al 1997) with surgical procedures such as radiofrequency neurotomies (Boswell et al 2007) being indicated in those with chronic and usually severe headaches which are recalcitrant to conservative care. The conservative physical therapies of manipulative therapy and specific therapeutic exercise have been shown to be effective in the management of cervicogenic headache (Jull et al 2002).

Accurate differential diagnosis is fundamental to successful management of any headache type. Diagnostic accuracy for cervicogenic headache is strengthened in the presence of a pattern of symptomatic features in association with a pattern of cervical musculoskeletal impairment. Cervicogenic headache is usually a benign disorder but caution is required in instances of acute onset severe headache. The vertebral artery in its upper course, as well as the spinal dura mater and the dura mater of the posterior cranial fossa, receive a nerve supply from the upper cervical nerves (Bogduk 2004). Hence occipital or suboccipital pain may accompany the acute onset of severe headaches of more sinister pathologies such as a spontaneous dissection of the vertebral artery (Sturzenegger 1994). Patients presenting with first time severe headache or headaches that are progressively worsening always require urgent medical review (Silberstein 1992).

The evidence supports a multimodal approach for management of cervical musculoskeletal disorders (Gross et al 2007). Conservative management may use several therapeutic strategies in the rehabilitation of the cervicogenic headache patient. One management program is outlined in Table 15.1 and is based on the evidence of the impairments presenting in the cervical musculoskeletal system. The program aims to reduce headache and associated symptoms and to prevent recurrences by rehabilitating the musculoskeletal impairments associated with headache and educating the patient on healthy work and lifestyle practices. Several of the intervention strategies have overlapping effects on the pain, motor and sensorimotor

Table 15.1 A multimodal approach to the management of cervicogenic headache.

Target	Intervention

Outcome measures	Patient centered
	    Headache frequency, intensity, duration
	    Neck Disability Index (Vernon & Silvano 1991)
	    Patient Specific Functional Scale (Westaway et al 1998)
	Physical
	    Quantitative evaluation of physical impairments e.g. ROM, CCFT

Pain management	Assurance, education and advice Medical management (pharmaceutical) Specific low load therapeutic exercise, emphasizing muscle control Manipulative therapy
Movement dysfunction	Manipulative therapy Specific active exercise directed to the segmental level
Muscle system	Re-education of muscle control of the craniocervical and cervicobrachial regions Re-education of craniocervical and cervicobrachial movement patterns Training of neck muscle endurance at different contraction intensities Training of neck muscle strength
Sensorimotor system	Re-education of kinesthetic awareness Re-education of balance Re-education of eye movement control
Neural system	Management of articular dysfunction Gentle mobilization of neural structures
Self management	Advice on ergonomic aspects of occupation and activities of daily living Strategies to prevent factors provocative of headache; adaptation to new work or movement strategies. Posture re-education for work and daily activities. Participation in specific exercise program.

ROM = range of motion; CCFT = Cranio-cervical flexion test.

systems. A brief description of this physical therapy approach to management is provided. It is presented in separate sections, although in clinical practice, these procedures are implemented concurrently as per the individual patient's needs and are progressed accordingly.

Pain management

The headache and neck pain is managed with several strategies often initially in association with analgesics (Pollmann et al 1997, Sjaastad et al 1997), with a reduction in their use being a positive outcome measure for the effects of rehabilitation. Good communication and patient education is essential. Assurance is provided on the benign nature of cervicogenic headache and education is given about the pathophysiology of pain and headache and its links with cervical impairments and provocative lifestyle factors. Understanding the condition and its features relieves anxiety and places the patient well to be an informed and active contributor in the rehabilitation process.

Therapeutic strategies such as manipulative therapy and specific exercise for both the motor and sensorimotor systems have been shown in controlled trials to have pain relieving effects as well as other physiological effects on the relevant systems (Hoving et al 2002, Jull et al 2002, Nilsson et al 1997, Revel et al 1994). Manipulative therapy procedures appear to act on multiple levels of the central nervous system to achieve their analgesic effects (Dishman & Burke 2003, Haavik-Taylor & Murphy 2007, Skyba et al 2003, Sterling et al 2001, Vicenzino et al 1998). Manipulative therapy and therapeutic exercise used singularly or in combination have been shown to reduce headache frequency and intensity in persons with cervicogenic headache (Jull et al 2002, Nilsson et al 1997, Schoensee et al 1995).

Movement dysfunction

As discussed in Chapter 14, the presence of painful dysfunction in the upper cervical joints and associated regions as well as restriction of cervical motion is pathognomic of cervicogenic headache. Both manipulative therapy and active exercise can be used in a complementary way to address these painful movement impairments. Several manipulative therapy approaches have been used in the management of cervicogenic headache including high velocity manipulative thrust techniques, low velocity passive mobilization techniques and techniques combining passive movement at the segmental level with active movement (Jull et al 2002, Mulligan 1995, Nilsson et al 1997, Schoensee et al 1995, Whittingham et al 1994). The choice of manipulative therapy technique is derived from the information gained about the nature and direction of the movement dysfunction in the physical examination as well as the pain response to movement and there are numerous texts describing such techniques. Suffice it to comment that both high velocity and low velocity manipulative therapy procedures have been shown to have benefit for cervicogenic headache (Jull et al 2002, Nilsson et al 1997, Schoensee et al 1995, Whittingham et al 1994). Debate in the future will likely continue on risk/benefit issues of the two forms of technique (Dabbs & Lauretti 1995, Ernst 2002, Haldeman et al 1999).

Active exercise is an essential reinforcement of movement gained with manipulative therapy procedures as some of the range gained from these passive treatments can be lost within 48 hours (Nansel et al 1990). The exercises should be directed to the dysfunctional segment(s) as well as regionally. For example, the exercise may focus on craniocervical movements with, for instance, the neck prepositioned in flexion so that head rotation can mobilize more specifically the C1–C2 articulation (Amiri et al 2003, Hall & Robinson 2004). Assistive straps can be used to apply a self-assisted mobilization to a particular spinal level (Mulligan 2003). The combined use of arm elevation and head rotation may assist mobilization of the often hypomobile cervicothoracic region (Stewart et al 1995).

Muscle system

Improved understanding of the complexity of the impairments in the muscle system and its control by the central nervous system in cervical disorders is continually shaping therapeutics. Some attention will be given to a brief description of one exercise approach based on the current evidence of the impairments in the muscle system. It seems unlikely that these muscle impairments will resolve spontaneously without specific intervention, even though pain may have subsided (Jull et al 2002, Sterling et al 2003). Restoring as normal function as possible in the muscle system would logically be concordant with the aim of intervening into

> ### Box 15.1
>
> **Exercise approach to management of muscle system impairment.**
> Stage 1: Specific activation of deep and postural supporting muscles
> Stage 2: Training endurance capacity
> Stage 3: Training movement patterns
> Stage 4: Higher level strength and endurance training

the chronic nature of this condition and preventing recurrent episodes of headache.

There are several ways that muscles can be exercised but evidence is emerging which supports the benefits of specificity of exercise relevant to the particular impairment (Falla et al 2007a & b, Jull et al 2007b). The exercise approach is summarized in Box 15.1; it emphasizes motor learning in the first instance (Jull et al 2004b). The program comprises progressive stages and patients progress through the different stages as they master each step. The progress is rapid for some (2–4 weeks) but may take 6–8 weeks in others.

Specific activation of deep and postural supporting muscles

An emphasis is placed initially on specific activation and training of the deep neck and scapular supporting muscles in formal exercises as well as incorporating their activity in their functional role of active postural support. This is in response to the reduced activation capacity and the changed movement strategies that patients have been shown to use in response to this deep muscle weakness (Falla et al 2004a, Jull et al 2004a).

In the therapeutics, attention is first placed on the patient achieving correct patterns of movement to ensure that the target muscles can be activated without substitution from inappropriate synergists. The re-education of

the deep cervical flexors, longus capitis and colli, commences with the patient learning to perform craniocervical flexion as a true rotation in the sagittal plane in a supine lying position. Feedback of the correct action is gained by the patient perceiving the cephalad-caudad slide of the back of the head on the supporting surface and a large range of movement is used initially for movement awareness. Self-palpation of the superficial flexors provides feedback to help the patient achieve the action without unwanted use of the superficial flexor muscles (Fig. 15.1).

Two sets of exercise are practiced for the neck extensors. The first is craniocervical rotation (which emphasizes the action of the obliquus capitis superior and inferior) and craniocervical extension (which emphasizes the action of the rectus capitis posterior major and minor). The second is active cervical extension maintaining the craniocervical position in a neutral position. While all neck extensors will contribute to this action, it emphasizes the cervical extensors (for example the semispinalis cervicis and multifidus rather than the extensors of the head (splenius capitis and semispinalis capitis)) (Fig. 15.2).

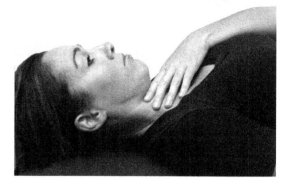

Figure 15.1 • Training the pattern of craniocervical flexion with the patient palpating the superficial neck flexors to ensure performance is with the deep longus capitis and colli. Downward and upward eye movement is used to help facilitate the flexors and extensors respectively.

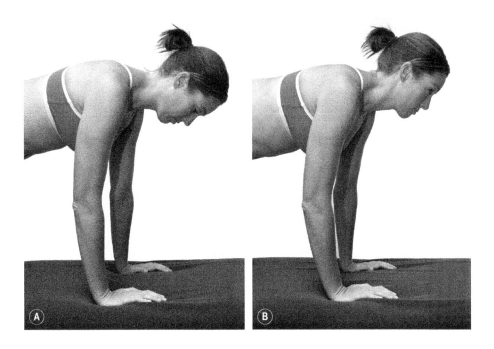

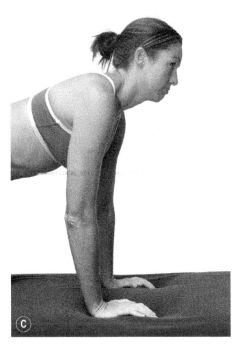

Figure 15.2 • Exercises in the four point kneeling position (A) starting position, (B) to emphasize the suboccipital extensors, (C) to emphasize the cervical extensors.

Scapular muscle re-education is commenced with the patient being taught to move and hold the scapulae in a neutral position on the chest wall, with appropriate interaction of the tripartite trapezius muscle and in particular the serratus anterior muscle, without unwanted activity of the latissimus dorsi, rhomboids or levator scapulae. Scapular muscle control is undertaken and practiced in sitting in tandem with correction of the upright spinal postural position so that regular practice can occur throughout the day. Training is also undertaken in a side lying or prone position where the clinician can provide specific facilitation to the scapular synergists. On occasions, axioscapular muscles such as the pectoralis minor or major may require lengthening to facilitate the scapular position training. In general, stretching of cervicobrachial muscles is not a priority in this management approach. Rather any muscle length changes are initially addressed by facilitating the correct scapular position and utilizing the effect of reciprocal relaxation to gain length changes in shortened and often tender muscles which often contribute to the scapular positional faults. This also respects any protective responses to mechanosensitive nerve tissues which may be accompanied by subtle tightness in the upper trapezius or scalene muscles for which stretching is ill advised. This approach is not to suggest that there is no indication for muscle stretching but uses an alternative to stretching exercises that may be more successful in the long term by addressing the reasons for the muscle shortness.

Patients are taught to assume a neutral upright postural position in sitting to activate the spinal postural supporting muscles functionally. Posture is corrected from the pelvis, drawing the pelvis to an upright neutral position with the formation of a low lumbar lordosis and activation of the lumbar multifidus. When performed precisely, this strategy also facilitates the longus capitis/colli (Falla et al 2007b).

A neutral thoracic position may be assumed automatically but may require a correction with a subtle sternal depression if the thoracic region is held in extension or conversely a subtle sternal lift if the thorax is in some flexion. The head-neck posture is corrected through a subtle active elongation of the neck and the patient practices sliding the scapulae to their neutral position on the chest wall. The process of learning to move to a neutral postural position may have to be sequentially taught if patients have problems assuming particular components. Frequent correction to an upright neutral posture serves two functions. It ensures a regular reduction of adverse loads on the cervical joints induced by poor spinal, cervical and scapular postures. It also trains the deep and postural stabilizing muscles in their functional postural supporting role.

Postural correction is practiced frequently throughout the day in the relearning process and the position is held for at least 10 seconds in each practice repetition. Repetition also aims for a change in postural habit. In addition, the patient should undertake practice of the formal exercises for the neck flexor, extensor and scapular muscles at least twice per day in a home exercise program.

Training endurance capacity

The holding capacity or endurance of muscles has been shown to be deficient at various contraction intensities, more so in the cervical flexors than extensors (Falla et al 2003b, Gogia & Sabbahi 1994, O'Leary et al 2007). Holding capacity is trained at low levels of maximum voluntary contraction (MVC) in the first instance. The deep cervical flexors are trained with the craniocervical flexion action. A pressure sensor is placed behind the neck to provide feedback, not only on the stage of craniocervical flexion able to be attained, but also whether the patient can successfully hold the position. Patients quickly learn the feel of the contraction and are able to practice at home without the feedback device. It is important that the patient continues to use the correct craniocervical flexion movement to train endurance at various test levels and does not revert to a retraction action with inappropriate muscle activity. Patients train over time to be able to progressively hold each inner range craniocervical flexion position, performing 10×10 second holds.

The scapular muscles are trained with repeated inner range holds in the neutral scapular position in prone or side lying. Training is also conducted in four-point kneeling, again with a neutral spine position and with activation of the serratus anterior to assist the holding of the neutral scapular position. The added advantage of the four-point kneeling position is the concomitant antigravity work that the neck extensors perform against head load. Appropriate scapular movement and control during arm elevation and lowering often requires facilitation and practice to avoid unnecessary loads on the cervical spine which may occur with poor scapular mechanics and muscle use (Behrsin & Maguire 1986).

Once activation of the deep neck flexors and extensors is achieved, exercises are introduced to train their co-contraction for support. This is achieved through the use of alternating isometrics performed with slight self-resistance in the rotation directions in an upright neutral sitting posture.

Training movement patterns

Once the activation capacity of the deep neck flexors has been achieved (the patient can perform and control inner range holding contractions of the longus capitis and colli at the highest level of the craniocervical flexion test (CCFT), the pattern of a craniocervical and then cervical extension and return to the neutral

position is practiced in sitting. This adds head load and gravity to the work of the flexors and trains them for eccentric control needed for functional use. The exercise is practiced with control and within pain free limits.

The work of the scapular muscles and trunk supporting muscles is increased using functional scenarios. The exercise is designed as appropriate to the patient's occupation or aggravating activities. For example, patients often report that computer work provokes their headache. Thus an exercise is designed to practice arm movements within $30°$ of arm elevation while maintaining correct head, neck, trunk as well as scapular position to maintain a non stressful posture while using the keyboard and mouse. If the patient is involved in light industry, light weights may be added to this exercise. Control of the trunk and scapulae is the most important feature of these exercises. Higher levels of fatigue have been found in the upper trapezius muscle in persons with neck pain during repetitive arm elevations (Falla & Farina 2005), indicating that endurance training is required especially for patients whose occupation requires repeated arm elevation.

Higher level strength and endurance training

Attention is directed towards strength and endurance deficits in the neck flexor and extensor muscles once the deep muscles are working appropriately in synergy with the superficial synergists (e.g. the patient can perform inner range craniocervical flexion holds with minimal work being contributed by the superficial flexors). Endurance is trained at various contraction intensities in accordance with the evidence of deficiencies at low and moderate levels of contraction intensity (O'Leary et al 2007). Progressive resistance exercises are introduced for the craniocervical flexors (resisted head flexion), the cervical flexors (head lift exercises with control of the craniocervical flexion position from a position of head support on two and then one pillow) as well as the neck extensors (e.g. resistance provided to the head by a resistive exercise band in the sitting or standing position). Strengthening regimens must not be provocative of symptoms and the levels of strength training should match the functional requirements of the patient.

Sensorimotor system

Evidence is emerging for the efficacy of specific exercise programs to address impairments identified within the sensorimotor system in reducing neck pain and other associated symptoms such as dizziness and unsteadiness (Humphreys & Ingrens 2002, Revel et al 1994). There are no known studies specific to cervicogenic headache. However, in a clinical trial testing manipulative therapy and specific exercise for the management of cervicogenic headache, it was shown that subjects with dizziness associated with their headache had lesser odds of achieving a successful outcome (Jull & Stanton 2005). No exercises were specifically directed towards the postural control system in this study and these results might provide a circuitous basis for their inclusion in clinical practice until more substantial research is conducted in the field.

The elements of the exercise program include head/neck relocation practice, balance, and oculomotor exercises. The tasks can be introduced early into the rehabilitation program and should be performed such that they do not produce pain or aggravate any symptoms of dizziness for prolonged periods of time.

Relocation practice. The patient practices relocating the head back to the natural head posture and to pre-determined positions in range in each movement plane. Practice is initially with the eyes open and then with eyes closed. The exercise is enhanced with feedback such as from a laser pointer attached to a headband or with practice of the task in front of a mirror.

Balance exercises. Balance exercises are progressed from comfortable stance to a narrow base stance, tandem stance or one foot stance. At each level the training progresses from eyes open, eyes closed to different supporting surfaces, for example standing on foam or an unstable surface.

Oculomotor exercises. The exercises include eye follow with a stationary head, eye-head coordination and gaze fixation with head movement (Revel et al 1994). They can be progressed by increasing speed of performance and the patient position, for example in lying, sitting and various standing postures. Exercise can be done to the point of dizziness, but exercise intensity should stop short of provoking prolonged periods of dizziness, increased pain and/or headache.

Neural system

Neural tissues can be allodynic and mechanosensitive in cervicogenic headache and in these cases treatment must progress with caution as such pain syndromes can easily be exacerbated. Movement based treatments have been evolving over the past two to three decades to manage neural tissue mechanosensitivity and the reader is referred to such sources for detailed description of treatment approaches (Butler 2000, Elvey 1979, 1997, Shacklock 2005). In the presence of neural tissue mechanosensitivity, exercises for the craniocervical flexors, and in some cases scapular posture training, may need modification as they can be provocative of symptoms. Neural tissue mechanosensitivity may resolve with management of the articular system but often a program using sequences of movement of the upper or lower limbs and neck is required to gently move or slide the nerve and nerve bed for proposed physiological effects of such movement on the neural tissues (Coppieters & Butler 2008).

Self-management regimen

Active participation by the patient in their management and goal setting is essential for its success. Patient compliance with the exercise regimen and other ergonomic advice and lifestyle strategies can be enhanced with a thorough explanation of the rationale for the exercise and other self help procedures. The exercise regimen has immediate as well as long term effects on the perception of palpable neck pain (Jull et al 2002). This link between the use of appropriate muscles and pain relief can be a powerful incentive for exercise compliance.

Conclusion

Evidence supports a multimodal approach for management of cervical musculoskeletal disorders including cervicogenic headache. Contemporary physiotherapy management of cervicogenic headache uses several therapeutic strategies based on the presenting musculoskeletal impairments. The program aims to reduce headache and associated symptoms and prevent recurrences by rehabilitating the detected impairments associated with headache and educating the patient on healthy work and lifestyle practices. Several of the intervention strategies have overlapping effects on the pain, motor, and sensorimotor systems.

References

Ahn Y, Lee S, Chung S et al 2005 Percutaneous endoscopic cervical discectomy for discogenic cervical headache due to soft disc herniation. Neuroradiol 47:924-930.

Alund M, Larsson SE, Ledin T et al 1991 Dynamic posturography in cervical vertigo. Acta Otolaryngol 481 (suppl):601-602.

Alund M, Ledin T, Odkvist L, Larsson SE 1993 Dynamic posturography among patients with common neck disorders. A study of 15 cases with suspected cervical vertigo. J Vestib Res 3:383-389.

Amiri M, Jull G, Bullock-Saxton J 2003 Measuring range of active cervical rotation in a position of full head flexion using the 3D Fastrak Measurement System: An intra-tester reliability study. Man Ther 8:176-179.

Amiri M, Jull G, Bullock-Saxton J et al 2007 Cervical musculoskeletal impairment in frequent intermittent headache. Part 2: Subjects with multiple headaches. Cephalalgia 27:891-898.

Antonaci F, Ghirmai S, Bono G et al 2001 Cervicogenic headache: evaluation of the original diagnostic criteria. Cephalalgia 21:573-583.

Bakker DA, Richmond FJ 1982 Muscle spindle complexes in muscles around upper cervical vertebrae in the cat. J Neurophysiol 48:62-74.

Bansevicius D, Sjaastad O 1996 Cervicogenic headache: The influence of mental load on pain level and EMG of shoulder-neck and facial muscles. Headache 36:372-378.

Barton PM, Hayes KC 1996 Neck flexor muscle strength, efficiency, and relaxation times in normal subjects and subjects with unilateral neck pain and headache. Arch Phys Med Rehabil 77:680-687.

Bartsch T, Goadsby P 2002 Stimulation of the greater occipital nerve induces increased central excitability of dural afferent input. Brain 125:1496-1509.

Bartsch T, Goadsby P 2003a The trigeminocervical complex and migraine: Current concepts and synthesis. Curr Pain Headache Rep 7:371-376.

Bartsch T, Goadsby P 2003b Increased responses in trigeminocervical nociceptive neurons to cervical input after stimulation of the dura mater. Brain 126:1801-1813.

Behrsin JF, Maguire K 1986 Levator scapulae action during shoulder movement. A possible mechanism of shoulder pain of cervical origin. Aust J Physiother 32:101-106.

Bogduk N 2004 The neck and headaches. Neurol Clin N Am 22:151-171.

Bogduk N 2005 Distinguishing primary headache disorders from cervicogenic headache: Clinical and therapeutic implications. Headache Currents 2:27-36.

Bogduk N, Marsland A 1988 The cervical zygapophysial joints as a source of neck pain. Spine 13:610-617.

Bolton PS, Tracey DJ 1992 Spinothalamic and propriospinal neurons in the upper cervical cord of the rat-Terminations of primary afferent fibers on soma and primary dendrites. Exp Brain Res 92:59-68.

Boswell M, Trescot A, Datta S et al 2007 Interventional techniques: evidence-based practice guidelines in the management of chronic spinal pain. Pain Physician 10:7-111.

Bovim G, Berg R, Dale LG 1992 Cervicogenic headache: anesthetic blockades of cervical nerves (C2-C5) and facet joint (C2/C3). Pain 49:315-320.

Boyd-Clark L, Briggs C, Galea M 2002 Muscle spindle distribution, morphology, and density in longus colli and multifidus muscle of the cervical spine. Spine 27:694-701.

Butler D 2000 The sensitive nervous system. NOIgroup Publications, Adelaide.

Chen J, Solinger AB, Poncet JF, Lantz CA 1999 Meta-analysis of normative cervical motion. Spine 24:1571-1578.

Chiu T, Law E, Chiu T 2005 Performance of the craniocervical flexion test in subjects with and without chronic neck pain. J Orthop Sports Phys Ther 35:567-571.

Coppieters M, Butler D 2008 Do 'sliders' slide and 'tensioners' tension? An analysis of neurodynamic techniques and considerations regarding their application. Man Ther (in press).

Corneil B, Olivier E, Munoz D 2002 Neck muscle responses to stimulation of monkey superior colliculus. I. Topography and manipulation of stimulation parameters. J Neurophysiol 88:1980-1999.

Coskun O, Ulcer S, Karakurum B et al 2003 Magnetic resonance imaging of patients with cervicogenic headache. Cephalalgia 23:842-845.

Dabbs V, Lauretti WJ 1995 A risk assessment of cervical manipulation Vs NSAIDs for the treatment of neck pain. J Manip Physiological Ther 18:530-536.

Dishman J, Burke J 2003 Spinal reflex excitability changes after cervical and lumbar spinal manipulation: a comparative study. Spine J 3:204-212.

Dreyfuss P, Rogers J, Dreyer S, Fletcher D 1994 Atlanto-occipital joint pain. A report of three cases and description of an intraarticular joint block technique. Reg Anesth 19:344-351.

Drottning M, Staff P, Sjaastad O 2002 Cervicogenic headache (CEH) after whiplash injury. Cephalalgia 22:165-171.

Dumas JP, Arsenault AB, Boudreau G et al 2001 Physical impairments in cervicogenic headache: traumatic vs. nontraumatic onset. Cephalalgia 21:884-893.

Dwyer A, Aprill C, Bogduk N 1990 Cervical zygapophyseal joint pain patterns: A study in normal volunteers. Spine 15:453-457.

Elvey R 1979 Brachial plexus tension test and the pathoanatomical origin of arm pain. In: Glasgow E, Twomey L (eds) Aspects of manipulative therapy: Institute of Health Sciences, Lincoln, p 105-110.

Elvey R 1997 Physical evaluation of the peripheral nervous system in disorders of pain and dysfunction. J Hand Ther 10:122-129.

Ernst E 2002 Manipulation of the cervical spine: a systematic review of case reports of serious adverse events, 1995-2001. Med J Aust 176:376-380.

Falla D 2004 Unraveling the complexity of muscle impairment in chronic neck pain. Man Ther 9:125-133.

Falla D, Farina D 2005 Muscle fiber conduction velocity of the upper trapezius muscle during dynamic contraction of the upper limb in patients with chronic neck pain. Pain 116:138-145.

Falla D, Jull G, Dall'Alba P et al 2003a An electromyographic analysis of the deep cervical flexor muscles in the performance of cranio-cervical flexion. Phys Ther 83:899-906.

Falla D, Rainoldi A, Merletti R, Jull G 2003b Myoelectric manifestations of sternocleidomastoid and anterior scalene muscle fatigue in chronic neck pain patients. Clin Neurophysiol 114:488-495.

Falla D, Jull G, Hodges P 2004a Neck pain patients demonstrate reduced activity of the deep neck flexor muscles during performance of the craniocervical flexion test. Spine 29:2108-2114.

Falla D, Bilenkij G, Jull G 2004b Chronic neck pain patients demonstrate altered patterns of muscle activation during performance of a functional upper limb task. Spine 29:1436-1440.

Falla D, Rainoldi A, Merletti R, Jull G 2004c Spatio-temporal evaluation of neck muscle activation during postural perturbations. J Electromyogr Kinesiol 14:463-474.

Falla D, Jull G, Hodges P 2004d Feedforward activity of the cervical flexor muscles during voluntary arm movements is delayed in chronic neck pain. Exp Brain Res 157:43-48.

Falla D, Jull G, O'Leary S, Dall'Alba P 2006 Further evaluation of an EMG technique for assessment of the deep cervical flexor muscles. J Electromyogr Kinesiol 16:621-628.

Falla D, Jull G, Russell T et al P2007a The effect of different neck exercise regimes on control of sitting posture in patients with chronic neck pain. Phys Ther 87:408-417.

Falla D, O'Leary S, Fagan A, Jull G 2007b Recruitment of the deep cervical flexor muscles during a postural correction exercise performed in sitting. Man Ther 12:139-143.

Feinstein B, Langton JNK, Jameson RM, Schiller F 1954 Experiments on referred pain from deep somatic tissues. J Bone Joint Surg 36A:981-987.

Fishbain D, Cutler R, Cole B et al 2001 International Headache Society headache diagnostic patterns in pain facility patients. Clin J Pain 17:78-93.

Fishbain D, Lewis J, Cole B et al 2003 Do the proposed cervicogenic headache diagnostic criteria demonstrate specificity in terms of separating cervicogenic headache from migraine. Cur Pain Headache Rep 7:387-394.

Fredriksen TA, Hovdal H, Sjaastad O 1987 Cervicogenic headache: clinical manifestations. Cephalalgia 7:147-160.

Fredriksen TA, Fougner R, Tangerud A, Sjaastad O 1989 Cervicogenic headache. Radiographical investigations concerning head/neck. Cephalalgia 9:139-146.

Fredriksen T, Stolt-Nielsen A, Skaanes K, Sjaastad O 2003 Headache and the lower cervical spine: long term, postoperative follow-up after decompressive neck surgery. Funct Neurol 18:17-28.

Frese A, Schilgen M, Edvinsson L et al 2005 Calcitonen gene-related peptide in cervicogenic headache. Cephalalgia 25:700-703.

Gdowski GT, McCrea RA 2000 Neck proprioceptive inputs to primate vestibular nucleus neurons. Exp Brain Res 135:511-526.

Gijsberts TJ, Duquet W, Stoekart R, Oostendorp R 1999a Pain-provocation tests for C0-4 as a tool in the diagnosis of cervicogenic headache. Abstract. Cephalalgia 19:436.

Gijsberts TJ, Duquet W, Stoekart R, Oostendorp R 1999b Impaired mobility of cervical spine as tool in diagnosis of cervicogenic headache. Abstract. Cephalalgia 19:436.

Gimse R, Tjell C, Bjorgen IA, Saunte C 1996 Disturbed eye movements after whiplash due to injuries to the posture control system. J Clin Exp Neuropsychol 18:178-186.

Gimse R, Bjorgen I, Tjell C et al 1997 Reduced cognitive functions in a group of whiplash patients with demonstrated disturbances in the posture control system. J Clin Exp Neuropsychol 19:838-849.

Gogia PP, Sabbahi MA 1994 Electromyographic analysis of neck muscle fatigue in patients with osteoarthritis of the cervical spine. Spine 19:502-506.

Govind J, King W, Bailey B, Bogduk N 2003 Radiofrequency neurotomy for the treatment of third occipital headache. J Neurol Neurosurg Psych 74:88-93.

Graff-Radford SB, Reeves JL, Jaeger B 1987 Management of chronic head and neck pain: Effectiveness of altering factors perpetuating myofascial pain. Headache 27:186 190.

Griegel-Morris P, Larson K, Mueller-Klaus K, Oatis CA 1992 Incidence of common postural abnormalities in the cervical, shoulder, and thoracic regions and their association with pain in two age groups of healthy subjects. Phys Ther 72:425-431.

Grimmer K 1997 An investigation of poor cervical resting posture. Aust J Physiother 43:7-16.

Gross A, Goldsmith C, Hoving J et al 2007 Conservative management of mechanical neck disorders: a systematic review. J Rheumatol 34:1083-1102.

Gurfinkel VS, Lipshits MI, Lestienne FG 1988 Anticipatory neck muscle activity associated with rapid arm movement. Neurosc Let 94:104-108.

Haavik-Taylor H, Murphy B 2007 Cervical spine manipulation alters sensorimotor integration: A somatosensory evoked potential study. Clin Neurophysiol 118:391-402.

Hack GD, Koritzer RT, Robinson WL et al 1995 Anatomic relation between the rectus capitis posterior minor muscle and the dura mater. Spine 20:2484-2486.

Haldeman S, Kohlbeck FJ, McGregor M 1999 Risk factors and precipitating neck movements causing vertebrobasilar artery dissection after cervical trauma and cervical manipulation. Spine 24:785-794.

Hall T, Robinson K 2004 The flexion-rotation test and active cervical mobility-A comparative measurement study in cervicogenic headache. Man Ther 9:197-202.

Headache Classification Committee of the International Headache Society 2004 The International Classification of Headache Disorders, 2nd edn. Cephalalgia 24(suppl 1):1-151.

Heikkila H, Astrom P 1996 Cervicocephalic kinesthetic sensibility in patients with whiplash injury. Scand J Rehabil 28:133-138.

Heikkila H, Wengren B 1998 Cervicocephalic kinesthetic sensibility, active range of cervical motion, and ocular function in patients with whiplash injury. Arch Phys Med Rehabil 79:1089-1094.

Heikkila H, Heikkila E, Eiseman M 1998 Predictive factors for the outcome of a multidisiciplinary pain rehabilitation programme on sick leave and life satisfaction in patients with whiplash trauma and other myofascial pain: a follow-up study. Clin Rehabil 12:487-496.

Hildebrandt J, Jansen J 1984 Vascular compression of the C_2 and C_3 roots-yet another cause of chronic intermittent hemicrania. Cephalalgia 4:167-170.

Hildingsson C, Wenngren B, Bring G, Toolanen G 1989 Oculomotor problems after cervical spine injury. Acta Orthop Scand 60:513-516.

Hildingsson C, Wenngren B, Toolanen G 1993 Eye motility dysfunction after soft-tissue injury of the cervical spine. Acta Orthop Scand 64:129-132.

Hinderaker J, Lord SM, Barnsley L, Bogduk N 1995 Diagnostic value of C2-3 instantaneous axes of rotation in patients with headache of cervical origin. Cephalalgia 15:391-395.

Hirai N, Hongo T, Sasaki S et al 1984 Neck muscle afferent input to spinocerebellar tract cells of the central cervical nucleus in the cat. Exp Brain Res 55:286-300.

Hoving JL, Koes BW, deVet HC et al 2002 Manual therapy, physical therapy or continued care by a general practitioner for patients with neck pain. Ann Int Med 136:713-722.

Humphreys B, Ingrens P 2002 The effect of a rehabilitation program on head repositioning accuracy and reported levels of pain in chronic neck pain subjects. J Whiplash Rel Disord 1:99-112.

Isa T, Sasaki S 2002 Brainstem control of head movements during orienting; organization of the premotor circuits. Prog Neurobiol 66:205-241.

Jaeger B 1989 Are cervicogenic headaches due to myofascial pain and cervical spine dysfunction. Cephalalgia 9:157-164.

Jansen J 2000 Surgical treatment of non responsive cervicogenic headache. Clin Exp Neurol 18:S67-S70.

Jansen J, Bardosi A, Hilderbrandt J, Lucke A 1989a Cervicogenic, hemicranial attacks associated with vascular irritation or compression of the cervical nerve root C2. Clinical manifestations and morphological findings. Pain 39:203-212.

Jansen J, Markakis E, Rama B, Hildebrandt J 1989b Hemicranial attacks or permanent hemicrania-a sequel of upper cervical root compression. Cephalalgia 9:123-130.

Jensen OK, Justesen T, Nielsen FF, Brixen K 1990 Functional radiographic examination of the cervical spine in patients with post-traumatic headache. Cephalalgia 10:295-303.

Jull G 1994 Headaches of cervical origin. In: Grant R (ed) Physical therapy of the cervical and thoracic spine. Churchill Livingstone, New York, p 261-285.

Jull GA 2000 Deep cervical neck flexor dysfunction in whiplash. J Musculoskel Pain 8:143-154.

Jull G 2002 The use of high and low velocity cervical manipulative therapy procedures by Australian manipulative physiotherapists. Aust J Physiother 48:189-193.

Jull G, Stanton W 2005 Predictors of responsiveness to physiotherapy treatment of cervicogenic headache. Cephalalgia 25:101-108.

Jull G, Bogduk N, Marsland A 1988 The accuracy of manual diagnosis for cervical zygapophysial joint pain syndromes. Med J Aust 148:233-236.

Jull G, Zito G, Trott P et al 1997 Inter-examiner reliability to detect painful upper cervical joint dysfunction. Aust J Physiother 43:125-129.

Jull G, Barrett C, Magee R, Ho P 1999 Further characterisation of muscle dysfunction in cervical headache. Cephalalgia 19:179-185.

Jull G, Trott P, Potter H et al 2002 A randomized controlled trial of exercise and manipulative therapy for cervicogenic headache. Spine 27:1835-1843.

Jull G, Kristjansson E, Dall'Alba P 2004a Impairment in the cervical flexors: a comparison of whiplash and insidious onset neck pain patients. Man Ther 9:89-94.

Jull G, Treleaven J, Falla D et al 2004b A therapeutic exercise approach for cervical disorders. In: Boyling J, Jull G, editors. Grieve's modern manual therapy of the vertebral column, 3rd edn. Churchill Livingstone, Edinburgh, p 451-470.

Jull G, Amiri M, Bullock-Saxton J et al 2007a Cervical musculoskeletal impairment in frequent intermittent headache. Part 1: Subjects with single headaches. Cephalalgia 27:793-802.

Jull G, Falla D, Treleaven J et al 2007b Retraining cervical joint position

sense: the effect of two exercise regimes. J Orthop Res 25:404-412.

Karlberg M, Persson L, Magnusson M 1995 Reduced postural control in patients with chronic cervicobrachial pain syndrome. Gait and Posture 3:241-249.

Karlberg M, Johansson R, Magnusson M, Fransson PA 1996 Dizziness of suspected cervical origin distinguished by posturographic assessment of human postural dynamics. J Vestib Res 6:37-47.

King W, Lau P, Lees R, Bogduk N 2007 The validity of manual examination in assessing patients with neck pain. Spine J 7:22-26.

Kogler A, Lindfors J, Odkvist L, Ledin T 2000 Postural Stability using different neck positions in normal subjects and patients with neck trauma. Acta Orthop Scand 120:151-155.

Kristjansson E, Dall'alba P, Jull G 2001 Cervicocephalic kinaesthesia: Reliability of a new test approach. Physiother Res Int 6:224-235.

Kristjansson E, Dall'Alba P, Jull G 2003 A study of five cervicocephalic relocation tests in three different subject groups. Clin Rehabil 17:768-774.

Kulkarni V, Chandy M, Babu K 2001 Quantitative study of muscle spindles in suboccipital muscles of human foetuses. Neurol India 49:355-359.

Lee H, Nicholson LL, Adams RD 2003 Cervical range of motion associations with subclinical neck pain. Spine 29:33-40.

Leone M, D'Amico D, Moschiano F et al 1995 Possible identification of cervicogenic headache among patients with migraine: An analysis of 374 headaches. Headache 35:461-464.

Leone M, D'Amico D, Grazzi L et al 1998 Cervicogenic headache: A critical review of current diagnostic criteria. Pain 78:1-5.

Liu J, Thornell L, Pedrosa-Domellof F 2003 Muscle spindles in the deep muscles of the human neck: A morphological and immunocytochemical study. J Histochem Cytochem 51:175-186.

Lord S, Bogduk N 2002 Radiofrequency procedures in chronic pain. Best Practice and Research in Clin Anaesthesiol 16:597-617.

Lord S, Barnsley L, Wallis B, Bogduk N 1994 Third occipital nerve headache: a prevalence study. J Neurol Neurosurg Psych 57:1187-1190.

Lord SM, Barnsley L, Bogduk N 1995 Percutaneous radiofrequency neurotomy in the treatment of cervical zygapophysial joint pain: a caution. Neurosurg 36:732-739.

Mayoux-Benhamou MA, Revel M, Vallee C et al 1994 Longus colli has a postural function on cervical curvature. Surg Radiol Anat 16:367-371.

McDonald GJ, Lord SM, Bogduk N 1999 Long-term follow-up of patients treated with cervical radiofequency neurotomy for chronic neck pain. Neurosurg 45:61-67.

Mitchell BS, Humphries BK, O'Sullivan E 1998 Attachments of ligamentum nuchae to cervical posterior dura and the lateral part of the occipital bone. J Manip Physiol Ther 21:145-148.

Montgomery M, Gordon S, Sickels JV, Harms S 1992 Changes in signs and symptoms following temporomandibular joint disc repositioning surgery. J Oral Maxillofac Surg 50:321-328.

Mulligan B 1995 Manual therapy 'NAGS', 'SNAGS', 'MWMS', 5th edn. Plane View Press, Wellington.

Mulligan B 2003 Self treatments for back, neck, and limbs, a new approach. Plane View Press, Wellington.

Nansel D, Peneff A, Cremata E, Carlson J 1990 Time course considerations for the effects of unilateral lower cervical adjustments with respect to the amelioration of cervical lateral-flexion passive end-range asymmetry. J Manip Physiol Ther 13:297-304.

Nederhand MJ, Hermens HJ, Ijzerman MJ et al 2003 Cervical muscle dysfunction in chronic whiplash-associated disorder grade 2: The relevance of the trauma. Spine 27:1056-1061.

Nilsson N 1995 The prevalence of cervicogenic headache in a random population sample of 20-59 year olds. Spine 20:1884-1888.

Nilsson N, Christensen HW, Hartvigsen J 1997 The effect of spinal manipulation in the treatment of cervicogenic headache. J Manip Physiol Ther 20:326-330.

O'Leary S, Vicenzino B, Jull G 2005 A new method of isometric dynamometry for the cranio-cervical flexors. Phys Ther 85:556-564.

O'Leary S, Jull G, Kim M, Vicenzino B 2007 Cranio-cervical flexor muscle impairment at maximal, moderate, and low loads is a feature of neck pain. Man Ther 12:34-39.

Ogince M, Hall T, Robinson K, Blackmore A 2007 The diagnostic validity of the cervical flexion-rotation test in C1/2-related cervicogenic headache. Man Ther 12:256-262.

Persson GCL, Carlsson JY 1999 Headache in patients with neck-shoulder-arm pain of cervical radicular origin. Headache 39:218-224.

Petersen S 2003 Articular and muscular impairments in cervicogenic headache: a case report. J Orthop Sports Phys Ther 33:21-30.

Peterson DI, Austin GM, Dayes LA 1975 Headache associated with discogenic disease of the cervical spine. Los Angeles Neurolog Soc 40:96-100.

Pfaffenrath V, Dandekar R, Pollmann W 1987 Cervicogenic headache-the clinical picture, radiological findings and hypotheses on its pathophysiology. Headache 27.495-499.

Pikus H, Phillips J 1995 Characteristics of patients successfully treated for cervicogenic headache by surgical decompression of the second cervical root. Headache 35:621-629.

Placzek JD, Pagett BT, Roubal PJ et al 1999 The influence of the cervical spine on chronic headache in women: A pilot study. J Man Manip Ther 7:33-39.

Pollmann W, Keidel M, Pfaffenrath V 1997 Headache and the cervical spine: a critical review. Cephalalgia 17:801-816.

Pool J, Hoving J, de Vet H et al 2004 The interexaminer reproducibility of physical examination of the cervical spine. J Manip Physiol Ther 27:84-90.

Radanov B, Di-Stefano G, Augustiny K 2001 Symptomatic approach to posttraumatic headache and its possible implications for treatment. Eur Spine J 10:403-407.

Revel M, Andre-Deshays C, Minguet M 1991 Cervicocephalic kinesthetic sensibility in patients with cervical pain. Arch Phys Med Rehabil 72:288-291.

Revel M, Minguet M, Gergoy P et al 1994 Changes in cervicocephalic kinesthesia after a proprioceptive rehabilitation program in patients with neck pain: A randomized controlled study. Arch Phys Med Rehabil 75:895-899.

Schoensee SK, Jensen G, Nicholson G et al 1995 The effect of mobilization on cervical headaches. J Orthop Sports Phys Ther 21:184-196.

Shacklock M 2005 Clinical neurodynamics. Elsevier, Edinburgh.

Shinoda Y, Sugiuchi Y, Futami T et al 1994 Input patterns and pathways from the six semicircular canals to motoneurons of neck muscles. I. The multifidus muscle group. J Neurophysiol 72:2691-2702.

Shumway-Cook A, Horak F 1986 Assessing the influence of sensory integration on balance. Phys Ther 66:1548-1550.

Silberstein S 1992 Evaluation and emergency treatment of headache. Headache 32:396-407.

Sjaastad O, Saunte C, Hovdahl H et al 1983 'Cervicogenic' headache. An hypothesis. Cephalalgia 3:249-256.

Sjaastad O, Fredriksen TA, Pfaffenrath V 1990 Cervicogenic headache: diagnostic criteria. Headache 30:725-726.

Sjaastad O, Fredriksen TA, Stolt-Nielsen A et al 1997 Cervicogenic headache: A clinical review with a special emphasis on therapy. Funct Neurol 12:305-317.

Sjaastad O, Fredriksen TA, Pfaffenrath V 1998 Cervicogenic headache: diagnostic criteria. The Cervicogenic Headache International Study Group.Headache 38:442-445.

Sjaastad O, Fredriksen T, Petersen H, Bakketeig L 2003 Features indicative of cervical abnormality. A factor to be reckoned with in clinical headache work and research? Funct Neurol 18:195-203.

Sjostrom H, Allum J, Carpenter M et al 2003 Trunk sway measures of postural stability during clinical balance tests in patients with chronic whiplash injury symptoms. Spine 28:1725-1734.

Skyba D, Radhakrishnan R, Rohlwing J et al 2003 Joint manipulation reduces hyperalgesia by activation of monoamine receptors but not opioid or GABA receptors in the spinal cord. Pain 106:159-168.

Solomon S 1997 Diagnosis of primary headache disorders: Validity of the International Headache Society criteria in clinical practice. Neurol Clin 15:15-26.

Solomon S, Lipton R 1993 A headache clinic-based approach to field trials of the International Headache Society criteria. Cephalalgia 12:63-65.

Sterling M, Jull G, Wright A 2001 Cervical mobilisation: Concurrent effects on pain, motor function and sympathetic nervous system activity. Man Ther 6:72-81.

Sterling M, Jull G, Vicenzino B et al 2003 Development of motor system dysfunction following whiplash injury. Pain 103:65-73.

Stewart S, Willems J, Ng J 1995 An initial analysis of thoracic spine motion with unilateral arm elevation in the scapular plane. J Man Manip Ther 3:15-21.

Sturzenegger M 1994 Headache and neck pain: the warning symptoms of vertebral artery dissection. Headache 134:187-193.

Szeto G, Straker L, Raine S 2002 A field comparison of neck and shoulder postures in symptomatic and asymptomatic office workers. Applied Ergon 33:75-84.

Szeto G, Straker L, Raine S 2003 The roles of upper trapezius and cervical erector spinae in controlling the neck-shoulder postures in symptomatic office workers

193

performing continuous keyboard work: towards developing an etiological model for work-related neck and upper limb disorders. IEA XVth Triennial Congress, Seoul, Korea, p 25-29.

Tjell C, Rosenhall U 1998 Smooth pursuit neck torsion test: A specific test for cervical dizziness. Amer J Otol 19:76-81.

Treleaven J, Jull G, Atkinson L 1994 Cervical musculoskeletal dysfunction in post-concussional headache. Cephalalgia 14:273-279.

Treleaven J, Jull G, Sterling M 2003 Dizziness and unsteadiness following whiplash injury-characteristic features and relationship to cervical joint position error. J Rehabil Med 35:36-43.

Treleaven J, Jull G, LowChoy N 2005a Standing balance in chronic whiplash-Comparison between subjects with and without dizziness. J Rehabil Med 37:219-223.

Treleaven J, Jull G, LowChoy N 2005b Smooth pursuit neck torsion test in whiplash associated disorders – relationship to self reports of neck pain and disability, dizziness and anxiety. J Rehabil Med 37:219-223.

Trevor-Jones R 1964 Osteoarthritis of the paravertebral joints of the second and third cervical vertebrae as a cause of occipital headache. S Afr Med J 38:392-394.

van Suijlekom JA, van Kleef M, Barendse GA et al 1998 Radiofrequency cervical zygapophyseal joint neurotomy for cervicogenic headache: A prospective study of 15 patients. Funct Neurol 13:297-303.

van Suijlekom H, Lame I, van den Berg SS 2003 Quality of life of patients with cervicogenic headache: a comparison with control subjects and patients with migraine or tension-type headache. Headache 43:1034-1041.

Vernon H, Silvano M 1991 The neck disability index: A study of reliability and validity. J Manip Physiol Ther 14:409-415.

Vicenzino B, Collins D, Benson H, Wright A 1998 An investigation of the interrelationship between manipulative therapy-induced hypoalgesia and sympathoexcitation. J Manip Physiol Ther 21:448-453.

Vincent M 1998 Validation of criteria for cervicogenic headache. Funct Neurol 13:74-75.

Watson DH, Trott PH 1993 Cervical headache: an investigation of natural head posture and upper cervical flexor muscle performance. Cephalalgia 13:272-284.

Westaway MD, Stratford PW, Blinkley JM 1998 The patient-specific functional scale: Validation of its use in persons with neck dysfunction. J Orthop Sports Phys Ther 27:331-338.

Whittingham W, Ellis WB, Molyneux TP 1994 The effect of manipulation (toggle recoil technique) for headaches with upper cervical joint dysfunction: a pilot study. J Manip Physiol Ther 17:369-375.

Xiaobin Y, Cook A, Hamill-Ruth R, Rowlingson J 2005 Cervicogenic headache in patients with presumed migraine: Missed diagnosis or misdiagnosis? J Pain 6:700-703.

Xiong G, Matsushita M 2001 Ipsilateral and contralateral projections from upper cervical segments to the vestibular nuclei in the rat. Exp Brain Res 141:204-217.

Zito G, Jull G, Story I 2006 Clinical tests of musculoskeletal dysfunction in the diagnosis of cervicogenic headache. Man Ther 11:118-129.

Zwart JA 1997 Neck mobility in different headache disorders. Headache 37:6-11.

16

Chiropractic approach

Grant Shevlin and Russell Mottram

People with headache frequently seek chiropractic care for symptom relief. In this chapter the authors, both chiropractors, provide an overview of the clinical and conceptual aspects of chiropractic practice as they relate to management of headache and temporomandibular disorders.

Chiropractors form the world's third largest regulated health care profession and are one of the most commonly utilized alternatives to medical care (Eisenberg 1998), with headache being one of the most frequent reasons for chiropractic consultation (Coulter 2002, Hurwitz 1998). Chiropractors practice within the scope of musculoskeletal management with a primary focus on spinal care. Chiropractic treatment typically involves the use of manual therapies including spinal manipulative therapy (SMT), which remains one of the most commonly employed techniques for the management of headache disorders (Fernandez de las Penas et al 2006). With training in manual therapies and their knowledge of spinal function, chiropractors are well positioned to manage cervicogenic headache (CGH), which has a distinct musculoskeletal component. However, some studies suggest that SMT may be useful in the management of other headache types including migraine (Nelson 1998)

and tension-type headache (TTH) (Boline 1995), even though these primary headaches are likely to have etiology in the central nervous system (CNS) rather than a peripheral musculoskeletal cause.

Central to chiropractic practice is the detection and correction of aberrant biomechanical function of spinal articulations which chiropractors refer to as a spinal or vertebral 'subluxation'. The World Health Organization (WHO 2005) defined chiropractic subluxation as: 'A lesion or dysfunction in a joint or motion segment in which alignment, movement integrity, and/or physiological function are altered, though contact between joint surfaces remains intact. It is essentially a functional entity, which may influence biomechanical and neural integrity.'

The term subluxation when used by chiropractors is distinct from medical use of the term, and refers to a conceptual model of spinal joint dysfunction. Several varied models of spinal subluxation exist (Kent 1996), though common to most models of spinal joint dysfunction is an acknowledgement of a complex of dysfunction beyond a purely biomechanical entity. Insights gained from biomechanical and neuroscientific investigations allow for the continual discussion and refinement of these models. Gatterman (1990) proposed a model comprising three key components:

- Kinesiopathology – changes in joint mobility
- Neuropathophysiology – facilitatory and/ or inhibitory effects on neural mechanisms at the spinal level and/or higher levels
- Histopathology – biochemical changes including inflammation and neuroimmune responses.

The etiology, pathophysiology, definition and clinical relevance of the subluxation continues to be investigated and debated by the chiropractic profession (Keating 2005), though in Keating's analysis 'the sum of the evidence is inconclusive and the clinical relevance of the subluxation is yet to be scientifically demonstrated'. The Association of Chiropractic Colleges Chiropractic Paradigm (2008) claims the effects of spinal subluxation to extend beyond merely musculoskeletal with influence on organ function and the greater well being of the patient. Seaman (1998) comments that claims of this nature are dogmatic rather than evidential and 'beyond the limits of supportive data'. He argues that the nature of the subluxation has traditionally been debated from a position of philosophy and theorizing rather than what has been scientifically demonstrated.

Integral to determining a headache patient's suitability for chiropractic management is the identification of spinal subluxation in the upper cervical region. With varying models of subluxation being utilized within the profession (Keating 2005), methods for detecting and correcting spinal subluxation are not entirely uniform and no 'gold standard' diagnostic indicator is evident. In order to identify, categorize and correct spinal subluxation, chiropractors pragmatically rely on: 'personal experience or the collective experience of the profession and the plausibility and consistency of chiropractic theory and technique with knowledge drawn from the basic sciences' (Grod 2001).

Consequently several diverse and varied approaches have been developed for detecting and treating subluxation (CCP 1998). Some of the more commonly utilized approaches include Applied Kinesiology (AK), sacro-occipital technique (SOT), Gonstead, and activator techniques. (Grazier 1998). Clinical signs of subluxation are generally reflective of the pathophysiological components of the subluxation, ie. kinesiopatholgy, neuropathophysiology, histopathology (Gatterman 1990). These may include: altered alignment, aberrant spinal joint motion, palpable soft tissue changes, localized/referred pain, muscle contraction or imbalance, focal joint tenderness, and altered physiological function (Association of Chiropractic Colleges 2008).

Walker (1997) determined the most commonly used methods for diagnosing subluxation as being; static palpation, pain description of the patient, orthopedic tests, motion palpation, visual posture analysis, leg length discrepancy, neurological tests and plain static X-rays. Motion palpation was regarded as the most reliable method. This technique involves palpating the spinal joints as they move through and reach the limit of their normal range of movement, allowing a qualitative assessment of joint mobility. An element of subjective interpretation is inherent in this approach. Though some studies report good intra-and inter-practitioner reliability (Humphreys et al 2004, Jull & Bullock 1987), a review of available studies by Seffinger et al (2003) observed that motion palpation shows at best fair to moderate intra-rater reliability and poor to fair inter-rater reliability. Some chiropractors utilize analysis of plain film spinal radiographs and electro-myographic evaluation of spinal musculature to attain a more objective diagnosis of subluxation, though the validity and reliability of these methods has been questioned (French et al 2000).

SMT, the cervical spine and head pain

An anatomical basis for the causal relationship between the cervical spine and head pain has been described by Bogduk (2001). He identified the convergence in the trigeminocervical nucleus between nociceptive afferents from the field of the trigeminal nerve and the receptive fields of the first three cervical nerves as the neurological mechanism by which cervical spinal pain is referred to the head from the upper cervical region. Muscles, joints and ligaments of the upper three cervical segments along with the dura mater of the spinal cord and posterior cranial fossa, and the vertebral artery are recognized as pain sensitive structures capable of causing headache. Injury or inflammation of these structures may lead to increased nociceptive activity in the peripheral afferent nerve fibers innervating these tissues, with subsequent transmission centrally to the trigemino-cervical nucleus.

Combining this anatomical knowledge and the theories of spinal joint dysfunction, it is possible to hypothesize several mechanisms by which subluxation may directly and indirectly contribute to head pain. They include:

- Altered mechanical loading of the upper cervical spinal articulations leading to irritation of intra articular pain sensitive structures and resultant nociceptive input to the trigeminocervical nucleus.
- Reflex arthrogenic muscle spasm occurring as a result of intra-articular nociception that may result in primary referred myofascial pain.

Secondary muscular involvement may include; compression of the C2 dorsal ramus by hypertonic cervical musculature (Pikus and Phillips 1995, Terret 2005), and, increased tension or spasm in the rectus capitis posterior minor muscle affecting the pain sensitive upper posterior cervical dura mater via a connective tissue bridge existing at the posterior atlanto-occipital level (Hack et al 1995, Hack & Halgren 2004). Meeker and Haldeman (2002) postulate the effects of SMT to include; increase of joint movement, change in joint kinematics, increase in pain threshold, increase in muscle strength, attenuation of alpha motor neuron activity, enhanced proprioceptive behaviour and release of beta-endorphins and substance P. By considering these effects of SMT in the context of the theories discussed, chiropractors can commence to appreciate the mechanisms by which SMT may influence head pain.

Evidence for SMT in headache management

The benefit of SMT in the treatment of headaches has been recognized anecdotally by chiropractors and patients alike for some time. However, like most aspects of patient care, the use of SMT as a treatment for headache is being held increasingly accountable to the principles of evidence-based practice. What follows is a brief review of studies that are of historical or scientific significance in the growing body of literature investigating SMT and headache management. Table 16.1 provides a summary of these studies.

Migraine

Some of the earliest studies to report a positive effect of chiropractic SMT on migraine were conducted by Wight (1978) and Parker (1978), although the studies were not scientifically rigorous enough by current standards to allow credible conclusions. Wight's study involved 87 patients with common and classic migraine who received between 1 and 74 SMT treatments over a 2 year period. The outcome

Table 16.1 Overview of studies investigating spinal manipulation and headache.

Headache type	Study design	Summary of results
Migraine		
Wight (1978)	N = 87. Between 1 and 74 tmts of SMT Self rated questionnaire 2 yrs post 1st tmt	74.7% HA ceased or improved. Success maintained 2 years post treatment
Tuchin (2000)	N = 127. RCT monitored 2 m pre and post tmt Max 16 tmt over 2 m period	50% reported significant improvement of morbidity of each episode. F/up study 20 months post tmt showed maintained cure or continued improvement.
Parker (1978)	RCT n = 85. Compared chiropractic, medical SMT and physiotherapy mob. 6 wk of tmt, F/up 3, 6, 12 m	HA frequency: ↓ 40% in chiro group, ↓ 13% in med group, ↓ 34% in physio group. HA severity also reduced in chiro group.
Stodolny & Chmielewski (1989)	N = 31. Diagnosed with cervical mig	32.3% reported complete cessation of HA 22.6% reported ↓ neck pain 58.1% reported ↓ dizziness
Nelson et al (1998)	N = 218. Prospective randomized parallel group comparison 8 wks tmt, 3 groups: 1. SMT, 2. amitriptyline, 3.combined	HA Index score derived from daily headache pain diary. % ↓ from pre-tmt baseline: SMT group: ↓ 40% during tmt, ↓ 42% post tmt Amitriptyline group: ↓ 49% during tmt, ↓ 24% post tmt Combined group: ↓ 41% during tmt, ↓ 25% post tmt
Cervicogenic		
Jull (2002)	N = 200. RCT, unblinded tmt, blind assessor. 6 wk tmt period, F/up assessment at 3, 6, 12 m	4 tmt groups: 1. SMT, 2. Exercise, 3. Combined, 4. Control At 12m SMT and Exercise groups had ↓ HA freq, intensity. 10% more of Px in combined group had relief.
Nilsson (1995)	N = 39. RCT, blind observer, SMT twice/ wk for 3 wk, compared to cervical laser + deep friction massage	Significant ↓ in analgesic use per day, headache intensity per episode, and number of headache hr/day. No significant difference between tmt groups
Nilsson et al (1997)	N = 53. Prospective RCT, blind observer, 2 tmt groups: 1. SMT twice/wk 3 wks, 2. STT /laser	36% ↓ in analgesic use in SMT group though not STT group. HA hours ↓. 69% SMT Group, 37% SST. HA intensity ↓ 37% in SMT group, ↓ 17% STT group
Tension-type		
Boline et al (1995)	N = 150. RCT – 2 wk base, 6 wk tmt, 4 wk post. 2 tmt groups: 1. SMT, 2. amitriptyline. Outcome Px reported	4 wk post. SMT group: 32% ↓ intensity, 42% ↓ freq, 30% ↓ med use, 16% imp functional health status. Amitriptyline group: no improvement on base values for all measures
Bove & Nilsson (1998)	N = 75. RCT 8 tmts in 4 wks. 2 groups: 1. SMT/STT, 2. STT/placebo laser (Control)	Both groups experienced significant reductions in HA hours and analgesic use. No change in HA intensity
Grunnet-Nilsson & Bove (2000)	N = 75. RCT 2 tmt groups. I. SMT/STT, 2. STT/laser cervical spine.	3 m f/up. Both groups showed significant improvement, no differences between groups. Study concluded that SMT had no effect on episodic TTH

HA = headache, TTH = tension-type headache, Mob = mobilization, N = number of subjects in study, Px = patient, RCT = randomized controlled trial, SMT = spinal manipulation, STT = soft tissue therapy, Tmt = treatment.

was based on a self-rated patient questionnaire and demonstrated that 33.3% of patients reported cessation of migraine 2 years following treatment while a further 41.4% reported their migraines as being much improved.

Parker (1978) conducted a randomized controlled trial (RCT) in which 85 migraine sufferers were allocated to one of three treatment groups: chiropractic manipulation, medical manipulation or physical therapy mobilization. There was no control group. Participants received an average of 7 treatments. In the chiropractic group headache frequency was reduced by 40%, by 13% in the medical group, and by 34% in the physical therapy group. The only measured outcome to reach statistical significance was a reduction of pain intensity in the chiropractic group, though the validity of statistical analysis method was questioned. A second more stringent analysis of data was undertaken (Parker 1980). This follow up publication failed to detect statistically significant outcomes, with a high likelihood of Type II errors due to the small sample size.

Higher quality studies have since been performed, most notably by Nelson (1998) and Tuchin (2000). Nelson conducted an RCT in which 218 patients with a diagnosis of migraine were allocated into 3 treatment groups. Following a 4-week pre-trial period, patients received an 8 week course of therapy involving SMT, amitriptyline, or a combination of both, followed by a 4 week follow up period. A headache index score was obtained from a daily headache pain diary during the last 4 weeks of treatment and the 4 week follow up period. Participants in the amitriptyline group recorded a 47% reduction of the headache index scores from the baseline period, while the SMT and combined groups showed 40% and 41% reductions respectively. Interestingly the SMT group demonstrated a greater reduction in the follow up period with a 42%

reduction compared to the amitriptyline group (24% reduction) and the combined group (25% reduction), suggesting a protracted benefit from SMT. Nelson concluded that SMT appeared to be as effective as amitriptyline for managing migraine patients.

Tuchin (2000) conducted a RCT in which 127 subjects with migraine diagnosed using International Headache Society criteria were allocated to an SMT group or control group of no treatment. Participants maintained a headache diary throughout a 2 month pre-treatment stage, a 2 month treatment stage and a further 2 month post-treatment stage. The treatment group received a maximum of 16 treatments in their course of therapy. The SMT group obtained statistically significant reductions in frequency, duration, disability and medication use compared to the control group.

Cervicogenic headache

Jull et al (2002) conducted an RCT in which 200 participants meeting the criteria for cervicogenic headache (CGH) were randomized to 1 of 3 treatment groups (SMT by physiotherapists, exercise therapy, and a combination of the two therapies plus medication) and a control group who were managed by their general practitioners with simple analgesics or non-steroidal anti inflammatory medication. Follow-ups were conducted at 3, 6, and 12 months. The primary outcome measure was headache frequency while changes in intensity, duration, patient satisfaction, medication use, and neck pain were also recorded. Both the SMT and exercise therapy groups showed significant reductions in headache frequency and intensity ($p < 0.05$). Though the combined therapy did not demonstrate statistically better outcomes than the other treatment groups, 10% more individuals in the combined group achieved either complete or 50% reduction in headache frequency.

Nilsson (1997) was also able to demonstrate a statistically significant benefit of SMT in treating CGH. SMT or combined laser and massage therapy was provided to 53 participants twice weekly for a three week period. The findings showed that analgesic use was reduced by 36% in the SMT group compared to no change in the soft-tissue group. Furthermore, headache hours per day decreased by 69% in the SMT group and 37% for the soft tissue group, and headache intensity per episode decreased 36% in the SMT group compared to 17% in the soft tissue group.

Tension-Type Headache

Boline (1995) conducted a RCT comparing the effectiveness of SMT and amitriptyline in 150 patients diagnosed with chronic Tension-Type Headache (TTH). Patients self-reported changes in daily headache intensity, weekly headache frequency, medication used, and functional health status (SF-36). Participants were randomly allocated to either therapy group during a 2 week pre-treatment phase, 6 week treatment period, and a 4 week post treatment period. During the treatment period participants in both groups achieved very similar improvements in measured outcomes, however substantial differences were observed at 4 weeks post cessation of treatment. The SMT group reported a 32% reduction in headache intensity, 42% reduction in headache frequency, 30% reduction in medication use and a 16% improvement in functional health status. In comparison the amitriptyline group showed a slight worsening from baseline values for all measures with 82% of participants in that group reporting of side effects that included dry mouth, weight gain and drowsiness. By comparison only 4.3% of participants in the SMT reported side effects, mainly neck soreness and stiffness. The findings appear to echo the Nelson et al (1998) study

demonstrating that SMT achieved a more sustained therapeutic benefit. Bove (1998) also investigated the efficacy of SMT as a treatment for episodic TTH, though no significant differences in outcomes between control and SMT groups were reported.

Systematic reviews

In recent years several systematic literature reviews have been undertaken to assess the scientific evidence supporting the use of SMT in headache management (Astin & Ernst 2002, Biondi 2005, Bronfort et al 2004, Fernandez-de-la-Penas et al 2006, Lensinck et al 2004). These reviews acknowledged that the available studies investigating SMT and headache showed a tendency toward benefits of treatment. However, it was noted that these studies often had inadequate patient numbers and/or methodological quality to demonstrate conclusive evidence for effectiveness. Most reviews concluded that there was a need for high quality randomized clinical trials to assess the effectiveness of SMT in headache management.

Chiropractic assessment of headache

Chiropractic management of headache primarily involves identifying and treating musculoskeletal dysfunction in the cervical and craniomandibular regions. Assessment may also be broadened further to include postural and functional assessment of any kinematically related regions that can influence neck and jaw function (Chaitow 2002, Janda 1986, Pederick 2005, Rocabado et al 1991, Walker 1998).

Of particular relevance in determining the suitability of chiropractic management of a patient with headache is the identification of contraindications to the use of SMT. Vertebral artery syndrome remains the most serious, albeit rare possible consequence of SMT (Licht 2003). Symptoms of vertebrobasilar-insufficiency (VBI) may be evident in the patient history and may be elicited by VBI provocation tests involving extension and rotation of the cervical spine, though much contention surrounds the predictive validity of these procedures (Licht 2000, Thiel & Rix 2005).

Chiropractic management of headache

Clinical decision making in chiropractic management has generally been governed by individual experience, clinical consensus, descriptive studies and interpretation of models of spinal dysfunction. Though some attempts have been made to standardize the approach to headache management (Campbell et al 1996, Nelson & Boline 1991), comprehensive evidence-based guidelines have not been established. Chiropractors to some extent approach headache treatment from the perspective of managing musculoskeletal dysfunction of the cervical spine, and as such, in the absence of comprehensive evidence-based guidelines specifically for headache, some relevance can be drawn from guidelines regarding musculoskeletal management of low back pain (NHMRC 2003) and neck pain (CCP 2007).

Though the available studies generally address SMT as an isolated treatment, in clinical practice chiropractors will often provide a comprehensive range of strategies to manage headache in recognition of the often multicausal nature of headache. Their use of SMT and other manual therapies with the intent of restoring functional spinal integrity does however remain the integral component of chiropractic headache management. Chiropractors refer to 'adjusting' a spinal segment in order to restore biomechanical integrity and spinal function. Traditionally an adjustment would

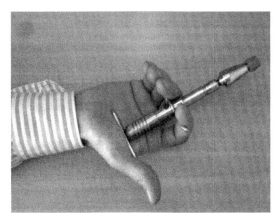

Figure 16.1 • Activator adjusting instrument.

involve SMT, though a wide variety of adjusting techniques are currently practiced by chiropractors, including the use of handheld mechanical devices (Fig. 16.1) which deliver a high velocity low amplitude (HVLA) impulse into the vertebral joint complex.

Chiropractic management of head pain may also address associated dysfunction of cervical musculature and the temporomandibular joint which are discussed later in this chapter and in Chapter 8. In order to address biomechanical dysfunction in the cervical spine comprehensively, chiropractors may employ other supportive measures such as instruction in exercise therapy, behavioral and lifestyle modification. To maintain ongoing benefit, a more comprehensive neuromusculoskeletal rehabilitative approach may be required to address chronic postural and/or movement pattern changes.

A headache diary (see Ch. 13) can be an invaluable tool for monitoring response to therapy, identifying factors that may be impeding recovery and allowing for further individualization of treatment. Using a similar format to those used in clinical research, it may be useful to record outcome measures such as headache frequency and duration, pain intensity and medication use and that described in the headache measurement chapter (Ch. 13).

Questionnaires such as the MIDAS (the migraine-specific disability assessment scale) and HIT (headache impact test) (see Ch.13) may also provide greater detail for monitoring. Studies of chiropractic management of headache have tended to investigate the efficacy of SMT as a preventive rather than a palliative treatment. In the authors' clinical experience, we are yet to determine any accurate predictors of whether a patient is likely to respond favorably to treatment. This approach must be determined on a patient to patient basis by reviewing the efficacy of intervention with patient specific outcome measures.

The chronicity of the patient's headaches and the continuing presence of aggravating or contributing factors may determine the length of the initial course of therapy and the need for ongoing care to maintain proper spinal function. The available clinical research generally follows treatment schedules ranging from 3 to 12 visits, over 3 to 6 week periods. A pilot study by Haas (2004) investigating dose response for chiropractic care for cervicogenic headache, showed substantial benefit to patients who had received 9 to 12 treatments over 3 weeks, compared to those who received 3 treatments over 3 weeks.

In recognition of the diverse needs of patients with headache, a multidisciplinary collaborative approach to management needs to be considered. Effective management of headache should also consider patient education and self participation as well as the establishment of reasonable patient expectations and effective communication' (Aukerman et al 2002).

One final relevant point of interest is that Lance and Goadsby (2004) consider the possibility that cervicogenic headache is a variety of migraine triggered from the upper cervical spine in a manner comparable with migraine triggered by other forms of afferent stimulation, such as glare and noise. Terret (2005) refers to this as 'cervical modulated' migraine and suggests that SMT could be utilized as a diagnostic tool as well as a treatment modality.

Craniomandibular disorder

Craniomandibular disorder (CMD) refers specifically to disorder resulting from dysfunction of the temporomandibular joint (TMJ) and biomechanically related structures. The term craniomandibular is preferred in this chapter as it implies the inclusion of anatomical structures that extend beyond just the temporomandibular joint. These include the cranium and its articulations, and the dental occlusion. The term temporomandibular disorders (TMD) is often used interchangeably with CMD.

Assessment and management

CMD may be a manifestation of a multifactorial disturbance in function of any of the following components:

- temporomandibular joint articular mechanism
- muscles of mastication
- the dental occlusion (providing mandibular positional stability and movement guidance)
- structural and biomechanical aspects of the cranial vault and facial bones
- myofascial structures that sustain postural relationships of the mandible, head, neck and shoulder regions
- afferent neural input from teeth, joints, muscles, fascia and ligaments of the craniomandibular anatomy and subsequent efferent responses
- centrally generated nervous system phenomena possibly responsible for bruxism, clenching and other oral habits.

The diversity of structures comprising this region, and the different health disciplines that offer treatment for these structures, may cause confusion in patients in determining the appropriate practitioner to approach for help when experiencing craniomandibular symptoms.

As stated earlier in the chapter, the chiropractic approach to the treatment of neuromusculoskeletal conditions focuses on the normalization of joint function. The temporomandibular joint, being a compound diarthrodial joint, is conceptually approached like other synovial joints in the application of chiropractic therapy. The anatomical characteristics of the TMJ, i.e., opposing cartilage covered bones, ligamentous joint capsule, associated myofascial structures and internal disc (meniscal) features, are not entirely unique. Consequently, diagnostic procedures that seek to discover joint and myofascial dysfunction, which are the mainstay of chiropractic analysis, can also be applied to this joint. Treatment strategies usually involve a combination of whole body biomechanical correction (based on the fundamental chiropractic concept of neuromusculoskeletal integration, described later in this chapter), combined with therapy to the TMJ itself (Table 16.2). These techniques are drawn from published material plus the authors' 25 years of clinical experience in treating CMD. They include:

- high velocity, low amplitude (HVLA) adjustments or manipulations to hypomobile joint structures (these may be applied manually or by using an adjusting instrument)
- transverse friction massage to capsuloligamentous restrictions
- myofascial trigger point therapy to muscles of mastication
- mobilizing, tractioning, gapping and stretching techniques to influence intra-articular disc position

and adhesion in cases of non-reducing displacement

- retraining exercises to attempt postural repositioning of the mandible and to equip patients with self-help tools for relieving pain and maintaining function
- electrotherapeutic modalities such as ultrasound, laser and electrical stimulation to assist in pain reduction and soft tissue rehabilitation.

Evidence-based research within the scientific literature is not extensive with respect to the effectiveness of these approaches for CMD. Most supporting literature consists of studies of relatively small sample size. A prospective study of nine individuals treated with an instrument delivering a measurable HVLA impulse to the TMJ was successful in relieving pain and improving mandibular opening amplitude in CMD (Devocht et al 2003).

A case study by Saghafi and Curl (1995) demonstrated benefits for a 21 year old subject with a four-year history of pain and clicking with an anteriorly displaced, adhesed articular disc. They applied a specific HVLA thrust over several treatments with good functional and symptomatic improvement. However, further research needs to be conducted since HVLA may theoretically cause hypermobility of the TMJ. Evidence also exists for the positive benefits to patients with CMD from laser therapy, pulsed radio frequency, manual therapy, exercise, and postural retraining (Al-Badawi 2004, Kulekcioglu 2003, Nicolakis et al 2001a & b).

Mandibular rest position and forward head posture

An important component of the physical assessment and management of CMD is mandibular rest position and its relationship to forward head posture. Curl (1994) presented a

Table 16.2 Protocol for management of range of motion disturbances of the TMJ.

Range of motion discrepancy	Possible etiology	Possible treatment strategy
Diminished jaw opening without deviation or deflection	1. Hypertonicity of mandibular elevator muscles bilaterally. (Softer end feel, reduced TMJ translation) 2. Bilateral closed lock (little translation of TMJ, hard end feel of TMJ) 3. Ligamentous restriction bilaterally (some translation, harder end feel)	1. MTP therapy to mandibular elevator muscles, MET, gentle self stretch techniques to point of no discomfort 2. Condylar reduction technique, TMJ mobilization 3. TFM of ligaments, TMJ mobilization, HVLA impulse adjustment
Diminished jaw opening with deviation	1. Unilateral hypertonicity of mandibular elevator muscles. (Soft end feel of TMJ, no clicking) 2. Unilateral disc derangement with closed lock 3. Unilateral ligamentous restriction. (Harder end feel of TMJ, no clicking)	1. MTP therapy, MET (lateral excursion and straight opening) 2. TMJ mobilization, condylar reduction 3. TFM, HVLA impulse adjustment
Diminished jaw opening with deflection 1. With click 2. Without click	1. Disc derangement 2a. Disc derangement (without click) 2b. Unilateral elevator muscle hypertonicity or ligamentous contracture causing delayed translation	1. MTP therapy to lateral pterygoid, TFM to joint capsule, Mandibular advancement dental splint to recapture disc 2a. As above 2b. MTP therapy, MET, TFM to myofascial structures
Diminished lateral excursion 1. Unilateral 2. Bilateral	1a. Disc derangement (especially if the clicking is in the contralateral TMJ to the side of diminished translation) 1b. Muscular or capsulo-ligamentous fixation (end feel to distinguish) 2a. Bilateral anterior disc derangement 2b. Bilateral muscle or ligamentous fixation	1a. MTP therapy to lateral pterygoid, joint mobilisation, occlusal splint 1b. MTP therapy especially to medial pterygoid, MET into lateral excursion especially, stretch with impulse to ligament 2a. Bilateral application of above 2b. As above

MTP = myofascial trigger point, MET = muscle energy technique, HVLA = high velocity low amplitude, TFM = transverse friction massage, TMJ = temporomandibular joint.

detailed description of the neuromuscular consequences of forward head posture, based partly on the work of Rocabado and Iglarsh (1991). In particular the relationship between craniocervical extension and increased jaw muscle activity in the temporalis, masseter and anterior digastric is described. In this scenario, the hyoid bone is repositioned superiorly and, together with the retruded mandible, causes the condyle to be habitually placed in a close packed position in the rear of the articular fossa. Curl speculated that this condylar position may induce microtrauma to the highly vascular and innervated retrodiscal tissues, thus causing inflammation, pain and deleterious effects on the disc/condylar mechanical integrity. This process is considered to be a common etiological factor in the eventual development of intra articular disc derangement and CMD (Simons 1999).

The consistent repositioning of the condylar head in a more anterior position is considered physiologically desirable and the object of a variety of treatment approaches (Simmons 2005). Dental appliances that seek to achieve this are widely used in CMD management (Simmons 2005). Olmos et al (2005) reviewed 51 patients who had received intra-oral appliance therapy to anteriorly reposition the mandibular condyle in the fossa. Pre- and post-treatment photographs showed on average a significant ($p < 0001$) 4.43 inch decrease in the measured slant between shoulder and the external auditory meatus on these patients, suggesting that optimizing condylar position could be important in the management of maladaptive head posture. A number of other studies have investigated the relationship between the cervical spine, the TMJ, and forward head posture (FHP). In a randomized controlled study of 60 patients with CMD (interventions of postural retraining of FHP) Wright et al (2000) produced significant functional and symptomatic improvements ($p < 0.005$). Higbie et al (1999) studied the effect of head position and mandibular opening in 40 adults and found a significant relationship between head position and mandibular opening amplitude. Kritsinelli and Shim (1992) showed a positive correlation between FHP and disorders of the TMJ in a study of 80 school children. Chiropractic therapy has been shown to influence cervical and lumbar spinal curvature and thereby head posture (Leach 1983, Banks 1983). Postural retraining to reduce musculoskeletal strain is a common management strategy for a variety of complaints seen in everyday chiropractic practice. It would seem reasonable to consider that the control of FHP in relation to mandibular position might be a worthwhile clinical strategy in the treatment of CMD. However the relationship between CMD and FHP is by no means established in the published literature (Valenzuela 2005, Visscher 2002). Further research needs to be conducted to evaluate the efficacy of improving postural awareness in patients with CMD.

Integration of neuromusculoskeletal components

As an illustration of this concept, the reader is asked to consider the following hypothetical clinical scenario:

Case study

A patient complaining of neck pain presents to the chiropractor who, finding biomechanical dysfunction of the upper cervical spine, commences a course of cervical spinal adjustment, gaining only temporary relief. Concurrently the patient is under the care of a dentist who has difficulty controlling tooth wear and recurrent issues related to fracture of a previously filled tooth. The patient meanwhile is complaining to their general practitioner (GP) of unremitting headache. The GP conducts extensive investigations to rule out intracranial pathology and then provides an array of palliative medications. These are of limited value because of an upset stomach and provide only short-term relief. On the advice of a friend, the patient enrolls in an exercise class and the instructor observes the habitual forward head carriage that characterizes the patient's posture. The Pilates program and the patient's home practice of improving posture eventually, over a period of several months, leads to a significant lasting diminution in headache, neck pain and bruxism.

Although this situation is hypothetical, it is based on similar clinical scenarios drawn from the authors' practice and seeks to illustrate the necessity to address beyond symptoms to wider influences. This situation is particularly important in attempting to manage biomechanical craniomandibular conditions. It is a basic tenet of chiropractic that the musculoskeletal system and its myriad proprioceptive neural connections is a highly integrated system (Seaman 1998).

The inter-relationship between the neck and TMJ is illustrated by the following three studies:

1. Hellstrom et al (2002) injected bradykinin into nociceptors in the TMJ of an anesthetized cat and recorded significant muscle spindle afferent responses in neck musculature, thus postulating a possible neurological mechanism for the sensory-motor disturbances in the neck region often seen in patients with TMJ disorders.

2. O'Reilly and Pollard (1996) were able to obtain pain relief in 12 CMD patients by the application of cervical spine manipulation and trigger point therapy to cervico-thoracic musculature without any direct treatment to the TMJ.

3. Alcantara (2002) described a 41 year old woman who was unsuccessfully treated for TMJ syndrome by dental and medical practitioners but was successfully treated with upper cervical spine SMT alone.

Many authors, including Rocabado and Iglarsh (1991), Janda (1986), and Chaitow (2002), allude to the connection between the shoulder girdle and the craniomandibular system, theorizing that ideal head and shoulder posture is necessary to establish biomechanical integrity of the mandible-head-neck-shoulder complex. In addition, Janda (1986) suggested that hyperextension of the knee joints, an increased pelvic tilt, hyperlordosis of the lumbar spine and a kyphotic thoracic spine (with associated muscular compensation patterns), could cause changes in FHP.

Pederick (2005) described several systems of postural and integrated kinematic assessment widely used within the chiropractic profession to detect and treat disorders of the craniomandibular system; sacro-occipital technique (SOT) and applied kinesiology (AK) are two of the most prominent. Walker (1998) coined the term 'chirodontics' to describe a diagnostic and management system that integrates chiropractic therapy, orofacial orthopedics and orthodontics with nutritional and postural therapy. These chiropractic management systems employ a variety of whole body analysis procedures to detect patterns of neuromusculoskeletal strain and propose a series of physical therapeutic interventions based on this information.

Cranial therapy

This term cranial therapy is used to describe a system of manual therapy directed at the osseous, membranous, and myofascial structures of the skull and face.

During the early part of the 20th century various osteopathic and chiropractic physicians became interested in the possible kinetic properties of the bones of the skull and the cranial sutures. Many histological, anatomical and kinesiological studies have since attested to the existence of patent cranial sutures into adult and even elderly life with subtle movements possible from sources both external (passive) and internal (generated by intracranial pressure fluctuations) (Kostopoulos & Keramidas 1992, Kovich 1976, Pick 1994). These sutures contain nerves and are conduits for connection between intra and extra cranial membranes. They are postulated to be possible sites of myofascial, neurological and kinesiological dysfunction with resultant clinical consequences including headache and CMD. For a comprehensive discussion of the theoretical models, research and clinical aspects of cranial therapy, readers are directed to Chaitow (2002). Within the chiropractic profession, two treatment systems (SOT and AK) make use of cranial therapy in the treatment of neuromusculoskeletal disorders including head and facial pain and TMJ syndrome (Pederick 2005). The use of cranial therapy in the treatment of head pain has some limited support in the scientific literature. Hanten and colleagues (1999) investigated the effectiveness of one particular cranial technique for Tension-type headache compared with two placebo interventions in a randomized controlled study of 60 patients. Improvement in pain intensity and the affective component of pain were significantly larger ($p < 0.05$) in the group that received the cranial technique.

Parikh et al (2001) conducted a randomized pilot study to test the effectiveness of cranial therapy compared to two other osteopathic techniques and a placebo in the treatment of sinus, tension and migraine headache. Pain was evaluated pre and post treatment. The findings demonstrated that all techniques provided more relief than placebo. Cranial therapy provided greater relief compared the osteopathic techniques, especially in migraine type headache. However, some reviews have highlighted the poor inter-examiner reliability of assessment procedures used in cranial therapy and therefore questioned the usefulness of this treatment approach (Hartman & Norton 2002).

Multidisciplinary considerations

The roles played by dental occlusion and 'parafunction' (central nervous system generated muscular activity) in the development of CMD need to be considered and are discussed in more detail in Chapters 19 and 20. The features of CMD that suggest dental malocclusion or significant psycho-emotional stress ought to be considered by the clinician. Curl (1994) stated that it should not be beyond the capacity of anyone working in the field of chronic pain to familiarize themselves with some of the basic premises of related disciplines. He suggested that clinicians seek to consistently maintain an attitude of 'holism' when confronted with the difficult task of diagnosis and treatment of the craniomandibular system. In the authors' experience a good inter-professional referral network and familiarity with diagnostic concepts and treatment protocols of each professional is worth cultivating. With respect to CMD, the chiropractor, medical practitioner, dentist and psychologist can all assist in the management of the CMD patient, either individually or in combination. To avoid the patient becoming confused or disillusioned by conflicting information, a consistent ongoing dialogue between practitioners should be pursued.

Conclusion

Headache represents a major health burden on society and remains a common reason for patient consultation with medical, complementary, and alternative health practitioners. Musculoskeletal dysfunction in the cervical and craniomandibular regions can contribute significantly to pain and needs to be considered in the assessment of patients with headache. Chiropractors are well placed to offer diagnosis and treatment and should be considered as part of a multidisciplinary approach to headache management. Some studies support the use of SMT in the management of headache. However, it is apparent that further high quality research is necessary to validate this treatment modality and to establish comprehensive evidence-based practice guidelines. Until guidelines are established, practitioners must exercise clinical judgment in determining the suitability of chiropractic involvement in managing headache.

References

Al-Badawi EA, Mehta N, Forgione AG et al 2004 Efficacy of pulsed radio frequency energy therapy in temporomandibular joint pain and dysfunction. Cranio 22(1):10-20.

Alcantara J 2002 Chiropractic care of a patient with temporomandibular disorder and atlas subluxation. J Manip Physiol Ther 25(1):63-70.

Association of Chiropractic Colleges 2008 Chiropractic Paradigm. [Retrieved 10th Feb 2008 from: http://www.chirocolleges.org/paradigm scopehtml]

Astin JA, Ernst E 2002 The effectiveness of spinal manipulation for the treatment of headache disorders a systematic review of randomized clinical trials. Cephalalgia 22(8):617-623.

Aukerman G, Knutson D, Miser W 2002 Management of acute migraine headache. Am Fam Physician 66:2123-2130, 2140-2141.

Banks SD 1983 Lumbar facet syndrome: spinographic assessment of treatment by spinal manipulative therapy. J Manipulative Physiol Ther 6(4):175-180.

Biondi DM 2005 Cervicogenic headache: a review of diagnostic and treatment strategies. J Am Osteopath Assoc. 105(4):16-22.

Bogduk N 2001 Cervicogenic headache: anatomic basis and pathophysiologic mechanisms. Curr Pain Headache Rep 5(4):382-386.

Boline PD, Kassak K, Bronfort G et al 1995 Spinal manipulation vs. amitriptyline for the treatment of chronic tension type headaches: a randomised clinical trial. J Manipulative Physiol Ther 18(3):148-154.

Bove G, Nilson N 1998 Spinal manipulation in the treatment of episodic tension-type headache: a randomised clinical trial. JAMA 280:1576-1579.

Bronfort G, Nilsson N, Haas M et al 2004 Non-invasive physical treatments for chronic/recurrent headache. Cochrane Database of Systematic Reviews. Issue 3. CD 001878.

Campbell JK, Penzien DB, Wall EM 2007 Evidence-based guidelines for migraine headache: behavioral and physical treatments. Compiled on behalf of The US Headache Consortium. [Retrieved 12th Feb 2008 from: www.americanheadachesociety.org/professionalresources/USHeadacheConsortiumGuidelines.asp]

CCP (Council on Chiropractic Practice) 1998 Clinical Practice guideline Number 1-Vertebral Subluxation in Chiropractic Practice. [Retrieved 12th Feb 2008 from: http://www.ccp-guidelines.org/guideline-1998.]

Chaitow L 2002 Cranial manipulation: theory and practice, 2nd edn. Churchill Livingstone, Edinburgh, p 242.

Coulter ID, Hurwitz EL, Adams AH, et al 2002 Patients using chiropractors in North America: who are they, and why are they in chiropractic care? Spine 27:291-298.

Crazier RB 1998 Most commonly used methods of detecting subluxation and the preferred term for its description: a survey of chiropractic in Victoria, Australia. J Manipulative Physiol Ther 21(6):428-429.

Curl DD 1994 Chiropractic approach to head pain. Williams and Wilkins, Baltimore, p 121.

Devocht JW, Long CR and Zeitler et al 2003 Chiropractic treatment of temporomandibular disorders using the activator adjusting instrument: a prospective case series. J Manipulative Physiol Ther 26(7):421-425. Eisenberg et al 1998 Trends in alternative medicine use in the United States, 1990-1997. JAMA 280:1569-1575.

Fernandez de las Penas C, Alonso-Blanco C, San-Roman J et al 2006 Methodological quality of randomized controlled trials of spinal manipulation and mobilization in tension-type headache, migraine, and cervicogenic headache. J Orthop Sports Phys Ther 36(3):160-169.

French SD, Green S, Forties A 2000 1998 Reliability of chiropractic methods commonly used to detect manipulable lesions in patients with chronic low-back pain. J Manipulative Physiol Ther 23 (4):231-238.

Gatterman MI 1990 Chiropractic management of spine related disorders. Williams and Wilkins, Baltimore.

Grod JP, Sikorski D, Keating JC 2001 Unsubstantiated claims in patient brochures from the largest state, provincial and national Chiropractic Associations and research agencies. J Manipulative Physiol Ther 24:514-519.

Grunnet-Nilsson N, Bove G 2000 Therapeutic manipulation of episodic tension type headache. A randomized, controlled clinical trial. Ugeskr Laeger 162:174-177.

Haas M, Groupp E, Aickin M et al 2004 Dose response for chiropractic care of chronic cervicogenic headache end associated neck pain: a randomised pilot study. J Manipulative Physiol Ther 27(9):547-553.

Hack GD, Koritzer RT and Robinson WL et al 1995 Anatomic relation between the Rectus Capitis posterior minor muscle and the dura mater. Spine 20(23):2484-2486.

Hack GD, Halgren RC 2004 Chronic headache relief after section of suboccipital muscle dural connections; a case report. Headache 44:84-89.

Hanten WP, Olson SL, Hodson JL et al 1999 The effectiveness of CV-4 and resting position techniques on subjects with tension-type headache. J Manual Manip Ther 7(2):64-70.

Hartman SE, Norton JM 2002 Interexaminer reliability and cranial osteopathy. The Scientific Review of Alternative Medicine 6(1):23-34.

Hawk C, Khorsan R, Lisi AJ et al 2007 Chiropractic care for non-musculoskeletal conditions: a systems review with implications for whole systems research. J Altern Complement Med 13(5):491-512.

Hellstrom F, Thunberg J, Berenheim M et al 2002 Increased intra-articular bradykinin in temporomandibular joint changes the sensitivity in muscle spindles in the dorsal neck muscles of the cat. Neurosc Res 42:91-99.

Higbie EJ, Seidel-Cobb D, Taylor LF et al 1999 Effect of head position on vertical mandibular opening. J Orthop. Sports Phys Ther 29(2):127-130.

Humphreys BK, Delahaye M, Peterson CK 2004 An investigation into the validity of cervical spine motion palpation using subjects with congenital block vertebra as a 'gold standard'. BMC Musculoskelet Disord 15:5-19.

Hurwitz EL, Morgenstern H, Harber P et al 1998 Use of chiropractic services from 1985 through 1991 in the United States and Canada. Am J Pub Health 88(5):771-776.

Janda V 1986 Extracranial causes of facial pain. J Prosth Dent 56 (4):484-487.

Jull G, Bullock M 1987 A motion profile of the lumbar spine in an ageing population assessed by manual examination. Physiotherapy Practice 3:70-81.

Jull G, Trott P, Potter H et al 2002 A randomised controlled trial of exercise and manipulative therapy for cervicogenic headache. Spine 27:1835-1843.

Keating JC, Charlton KH, Grod JP et al 2005 Subluxation: dogma or science. Chiropr Osteopat 13:17.

Kent C 1996 Models of vertebral subluxation: a review. J Vertebral Subluxation Research 1(1):1-7.

Kostopoulos DC, Keramidas G 1992 Changes in elongation of falx cerebri during craniosacral therapy techniques applied on the skull of an embalmed cadaver. Cranio 10(1): 9-12.

Kovich VG 1976 Age changes in the frontozygomatic suture from 29-95 years. Am J Orthodontics 69:411-430

Kritsineli M, Shim YS 1992 Malocclusion, body posture and temporomandibular disorder in children with primary and mixed dentition. J Clin Pediatr Dent 16(2):86-93.

Kulekcioglu S, Sivrioglu K, Ozcan O et al 2003 Effectiveness of low-level laser therapy in temporomandibular disorder. Scand J Rheumatol 32(2):114-118.

Lance J, Goadsby P 2004 Mechanism and management of headache, 7th edn. Butterworth-Heinemann, Oxford, p 325.

Leach RA 1983 An evaluation of the effect of chiropractic manipulative therapy on hypolordosis of the cervical spine. J Manipulative Physiol Ther 6(1):17-23.

Lenssinck MLB, Damen L and Verhagen AP et al 2004 The effectiveness of physiotherapy and manipulation in patients with tension-type headache: a systematic review. Pain 112:381-388.

Licht PB Christensen HW and Hoilund-Carlsen FP 2000 Is there a role for premanipulative testing before cervical manipulation? J Manipulative Physiol Ther 23(3):115-179.

Licht PB, Christensen HW, Hoilund-Carlsen FP 2003 Is cervical spinal manipulation dangerous? J Manipulative Physiol Ther 26(1):48-52.

Meeker WC, Haldeman S 2002 Chiropractic: A profession at the crossroads of mainstream and alternative medicine. Annals of Internal medicine 136:216-227.

Nelson C, Boline PD 1991 A consensus on the assessment and treatment of headache. Chiropractic Technique 3(4):151-167.

Nelson CF 1998a Principles of effective headache management. Topics in clinical chiropractic. 5(1):55-61.

Nelson CF, Bronfort G and Evans R 1998b The efficacy of spinal manipulation, amitriptyline and the combination of both therapies for the prophylaxis of migraine headache. J Manipulative Physiol Ther 21(8):511-519.

NHMRC (Australian Government National Health and Medical Research Council) 2003 Evidence-based management of acute musculoskeletal pain: A guide for clinicians. Australian Academic Press, Brisbane.

Nicolakis P, Burak EC, Kollmitzer J 2001a An investigation of the effectiveness of exercise and manual therapy in treating symptoms of TMJ osteoarthritis. Cranio 19(1):26-32.

Nicolakis P, Erdogmus B, Kopf A et al 2001b Effectiveness of exercise therapy in patients with internal derangement of the temporomandibular joint. J Oral Rehabil 28(12):1158-1164.

Nilsson N 1995 The prevalence of cervicogenic headache in a random population sample of 20-59 year olds. Spine 20:1884-1888.

Nilsson N, Christensen HW, Hartvigsen J 1997 The effect of spinal manipulation in the treatment of cervicogenic headache. J Manipulative Physiol Ther 20:326-330.

Olmos SR, Silverman D, Halligan WM 2005 The effects of condyle fossa relationships on head posture. J Craniomandibular Pract 23(1):48-52.

O'Reilly A, Pollard H 1996 TMJ and chiropractic adjustment-a pilot study. Chiropr J Aust 26:125-129.

Parikh AS, Stouch B, Coughlin PM 2001 The effects of OMT on vital signs during headache [meeting abstract]. Journal of the American Osteopathic Association 101(8):475.

Parker GB, Pryor DS, Tupling H 1980 Why does migraine improve during a clinical trial? Further results from a trial of cervical manipulation for migraine. ANZ J Med 10:192-198.

Parker GB, Tupling H, Pryor DS 1978 A controlled trial of cervical manipulation for migraine. ANZ J Med 8:589-593.

Pederick F 2005 Chiropractic in the cranial field. In: Chaitow L (ed) Cranial manipulation theory and practice, 2nd edn. Churchill Livingstone, Edinburgh, p 111.

Pick MG 1994 A preliminary single case MRI investigation into maxillary fronto-parietal manipulation and its short term effect upon the inter-cranial structures of an adult human brain. J Manipulative Physiol Ther 17(3):168-173.

Pikus HJ, Phillips JM 1995 Characteristics of patients successfully treated for cervicogenic headache by surgical decompression of the second cervical nerve root. Headache 35:621-629.

Rocabado M, Iglarsh ZA 1991 Musculoskeletal approach to maxillofacial pain. Lippincott, Philadelphia, p 70.

Saghafi D, Curl DD 1995 Chiropractic manipulation of anteriorly displaced temporomandibular disc with adhesion. J Manipulative Physiol Ther 18(2):98-104.

Seaman DR 1998 Philosophy and Science versus dogmatism in the practice of chiropractic. J Chiropr Humanities 8:55-66.

Seffinger M, Adams A, Najm W et al 2003 Spinal palpatory diagnostic procedures utilized by practitioners of spinal manipulation: annotated bibliography of content validity and reliability studies. J Can Chiropr Assoc 47:93-109.

Simmons HC 2005 Guidelines for anterior repositioning appliance therapy for the management of craniofacial pain and TMD. Cranio 23(4):300-305.

Simons D, Travell J, Simons LS 1999 Myofascial pain and dysfunction: the trigger point manual, Vol 1, 2nd edn. Williams and Wilkins, Baltimore.

Stodolny J, Chmielewski H 1989 Manual therapy in the treatment of patients with cervical migraine. Manual Med 4:49-51.

Tenet A 2005 Correction of upper cervical subluxations in the treatment of migraine and migraine variants. Commentary published in The Australian Chiropractor (Newsletter of the Chiropractic Association of Australia) May 2005, p 11, 24-25.

Thel H, Rix G 2005 Is it time to stop functional pre-manipulation testing of the cervical spine? Man Ther 10(2):154-158.

Tuchin PJ, Pollard H, Bonello R 2000 A randomised controlled trial of chiropractic spinal manipulative therapy for migraine. J Manipulative Physiol Ther 23(2):91-95.

Valenzuela S, Miralles R, Ravera HJ et al 2005 Does head posture have a significant effect on the hyoid bone position and sternocleidomastoid electromyographic activity in young adults? Cranio 23(3):204-271.

Visscher CM, De Boer W and Lobbezoo F et al 2002 Is there a relationship between head posture and craniomandibular pain? J Oral Rehabil 29(11):1030-1036.

Walker BF 1997 Most commonly used methods of detecting spinal subluxation and the preferred term for its description: a survey of chiropractors in Victoria, Australia. J Manipulative Physiol Ther 20(9):583-589.

Walker R 1998 Chirodontics: A treatment paradigm for the new millennium. Funct Orthod 15 (4):12-I5.

Wight JS 1978 Migraine: a statistical analysis of chiropractic treatment. ACA J Chiropractic 15(9):S63-S67.

World Health Organization 2005 WHO guidelines on the basic training and safety in chiropractic. WHO Press Geneva. Glossary p 4.

Wright EF, Domenech MA, Fischer JR Jr 2000 Usefulness of posture training for patients with temporomandibular disorders. J Am Dent Assoc 131(2):202-210.

Chapter Seventeen

17

Osteopathic approach

Philip Tehan and Peter Gibbons

Headache, with or without spinal pain, is a common presenting complaint to osteopaths. In this chapter the authors, both osteopaths, describe the principles of osteopathy and the osteopathic approach to patient assessment with reference to the cervical region and headache.

While many primary care providers may view their headache patients from a holistic perspective, the osteopathic approach pays particular attention to: dysfunction in the whole of the musculoskeletal system and not just the cervical spine, the influence of the autonomic nervous system, and the impact of dysfunction on fluid and lymphatic drainage.

Osteopathic principles

Health is based on the natural capacity of the human organism to resist and combat noxious influences in the environment and to compensate for their effects; to meet, with adequate reserve, the stresses of daily life and the occasional stresses imposed by extremes of environment and activity. Osteopathic medicine recognizes that many factors impair this capacity primarily local disturbances or lesions of the musculoskeletal system (Special Committee on Osteopathic Principles and Osteopathic Technic 1953).

The philosophy underpinning the osteopathic approach can be reduced to a number of simple principles that are described in Box 17.1.

The distinguishing feature of the osteopathic approach to the treatment of headaches is a focus upon identifying and treating altered function in one or more body systems.

In headache syndromes osteopaths seek to identify and treat:

- Dysfunction in the whole musculoskeletal system
- Dysfunction within the cervical spine
- Dysfunction of the autonomic nervous system
- Dysfunction of fluid and lymphatic drainage.

The osteopath aims to determine the significance of any identified dysfunction in relation to the patient's symptoms. If appropriate, osteopathic manipulative therapy can then be utilized to treat the identified dysfunction.

Dysfunction in the whole musculoskeletal system

The osteopathic approach commences with a screening examination to evaluate the total musculoskeletal system. Greenman proposes a 12 step screening process (Greenman 2003).

Principles underpinning the osteopathic approach.

- The body is a self-regulating organism whose homeostatic mechanisms provide an inherent capacity for healing and repair.
- The body is an integrated unit and its structure and function are inter-dependent.
- Dysfunction of the neuromusculoskeletal system can affect a patient's overall health status and the ability to recover from injury and disease.
- Free and unhindered fluid interchange and drainage are necessary for the maintenance of health, e.g. blood, interstitial fluid, lymph, synovial fluid and cerebrospinal fluid.
- Osteopathic manipulative therapy can be used to assist recovery from injury and disease.

1. Gait analysis in multiple directions

2. Static posture and palpation of paired anatomic landmarks

3. Dynamic trunk sidebending in standing

4. Standing flexion test

5. Stork test

6. Seated flexion test

7. Screening test of upper extremities

8. Trunk rotation

9. Trunk sidebending in sitting

10. Head and neck mobility

11. Respiration of thoracic cage

12. Lower extremity screening (Greenman 2003)

The aim of this examination is to identify areas of dysfunction within the musculoskeletal system that may contribute to symptoms and which require further evaluation.

This approach is based upon the concept that mechanical and structural dysfunction can result from single incidences of trauma or from microtrauma occurring over time as a result of postural imbalance or occupational and environmental stresses. Cumulative microtrauma can lead to a breakdown of the body's normal compensatory mechanisms with resultant development of dysfunction and pain.

This biomechanical model requires the osteopath to restore maximum function to the musculoskeletal system with the aim of enhancing the body's ability to compensate for external mechanical stresses and postural imbalance. The aim of osteopathic treatment is to regain optimal function within joints, ligaments, muscle and fascia.

Dysfunction within the cervical spine

Headache arising from dysfunction within the cervical spine is termed cervicogenic headache. This type of headache may follow cervical spine trauma or may occur spontaneously and can be confused with other types of headache, e.g. tension type headache or migraine.

Patients with cervicogenic headache often present with restricted range of neck motion (Hall & Robinson 2004). Familiar headache symptoms may be elicited by active or passive movements and/or local palpation in the upper and mid cervical spine. Neurological assessment demonstrates no evidence of any radiculopathy. Diagnostic imaging cannot confirm a diagnosis of cervicogenic headache but is used to identify the extent of any degenerative change and the presence of disc protrusions, serious pathology or arteriovenous malformation.

The dorsal rami of C1, C2 and C3 innervate apophyseal joints of the upper cervical spine and dysfunction or local pathology of the upper three cervical segments is postulated as a potential cause of cervicogenic headache. Sensory fibers from the upper cervical roots interact with sensory nerve fibers in the descending tract of the trigeminal nerve in the trigeminocervical nucleus in the upper cervical spinal cord. It is postulated that this convergence of trigeminal and upper cervical sensory pathways might allow referral of pain between the cervical spine and the head. Similarly, sensory afferent nerve fibers from upper cervical regions have been observed to enter the spinal column by way of the spinal accessory nerve (Bremner-Smith et al 1999, Fitzgerald et al 1982). It is believed that the convergence of sensorimotor fibers in the spinal accessory nerve and upper cervical nerve roots with the descending tract of the trigeminal nerve may also be responsible for the referral of pain to the head arising from the cervical spine. However it is important to note that discectomy as low as C5–C6 has been associated with relief of chronic headache (Fredriksen et al 1999, Michler et al 1991).

Osteopaths identify and treat both joint and soft tissue dysfunction using a variety of manual approaches and exercise. A Cochrane review of manipulation and mobilization for mechanical neck pain concluded that, when combined with exercise, mobilization and/or manipulation is beneficial for persistent mechanical neck disorders with or without headache, providing strong evidence for using a multi-modal treatment approach (Gross et al 2004).

Dysfunction of the autonomic nervous system

Osteopaths believe that disturbances in the balance and integration of activity between the sympathetic and parasympathetic systems may lead to somatic dysfunction (Stone 1999). The autonomic nervous system (ANS) plays a role in regulating the internal environment of the body and has many links with the musculoskeletal system. It is thought that it is via this interaction that physical interventions may produce modification of ANS function.

Sympathetic innervation of the head and neck (Fig. 17.1) originates from the intermediolateral

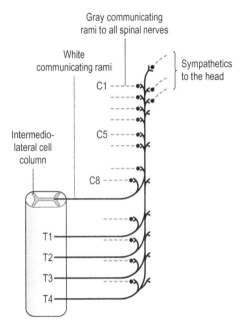

Figure 17.1 • Sympathetic innervation of the head and neck. C = cervical vertebrae, T = thoracic vertebrae.

nucleus of the upper thoracic segments (T1–T4) and enters the head via the sympathetic chain and superior cervical ganglion following the course of the carotid and vertebral arteries and the jugular vein (Willard 2003). Osteopaths often treat dysfunction in the upper and mid thoracic spine in patients with headaches.

Dysfunction of fluid and lymphatic drainage

Osteopaths believe that optimal lymphatic drainage of tissues is an essential component of normal tissue activity and metabolism and is of particular importance for the maintenance of a proper immunologic environment (D'Alonzo & Krachman 2003).

Lymphatic drainage from the head (Fig. 17.2) passes through the neck, cervical fascia and thoracic inlet and dysfunction in any of these structures may lead to lymphatic congestion.

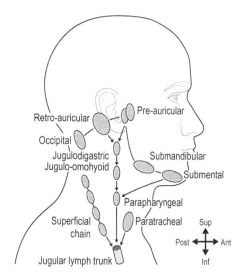

Figure 17.2 ● Lymphatic drainage from the head and neck.

The smooth muscle of the larger lymphatic vessels of the head and neck is supplied by the sympathetic nervous system. Increased sympathetic stimulation associated with upper thoracic and cervical spine dysfunction can constrict these vessels leading to decreased lymphatic drainage (Kappler & Ramey 2003).

Osteopathic diagnosis

Osteopaths follow a clinical decision making process when assessing a patient. These include identifying contraindications (red flags), determining the influence of psychosocial issues (yellow flags), and identifying the presence of any areas of dysfunction that may be amenable to osteopathic manipulative therapy.

Somatic dysfunction

Osteopaths commonly refer to the treatable lesion or area of dysfunction as somatic dysfunction, defined in the Glossary of Osteopathic Terminology as an impaired or altered function of

related components of the somatic (body framework) system: skeletal, arthrodial and myofascial structures, and related vascular, lymphatic, and neural elements (The Glossary Review Committee of the Educational Council on Osteopathic Principles 1993).

Osteopaths diagnose somatic dysfunction by assessing function within the somatic system including the cranium (Kappler 2003). Diagnosis is based on a number of positive findings from palpation. Specific criteria in identifying areas of dysfunction have been developed and relate to the observational and palpatory findings of tissue texture changes, asymmetry, altered range of motion, and tenderness (DiGiovanna & Schiowitz 1997, Greenman 2003, Kappler 2003). Pain provocation and reproduction of familiar symptoms should be used to localize somatic dysfunction.

Information gained from a thorough patient history and patient feedback during assessment should also be used to determine the presence of somatic dysfunction. Somatic dysfunction is identified using the S-T-A-R-T approach (Box 17.2).

Somatic dysfunction may be asymptomatic but most commonly exists within the context of presenting symptoms. Pain and **symptom reproduction** or provocation are, therefore, essential components of the physical examination.

The identification of **tissue texture change** is important in the diagnosis of somatic dysfunction. Palpable changes may be noted in superficial, intermediate and deep tissues.

Box 17.2
The S-T-A-R-T approach to diagnosis.

S	relates to symptom reproduction.
T	relates to tissue texture changes.
A	relates to asymmetry.
R	relates to range of motion.
T	relates to tissue tenderness

DiGiovanna links the criteria of **asymmetry** to a positional focus stating that the 'position of the vertebra or other bone is asymmetrical' (DiGiovanna & Schiowitz 1997) but the concept of asymmetry has been broadened to include functional and structural asymmetry (Greenman 2003).

Alteration in **range of motion** can apply to a single joint, several joints or a region of the musculoskeletal system. The abnormality may include a change in mobility or quality of movement and 'end feel'.

Undue **tissue tenderness** may also be present and must be differentiated from reproduction of the patient's familiar pain.

The diagnosis of somatic dysfunction using the S-T-A-R-T approach is determined by identification of a number of positive findings that are consistent with the patient's clinical presentation. For example, a patient who presents with occipital headaches might have restricted active and passive rotation range of movement in the cervical spine and segmental examination may identify localised movement restriction accompanied by muscular hypertonicity. Palpation of soft tissues and/or apophyseal joints may reproduce the patient's familiar head pain and be accompanied by undue tenderness. This clinical presentation of somatic dysfunction consists of a number of positive findings consistent with a patient presenting with occipital headaches and related musculoskeletal dysfunction.

Osteopathic manipulative prescription

Once symptoms of somatic dysfunction are established, consideration is then given to the most suitable treatment approach. Many factors can influence the final selection of manipulative techniques and the frequency of treatment. The osteopath takes account of factors such as the patient's age, the acuteness or chronicity of the presenting complaint, general health, response to previous treatment and the osteopath's own training and expertise in the delivery of specific osteopathic approaches.

When formulating the osteopathic manipulative prescription, the osteopath has a wide range of techniques to draw upon (Box 17.3).

Some techniques are named according to the activating forces used, e.g. muscle energy, springing, or high velocity low amplitude thrust. Whereas other techniques, e.g. strain/counterstrain, myofascial release and osteopathy in the cranial field, refer to a concept of treatment (Jones & Kappler 2003). Techniques are also classified as either direct or indirect techniques. Direct techniques involve the application of force to engage the restrictive barrier, whereas indirect techniques utilize identification of 'freedom' or 'ease' of movement by moving away from the restrictive barrier (Greenman 2003).

In practice the most commonly used osteopathic manipulative treatment techniques are soft tissue, articulatory, counterstrain, myofascial/

Box 17.3

Osteopathic manipulative techniques.

Articulatory techniques
Balanced ligamentous tension
Chapman's reflexes
Facilitated positional release
Fascial ligamentous release
Functional techniques
High velocity low amplitude thrust
Integrated neuromuscular release and myofascial release
Lymphatic techniques
Muscle energy techniques
Myofascial trigger point
Osteopathy in the cranial field
Progressive inhibition of neuromuscular structures
Soft tissue techniques
Strain and counterstrain
Visceral

neuromuscular release, muscle energy, and high velocity low amplitude thrust (Johnson & Kurtz 2003). An understanding of spinal biomechanics and coupled motion is a prerequisite for the safe and effective utilisation of osteopathic manipulative techniques applied to the spine but especially for the application of muscle energy and high velocity low amplitude (HVLA) thrust techniques.

Soft tissue techniques

Soft tissue techniques are direct techniques that treat the muscular and fascial structures of the body and associated neurovascular elements. Soft tissue techniques can be used alone but are more commonly used in combination with other osteopathic techniques (Ehrenfeuchter et al 2003).

Suboccipital inhibition (Fig. 17.3) is an example of a soft tissue technique which might be used in patients presenting with headache and who have associated suboccipital muscular hypertonicity.

Articulatory techniques

Articulatory techniques applied to the spine, thorax and pelvis, are direct techniques that rhythmically address any restrictive barrier with the intent of reducing the resistance and

improving physiological motion. Forces can be applied to a region or may be used more specifically to restore range of motion at a particular segment. Articulatory techniques stretch shortened soft tissues e.g. muscles, ligaments and joint capsules. Osteopaths believe these techniques often enhance lymphatic flow and stimulate increased circulation (Patriquin & Jones 2003). Articulatory techniques can be used alone but are more commonly used in combination with other osteopathic techniques. Cervicothoracic sidebending articulation (Fig. 17.4A & B) is an example of this type of technique.

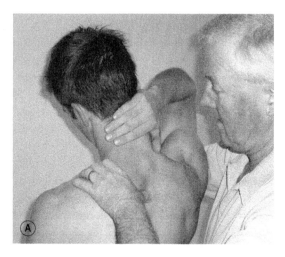

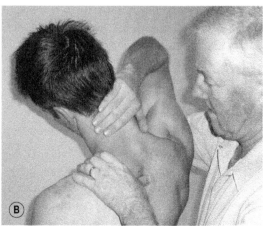

Figure 17.4 • Cervicothoracic sidebending articulation in A, early and B, mid-range.

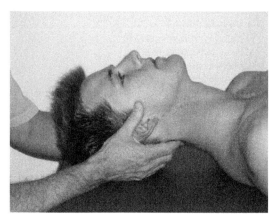

Figure 17.3 • Suboccipital inhibition.

Counterstrain

Counterstrain is a gentle indirect technique where patients are positioned away from restrictive barriers in the direction of comfort and ease (Jones et al 1995). When treating somatic dysfunction of the spine the osteopath identifies both anterior and posterior tender points. The osteopath gently positions the patient in the optimal position of release which is indicated by a local decrease in tissue tension and relief of tenderness on palpation. Patients are not required to generate any force from their own muscle contraction. The position of maximum comfort is usually held for approximately 90 seconds or until the osteopath feels a release in the tissues. The patient is then returned to a neutral position with the osteopath checking for decreased tenderness. Counterstrain can be used alone but is more commonly used in combination with other osteopathic techniques. An anterior C2, C3, C4, C5, C6 technique is an example of the counterstrain approach (Fig. 17.5). In this technique tender points are located on the anterior surface of the transverse processes of the cervical vertebra and the head and neck are positioned in flexion with the operator applying equal amounts of sidebending and rotation away from the tender side.

Myofascial/neuromuscular release

The osteopathic literature describes a wide variety of myofascial and neuromuscular release techniques. In practice the use of these techniques is highly individualised with the techniques often being integrated to treat patterns of dysfunction. The aim is to stretch and reflexively release both soft tissue and articular restrictions. Direct and indirect methods are used. The osteopath identifies and treats patterns of 'tightness' and 'looseness'. These treatment techniques often combine compression, traction and twisting maneuvers that address both static and dynamic movement barriers.

Myofascial and neuromuscular release techniques can be used alone but are commonly used in combination with other osteopathic techniques. Greenman (2003) describes a myofascial release technique for the thoracic inlet that may be useful for headache patients. The final hand placement and patient positioning used in this technique is demonstrated in Figure 17.6.

Muscle energy technique

Muscle energy technique is a direct technique that requires the patient to actively generate

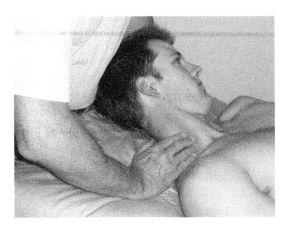

Figure 17.5 • Anterior C2–C6 counterstrain technique.

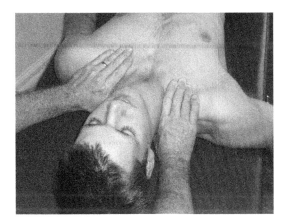

Figure 17.6 • Myofascial release technique for the thoracic inlet.

the corrective force in the form of a muscle contraction in a specific direction against a precisely executed counterforce applied by the osteopath. The spinal positioning from which the technique is executed is predicated upon the diagnosis of somatic dysfunction using the Type 1 and Type 2 models of spinal movement. Some osteopaths use muscle energy techniques as a stand alone approach to treat somatic dysfunction (Ehrenfeuchter & Sandhouse 2003) in headache patients but this approach can also be used in combination with other osteopathic techniques.

Figure 17.7 shows a muscle energy technique used for the treatment of upper thoracic Type 2 somatic dysfunction in headache (restriction of flexion, right rotation and right sidebending at T4).

High velocity low amplitude thrust techniques

High velocity low amplitude (HVLA) thrust techniques of the cervical and cervicothoracic spine are commonly used by osteopaths in the treatment of headache syndromes. The

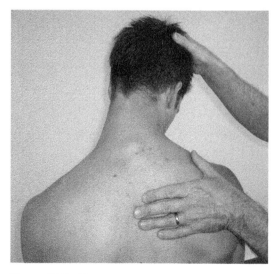

Figure 17.7 • Muscle energy technique for upper thoracic Type 2 dysfunction.

osteopath applies a rapid thrust aiming to achieve joint cavitation that is accompanied by an audible 'popping' or 'cracking' sound. This audible release distinguishes HVLA thrust techniques from other osteopathic manipulative techniques.

An understanding of spinal coupling behavior is necessary for the safe and effective application of HVLA thrust techniques to the cervical and cervicothoracic spine. Spinal locking is particularly important when using HVLA thrust techniques to localize forces and achieve cavitation at a specific vertebral segment (Beal 1989, Downing 1985, Gibbons & Tehan 2006, Greenman 2003, Hartman 1997, Kappler 1989, Nyberg 1993, Stoddard 1972).

The principle of facet apposition locking is to apply leverages to the spine that cause the facet joints of uninvolved segments to be apposed and consequently locked. To achieve locking by facet apposition, the spine is placed in a position opposite to that of normal coupling behavior. The vertebral segment at which cavitation is desired should never be locked.

Osteopathy commonly uses a model of physiologic movements of the spine to assist in the diagnosis of somatic dysfunction and the application of treatment techniques.

Below C2, normal coupling behavior in the cervical spine is that sidebending and rotation occur to the same side (Bennett et al 2002, Greenman 2003, Mimura et al 1989, Stoddard 1969). To generate facet apposition locking for HVLA thrust techniques in the cervical and cervicothoracic spine the spine is positioned in sidebending in one direction and rotation in the opposite direction, i.e. the opposite to normal coupling behavior. This positioning locks the segments above the joint to be cavitated and enables a thrust to be applied to one vertebral segment. The amount or degree of sidebending and rotation is dependent upon whether the osteopath is attempting to thrust in an upslope (Fig. 17.8) or downslope (Fig. 17.9) direction.

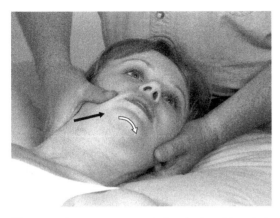

Figure 17.8 • HVLA thrust technique in the mid cervical spine using upslope thrust.

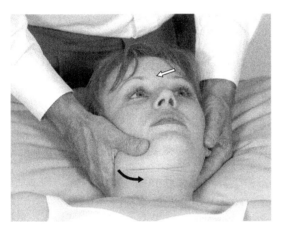

Figure 17.9 • HVLA thrust technique in the mid cervical spine using downslope thrust.

HVLA thrust techniques are rarely used alone by osteopaths and are more commonly used in combination with other osteopathic techniques, e.g. soft tissue and articulatory techniques.

It is often stated that HVLA thrust techniques applied to the spine are associated with a higher level of risk than other direct and indirect techniques. The potential benefits (Hurwitz et al 1996, Spitzer et al 1995) for the patient must be weighed against the risks associated with HVLA thrust techniques of the cervical spine. There are currently no high quality data

to enable accurate estimation of the risk of stroke following cervical HVLA thrust techniques (Breen 2002). While the data identify a temporal relationship between cervical thrust techniques and stroke, it is possible that in a number of instances the cause of the vertebral artery dissection may have preceded the patient's attendance for treatment and not be a consequence of the manipulation. While there is a potential for serious sequelae, the risk appears to be extremely low (Clubb 2002, Rivett 1995). Nonetheless, it is imperative to take all necessary precautions to avoid an adverse event resulting from compromise of the vertebral artery.

Vertebrobasilar insufficiency

There is a risk of serious adverse reactions arising from any osteopathic technique applied to the cervical and cervicothoracic spine in a patient who presents with symptoms arising from vertebrobasilar insufficiency (VBI). The vertebrobasilar system comprises the two vertebral arteries and their union to form the basilar artery (Fig. 17.10).

Most of the literature relates to serious injury arising from cervical spine manipulation. There is wide variation in the estimated incidence of serious adverse reactions arising from cervical manipulation. A number of authors have attempted to estimate the incidence of iatrogenic stroke following cervical spine manipulation with estimates varying between 1 incident in 10 000 cervical spine manipulations, to 1 incident in 5.85 million cervical spine manipulations (Carey 1993, Dabbs & Lauretti 1995, Dvorak & Orelli 1985, Dvorak et al 1993, Gutmann 1983, Haldeman et al 2002, Haynes 1994, Jaskoviak 1980, Klougart et al 1996, Lee et al 1995, Patijn 1991, Rivett & Milburn 1996, Rivett & Reid 1998). It is not clear what type of neck manipulation techniques were applied or the competence

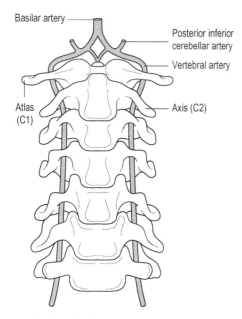

Basilar artery

Posterior inferior
cerebellar artery

Vertebral artery

Atlas
(C1)

Axis (C2)

Figure 17.10 ● Relationship of the cervical spine to the vertebral artery.

and training of the practitioner (Reid & Hing 2001).

In patients presenting with head and neck pain, especially sudden and severe symptoms, it is important to determine if there is associated dizziness and/or signs of brain stem ischemia such as nausea and/or vomiting as these symptoms may indicate a vertebral artery dissection syndrome.

One difficulty in recognising the symptoms of VBI is that many of the common symptoms, e.g. headache, pain and stiffness in the cervical spine, are similar to those for mechanical non-specific neck pain (Schievink 2001, Silbert et al 1995).

Pre-manipulative testing for VBI has been advocated as a means of risk management with a view to minimizing patient harm (Barker et al 2000). There are many physical tests that have been described for determining the presence or absence of VBI (Chapman-Smith 1999, Grant 1994, Maigne 1972, Maitland 1973, Oostendorp 1988, Terrett 1988). However these tests have

been reported to have low sensitivity and specificity for predicting cerebral ischemia prior to neck manipulation (Bolton et al 1989) and the value of such tests in determining VBI has been questioned (Cote et al 1996, Haldeman et al 1999, Licht et al 2002, Oostendorp 1988, Rivett et al 1998, Thiel et al 1994, Westaway et al 2003).

Screening tests should be both valid and reliable predictors of risk. VBI testing movements have neither of these qualities, with available scientific evidence failing to show predictive value (Bolton et al 1989, Di Fabio 1999, Licht et al 2000, Thiel & Rix 2005). Screening should also not be harmful. It has been suggested that the tests themselves may hold certain risks and could have morbid effects on the vertebral artery (Grant 1996). Minor adverse events associated with examination procedures involving rotation, including those related to the use of an established VBI testing protocol, have been documented (Magarey et al 2004).

It is difficult to support the continuing use of VBI screening tests or protocols in isolation as none of the rotation, extension or combination test movements have been shown to be valid or reliable predictors of risk. Is it possible through physical examination or screening procedures to identify patients at risk of vertebrobasilar injury from cervical and cervicothoracic techniques? Current evidence would suggest that the answer is no (McDermaid 2002, Terrett 2002, Thiel et al 1994).

Osteopathic practice in the past has placed an emphasis on pre-manipulative screening tests to minimise the risk of vertebrobasilar complications particularly when high velocity low amplitude (HVLA) thrust techniques are used as part of a treatment regime (Gibbons & Tehan 2006). With regard to the safe use of osteopathic treatment techniques, emphasis should be placed on a combination of a thorough patient history, a comprehensive physical examination and the need for a high level of technical skill in the application of whichever osteopathic technique is used.

A review of the literature, relating to the risk of neurovascular compromise complicating cervical spine high velocity manipulation, concluded that the risk and benefit analysis supported the continued judicial use of cervical spine HVLA thrust techniques by prudent and appropriately trained practitioners (Rivett 1995).

Evidence supporting practice

Best practice requires osteopaths to embrace the principles of evidence-based medicine that integrates the best results from clinical and epidemiological research with individual clinical experience and expertise whilst taking account of patient preferences (Pedersen et al 2001, Sackett et al 1997).

Since 1979 there have been over 50 mostly qualitative, non-systematic reviews published relating to manipulation and mobilization treatment for back and neck pain (Bronfort et al 2004). A number of systematic reviews and meta-analyses have also been undertaken in an attempt to determine the efficacy of spinal manipulation on back and neck pain (Bronfort et al 2004, Mior 2001), neck pain (Gross et al 2002, 2004, Hurwitz et al 1996), and chronic headache (Bronfort et al 2001).

A Cochrane review of manipulation and mobilization for mechanical neck pain concluded that when combined with exercise, mobilization and/or manipulation is beneficial for persistent mechanical neck disorders with or without headache, providing strong evidence for using a multimodal treatment approach (Gross et al 2004). A systematic review of the efficacy of spinal manipulation for chronic headache concluded that spinal manipulative therapy has an effect comparable to commonly prescribed prophylactic tension headache and migraine medications (Bronfort et al 2001).

Conclusion

The osteopathic approach to the treatment of headache not only addresses somatic dysfunction within the cervical spine but also takes into account dysfunction in other areas of the musculoskeletal system and disturbances in autonomic, lymphatic, and fluid systems. When formulating the osteopathic manipulative prescription the clinician has a wide range of direct or indirect techniques to draw upon. Substantive research has been undertaken into HVLA thrust techniques, often combined with mobilization and exercise, with increasing evidence of efficacy. However, many of the commonly-used osteopathic manipulative treatment techniques, e.g. soft tissue, articulatory, counterstrain, myofascial/neuromuscular release, and muscle energy technique, have not yet been subjected to well-designed research studies. The justification for the use of many of these techniques, either alone or in combination, is largely dependent upon osteopathic convention, anatomical knowledge, biomechanical analysis, and clinical experience, whilst taking account of patient preferences.

References

Barker S, Kesson M, Ashmore J et al 2000 Guidance for pre-manipulative testing of the cervical spine. Manual Therapy. 5(1):37-40.

Beal MC 1989 Teaching of basic principles of osteopathic manipulative techniques. In: Beal MC (ed) The principles of palpatory diagnosis and manipulative technique. American Academy of Osteopathy, Newark, p 162-164.

Bennett SE, Schenk R, Simmons E 2002 Active range of motion utilized in the cervical spine to perform daily functional tasks. Journal of Spinal Disorders & Techniques 15 (4):307-311.

Bolton P, Stick P, Lord R 1989 Failure of clinical tests to predict cerebral ischaemia before neck manipulation. Journal of Manipulative and Physiological Therapeutics 12:304-307.

Breen A 2002 Manipulation of the neck and stroke: time for more rigorous evidence. Medical Journal of Australia 176:364-365.

Bremner-Smith AT, Unwin AJ, Williams WW 1999 Sensory pathways in the spinal accessory nerve. J Bone Joint Surg Br 81:226-228.

Bronfort G, Assendelft W, Evans R et al 2001 Efficacy of spinal manipulation for chronic headache: a systematic review. J Manipulative Physiol Ther 24(7):457-466.

Bronfort G, Hass M, Evans R, Bouter L 2004 Efficacy of spinal manipulation and mobilization for low back and neck pain: A systematic review and best evidence synthesis. Spine 4(3):335-356.

Carey P 1993 A report on the occurrence of cerebral vascular accidents in chiropractic practice. Journal of the Canadian Chiropractic Association 37:104-106.

Chapman-Smith D 1999 Cervical adjustment. The chiropractic report 13(4):1-7.

Clubb D 2002 Cervical manipulation and vertebral artery injury: a literature review. Journal of Manual & Manipulative Therapy 10(1):11-16.

Cote P, Kreitz B, Cassidy J, Thiel H 1996 The validity of the extension-rotation test as a clinical screening procedure before neck manipulation: a secondary analysis. Journal of Manipulative and Physiological Therapeutics 19(3):159-164.

D'Alonzo G, Krachman S 2003 Pulmonology. In: Ward R (ed) Foundations for osteopathic medicine, 2nd edn. Lippincott Williams & Wilkins, Philadelphia, ch 34.

Dabbs V, Lauretti W 1995 A risk assessment of cervical manipulation vs NSAIDs for the treatment of neck pain. Journal of Manipulative and Physiological Therapeutics 18: 530-536.

Di Fabio RP 1999 Manipulation of the cervical spine: risks and benefits. Physical Therapy 79(1):51-65.

DiGiovanna EL, Schiowitz S 1997 An osteopathic approach to diagnosis and treatment, 2nd edn. Lippincott Williams & Wilkins, Philadelphia.

Downing CH 1985 Principles and practice of osteopathy. Tamor Pierston, London.

Dvorak J, Orelli F 1985 How dangerous is manipulation to the cervical spine? Journal of Manual Medicine 2:1-4.

Dvorak J, Loustalot D, Baumgartner H, Antinnes J 1993 Frequency of complications of manipulations of the spine. A survey among the members of the Swiss medical society of manual medicine. European Spine Journal 2:136-139.

Ehrenfeuchter W, Sandhouse M 2003 Muscle energy techniques. In: Ward R (ed) Foundations for osteopathic medicine, 2nd edn. Lippincott Williams & Wilkins, Philadelphia, ch 57.

Ehrenfeuchter W, Heilig D, Nicholas A 2003 Soft tissue techniques. In: Ward R (ed) Foundations for osteopathic medicine, 2nd edn. Lippincott Williams & Wilkins, Philadelphia, ch 54.

Fitzgerald MJ, Comerford PT, Tuffery AR 1982 Sources of innervation of the neuromuscular spindles in sternomastoid and trapezius. J Anat 134(pt 3):471-490.

Fredriksen TA, Salvesen R, Stolt-Nielsen A, Sjaastad O 1999 Cervicogenic headache:long-term postoperative follow-up. Cephalalgia 19:897-900.

Gibbons P, Tehan P 2006 Manipulation of the spine thorax and pelvis, 2nd edn. Churchill Livingstone Elsevier, Edinburgh.

Grant R 1994 Vertebral artery insufficiency: A clinical protocol for pre-manipulative testing of the cervical spine. In: Boyling J, Palastanga N (eds) Grieves modern manual therapy, 2nd edn. Churchill Livingstone, Edinburgh, p 371-380.

Grant R 1996 Vertebral artery testing – the Australian Physiotherapy Association Protocol after 6 years. Manual Therapy 1(3):149-153.

Greenman PE 2003 Principles of Manual Medicine, 3rd edn. Lippincott Williams & Wilkins, Philadelphia.

Gross A, Hoving J, Haines T et al 2004 A Cochrane review of manipulation and mobilization for mechanical neck disorders. Spine 29(14):1541-1548.

Gross A, Kay T, Hondras M et al 2002 Manual therapy for mechanical neck disorders: a systematic review Manual Therapy 7(3):131-149.

Gutmann G 1983 Injuries to the vertebral artery caused by manual therapy. Manuelle Medizin 21:2-14.

Haldeman S, Kohlbeck F, McGregor M 1999 Risk factors and precipitating neck movements causing vertebrobasilar artery dissection after cervical trauma and spinal manipulation. Spine 24(8):785-794.

Haldeman S, Kohlbeck F, McGregor M 2002 Unpredictability of cerebrovascular ischemia associated with cervical spine manipulation therapy: a review of sixty four cases after cervical spine manipulation. Spine. 27(1):49-55.

Hall T, Robinson K 2004 The flexion-rotation test and active cervical mobility – a comparative measurement study in cervicogenic headache. Man Ther 9:197-202.

Hartman L 1997 Handbook of osteopathic technique, 3rd edn. Chapman and Hall, London.

Haynes M 1994 Stroke following cervical manipulation in Perth. Chiropractic Journal of Australia 24:42-46.

Hurwitz E, Aker P, Adams A et al 1996 Manipulation and mobilization of the cervical spine: a systematic review of the literature. Spine 21 (15):1746-1760.

Jaskoviak P 1980 Complications arising from manipulation of the cervical spine. Journal of Manipulative and Physiological Therapeutics 3: 213-219.

Johnson S, Kurtz M 2003 Osteopathic manipulative treatment techniques preferred by contemporary osteopathic physicians. Journal of the American Osteopathic Association 103(5):219-224.

Jones J, Kappler R 2003 Osteopathic considerations in palpatory diagnosis and manipulative treatment. In: Ward R (ed) Foundations for osteopathic medicine, 2nd edn. Lippincott Williams & Wilkins, Philadelphia, Section VII.

Jones L, Kusunose R, Goering E 1995 Jones Strain-Counterstrain. Jones Strain-Counterstrain Inc, Boise, ID 83706.

Kappler RE 1989 Direct action techniques. In: Beal MC (ed) The principles of palpatory diagnosis and manipulative technique. American Academy of Osteopathy, Newark, p 165-168.

Kappler RE 2003 Palpatory skills and exercises for developing the sense of touch. In: Ward R (ed) Foundations for osteopathic medicine, 2nd edn. Lippincott Williams & Wilkins, Philadelphia, ch 38.

Kappler R, Ramey K 2003 Head: diagnosis and treatment. In: Ward R (ed) Foundations for osteopathic medicine, 2nd edn. Lippincott Williams & Wilkins, Philadelphia, ch 45.

Klougart N, Leboeuf -Yde C, Rasmussen LR 1996 Safety in chiropractic practice, part 1: the occurrence of cerebrovascular accidents after manipulation to the neck in Denmark from 1978 - 1988. Journal of Manipulative and Physiological Therapeutics 19:371-377.

Lee K, Carlini W, McCormick G, Albers G 1995 Neurologic complications following chiropractic manipulation: a survey of California neurologists. Neurology 45:1213-1215.

Licht P, Christensen H, Hoilund-Carlsen P 2002 Carotid artery blood flow during premanipulative testing. Journal of Manipulative and Physiological Therapeutics 25 (9):568-572.

Licht P, Christensen H, Hoilund-Carlsen P 2000 Is there a role for pre-manipulative testing before cervical manipulation. Journal of Manipulative and Physiological Therapeutics 23:175-179.

Magarey M, Rebbeck T, Coughlan B et al 2004 Pre-manipulative testing of the cervical spine: review, revision and new clinical guidelines. Manual Therapy 9(2):95-108.

Maigne R 1972 Orthopaedic medicine: a new approach to vertebral manipulation. Charles C Thomas, Illinois.

Maitland G 1973 Vertebral manipulation, 3rd edn. Butterworths, London.

McDermaid C 2002 Vertebrobasilar incidents and spinal manipulative therapy of the cervical spine. In; Vernon H (ed) Chapter 14. The cranio-cervical syndrome. Butterworth Heinemann, London.

Michler RP, Bovim G, Sjaastad O 1991 Disorders in the lower cervical spine. A cause of unilateral headache? Headache 31:550-551.

Mimura M, Moriya H, Watanabe T et al 1989 Three dimensional motion analysis of the cervical spine with special reference to the axial rotation. Spine 14(11):1135-1139.

Mior S 2001 Manipulation and mobilization in the treatment of chronic pain. Clinical Journal of Pain 17(4):S70-S76.

Nyberg R 1993 Manipulation: definition, types, application. In: Basmajian J, Nyberg R (eds) Rational manual therapies. Williams and Wilkins, Baltimore, ch 3.

Oostendorp R 1988 Vertebrobasilar insufficiency. Proceedings of the International Federation of Orthopaedic Manipulative Therapists Congress, Cambridge, p 42-44.

Patijn J 1991 Complications in manual medicine: a review of the literature. Journal of Manual Medicine 6:89-92.

Patriquin D, Jones J 2003 Articulatory techniques. In: Ward R (ed) Foundations for osteopathic medicine, 2nd edn. Lippincott Williams & Wilkins, Philadelphia, ch 55.

Pedersen T, Gluud C, Gotzsche P et al 2001 What is evidence-based medicine? Ugeskr Laeger 163 (27):3769-3772.

Reid D, Hing W 2001 AJP Forum: Pre-manipulative testing of the cervical spine. Australian Journal of Physiotherapy 47:164.

Rivett D 1995 Neurovascular compromise complicating cervical spine manipulation: What is the risk?

Journal of Manual & Manipulative Therapy 3(4):144-151.

Rivett D, Milburn P 1996 A prospective study of cervical spine manipulation. Journal of Manual Medicine 4:166-170.

Rivett D, Reid D 1998 Risk of stroke for cervical spine manipulation in New Zealand. New Zealand Journal of Physiotherapy 26:14-17.

Rivett D, Milburn P, Chapple C 1998 Negative pre-manipulative vertebral artery testing despite complete occlusion: a case of false negativity. Manual Therapy 3 (2):102-107.

Sackett D, Richardson W, Rosenberg W, Haynes R 1997 Evidence-based medicine. How to practice & teach EBM. Churchill Livingstone, New York.

Schievink W 2001 Spontaneous dissection of the carotid and vertebral arteries. New England Journal of Medicine 344: 898-906.

Silbert P, Mokri B, Schievink W 1995 Headache and neck pain in spontaneous internal carotid and vertebral artery dissections. Neurology 45:1517-1522.

Special Committee on Osteopathic Principles and Osteopathic Technic, Kirksville College of Osteopathy and Surgery. 1953 An interpretation of the osteopathic concept. Tentative formulation of a teaching guide for faculty, hospital staff and student body. Journal of Osteopathy 60: 8-10.

Spitzer W, Skovron M, Salmi L et al 1995 Monograph of the Quebec Task Force on Whiplash Associated Disorders: Redefining Whiplash and its Management. Spine 20:8S.

Stoddard A 1969 Manual of osteopathic practice. Hutchinson Medical Publications, London.

Stoddard A 1972 Manual of osteopathic technique, 2nd edn. Hutchinson Medical Publications, London.

Stone C 1999 Science in the art of osteopathy – osteopathic principles and practice. Stanley Thornes, Cheltenham, UK.

Terrett A 1988 Vascular accidents from cervical spine manipulation: the mechanisms. Australian Chiropractors Association. Journal of Chiropractic 22(5):59-74.

Terrett A 2002 Did the SMT practitioner cause the arterial injury? Chiropractic Journal of Australia 32 (3):99-119.

The Glossary Review Committee of the Educational Council on Osteopathic Principles 1993 Glossary of osteopathic terminology. In: Allen TW (ed) AOA Yearbook and Directory of Osteopathic Physicians. American Osteopathic Association, Chicago.

Thiel H, Rix G 2005 Is it time to stop functional pre-manipulation testing of the cervical spine? Manual Therapy 10(2):154-158.

Thiel H, Wallace K, Donat J, Yong-Hing K 1994 Effect of various head and neck positions on vertebral artery flow. Clinical Biomechanics 9:105-110.

Westaway M, Stratford P, Symons B 2003 False-negative Extension/Rotation pre-manipulative screening test on a patient with an atretic and hypoplastic vertebral artery. Manual Therapy 8(2):120-127.

Willard FH 2003 Autonomic nervous system. In: Ward R (ed) Foundations for osteopathic medicine, 2nd edn. Lippincott Williams & Wilkins, Philadelphia, ch 6.

Integrative medicine approach

Iggy Soosay

Effective assessment and treatment of headache or migraine depends on a good history. In some cases a dietary history is important as food allergy or sensitivities can be a key factor in the precipitation of headache. In this chapter the author, a general practitioner, addresses the effect of food allergy and tyramine-rich foods on headache. The chapter also discusses dietary modification to reduce the incidence, frequency, and duration of headaches.

Headache, including migraine, is a common health problem and can be a challenge to the treating practitioner. A number of etiological factors such as food sensitivities or allergies, nutritional deficiencies, or neuroendocrine imbalances can be involved. Hence, the challenge of effecting a cure rather than symptom management involves the identification of causes and contributing factors specific to each presenting patient. Whilst this may not always be possible, unless one starts with the aim of exploring possible causes the practitioner may miss the opportunity to effect a cure.

Integrative medicine

Effective management of headache requires an integrative approach. Integrative medicine has been found to be a scientifically accurate approach to healing that focuses on the whole person (not merely on disease or symptoms),
treats the patient as a unique individual (both in assessment and treatment), and emphasizes health promotion (Pizzorno 2003).

Careful assessment is made of lifestyle patterns as they relate to sleep, nutrition, exercise, and stress management. Where applicable, improvement of eating and sleeping habits can have a significant beneficial effect on headache frequency.

This chapter looks first at specific dietary causes of headache and migraine, while the second part addresses toxic overload, focusing on the effect this may have on the gut and the liver. The information is referenced where evidence exists; nutritional medicine is an evolving field and whilst evidence is increasing it is not complete. Treating the patient with headache can be a challenge. With some difficult patients it is the failure of conventional medicine that leads them to seek help from alternative medicine practitioners. The author has been practicing and lecturing in this form of medicine for over 25 years and draws on clinical experience to present this approach to treating a patient with headache or migraine.

Dietary factors

Allergy and food sensitivities can trigger various types of headaches. In one study over 70% of migraine sufferers exhibited at least one reaction induced by food (Mansfield et al 1985). In another study, 93% of children with migraine improved with a diet that avoided offending foods (Egger et al 1983). Whilst there is no conclusive evidence as to which chemicals in foods trigger headaches, it is thought that vasoactive amines such as tyramine and other amines including phenylethylamine and histamine are responsible.

Tyramine is found in cheese, especially aged, strong, and cheddar varieties. Phenylethylamine is found in chocolate, octopamine in citrus fruits, and histamine in red wine and beers. Caffeine addiction and withdrawal can be associated with headaches and exacerbation of migraine (Scher et al 2004). Fasting or skipping meals leading to hypoglycemia can also trigger migraines (Jacome 2001).

Chocolate is a common trigger and the chemicals in this food are, phenylethylamine, theobromine, and caffeine. The postulated cause is an alteration of blood flow and the release of norepinephrine (Martin & Behbehani 2001). A proposed mechanism by which caffeine can cause headaches presumes a vasoconstrictive action on the cerebral arteries. When caffeine consumption is reduced or ceases, the blood vessels dilate and the increased cerebral blood flow results in headaches in susceptible individuals.

Alcohol also has a vasodilator effect on cranial blood vessels. However the alcohol itself is probably not the migraine-provoking chemical, but rather the tyramine and histamine contained in red wines and beers.

Headache can be induced by histamine in wine and some foods in patients suffering from histamine intolerance. Histamine is degraded by the enzyme diamine oxidase in the small bowel. Hence, a reduced level of activity or lack of this enzyme can trigger a headache when a histamine-containing food is consumed.

A histamine-free diet is the treatment of choice for patients with histamine intolerance and chronic headache. Treatment is started with an H1 blocker antihistamine for 14 days as well

Box 18.1

Histamine-rich foods (partial list).

Anchovies
Beer
Cheeses
Ciders
Eggplant
Fermented foods
Processed meats
Sardines
Tomatoes
Wines
Yeast extract
Yoghurt

as a histamine-free diet for at least 4 weeks. Box 18.1 lists the major histamine-rich foods. As supportive treatment, vitamin B6 (pyridoxal phosphate) is also suggested, as pyridoxal phosphate seems to be crucial for diamine oxidase activity (Jarisch & Wantke 1996).

Nitrates as food additives are another cause of headache. Cured meats such as ham, bacon, salami and hot dogs contain nitrates.

Aspartame is a sweetener cleared for general consumption except for children with phenylketonuria. This additive is approved for use in pharmaceutical products and, as well as its use as a sweetener in many foods, is being used increasingly in chewable tablets and sugar-free formulations. Headache is the most common adverse effect attributed to aspartame. Aspartame in chewing gum has been reported to be a cause of headaches (Blumenthal & Vance 1997), while up to 11% of patients with chronic migraine reported headaches triggered by aspartame (Lipton et al 1989). However a double-blind challenge with three doses of 10 mg/kg given every 2 hours triggered no more headaches than did placebos in patients with vascular headaches believed to be exacerbated by aspartame (Schiffman et al 1987). A small, double-blind, trial showed an increase in frequency of headaches after ingestion of 1200 mg/day over a four weeks, indicating that a longer challenge period may be necessary (Koehler & Glaros 1988). Many scientists have expressed caution concerning the use of aspartame in patients with migraine, epilepsy, and psychiatric disorders (Millichap 2001, Newman & Lipton 2001).

An under-recognized cause of migraine is gluten sensitivity. Classical celiac disease is a gluten-sensitive enteropathy where small bowel villous atrophy is associated with malabsorption, steatorrhea, and weight loss. This disease affects different people differently and there are no typical signs and symptoms. Most people with celiac disease have general complaints such as intermittent diarrhea, abdominal pain and bloating; some have no gastrointestinal symptoms at all. The symptoms of this disease may also mimic other conditions such as irritable bowel syndrome, Crohn's disease, or skin disorders.

Clinical experience suggests that most patients with celiac disease present with non-specific or trivial complaints (Box 18.2), with the diagnosis only inferred from abnormalities in routine blood tests, e.g. anemia, iron, and/or vitamin B12 deficiency. Gluten is found in foods containing wheat, rye, barley, and oats. The 'gold standard' for the diagnosis of celiac disease is small bowel biopsy but antibody testing is a useful first line investigation.

Box 18.2

Symptoms of celiac disease.

Weight loss
Diarrhea/constipation
Recurring abdominal bloating and pain
Fatigue
Pale, foul smelling stools
Iron deficiency anemia not responding to iron
  therapy
Joint pain
Paresthesia in the legs
Mouth sores
Skin rash
Stunted growth (in children)
Osteopenia or osteoporosis

It is only relatively recently that gluten sensitivity has been recognized as a cause of neurological illness (Hadjivassiliou et al 2002). It has been estimated that 10% of patients with celiac disease develop neurological complications (Finelli et al 1980). Retrospective analysis of data from a hospital in the UK found that neurological and psychiatric conditions occurred in 189 out of 620 patients with celiac disease. The three most common conditions were depression, epilepsy, and migraine (Pengiran Tengah et al 2002).

In a study of 90 patients with migraine, 4.4% were found to have celiac disease compared with 0.4% of blood donor controls. During 6 months on a gluten-free diet there was a significant lessening of the frequency, duration, and intensity of migraine (Gabrielli et al 2003). In adolescents with celiac disease there is an increased incidence of migraine and tension headaches (Roche Herrero et al 2001).

Asymptomatic patients with an enteropathy characteristic of celiac disease are considered to have 'silent celiac disease' and those with apparently normal small bowel biopsy who develop typical histological features later in life are regarded as having 'latent celiac disease'. These observations have led to the concept of a 'celiac disease iceberg' made up of a visible part of those who are diagnosed clinically and a far larger submerged portion that includes all individuals who are undiagnosed because of atypical, latent, or silent disease (Pengiran Tengah et al 2002).

Management of food-induced migraine

Treatment involves keeping a headache and diet diary, and the selective avoidance of food presumed to trigger attacks. Headache diaries can be downloaded from the internet. Figure 18.1 is an example of the diaries that can be found on the site of The American Council of Headache Education.

Daily Diary

Date of headache: ....

Type of headache: migraine   tension-type   other: ....

	Comment
Description of prodrome (symptoms prior to onset of pain)	
Presence of aura	
Time of headache onset	
Severity of worst pain (0 = no pain: 10 = severe pain)	
Symptoms (e.g. nausea, vomiting, photophobia, throbbing, disability)	
Medication 1 taken	Type of medicine: Dose: Time of dose:
Medication 2 taken	Type of medicine: Dose: Time of dose:
Time of headache relief	
Noted triggers of factors that may cause headache (e.g. caffeine, menstruation, fasting, sleep deprivation, other)	
Other comments	
Questions about your headache or medication	

Figure 18.1 ● A daily headache diary. (Daily, weekly, and monthly diaries are available for download from http://www.achenet.org/)

A universal migraine diet with simultaneous elimination of all potential triggers is generally not advised in practice as it can be extremely difficult to adhere to and there is a danger of developing nutrient deficiencies. Dietary advice should therefore only be given by an experienced professional. A well balanced diet is encouraged with avoidance of fasting. This approach to identifying and eliminating food triggers should be attempted prior to long-term prophylactic drug therapy.

Both Omega-3 polyunsaturated fatty acids and olive oil supplements have been shown to reduce the frequency and severity of migraines in adolescents (Harel et al 2002).

Coenzyme Q10

In some patients mitochondrial dysfunction resulting in impaired oxygen metabolism has been implicated in migraine pathogenesis (Montagna et al 1994). Coenzyme Q10 is a naturally occurring substance and an essential element in the mitochondrial electron transport chain. An open label study (Rozen et al 2002) using 150 mg per day of Coenzyme Q10 was trialed as a preventive for migraine. Mean reduction in migraine frequency after one month of treatment was 13% and this increased to 55% by the end of 3 months. There were no side effects noted with Coenzyme Q10. Another study (Sandor et al 2005) compared Coenzyme Q10, 100 mg three times daily, and placebo in 42 migraine patients in a double-blind placebo-controlled trial. Coenzyme Q10 was superior to placebo in reducing attack frequency, headache days, and days with nausea. Tolerability was excellent with one adverse effect to the Coenzyme Q10 being cutaneous allergy.

Coenzyme Q10 has been suggested as effective in the prevention of pediatric and adolescent migraine. In this study (Herskey et al 2007), one-third of the study population of 1550 patients was found to be deficient in Coenzyme Q10. Treatment with a dose of 1 to 3 mg/Kg per day of Coenzyme Q10 resulted in significant reduction in migraine frequency and disability over 100 days

Magnesium and fish oil

Both magnesium and fish oil (Box 18.3) have been associated with inhibition of platelet aggregation and inhibition of vasospasm. Magnesium is also thought to stabilize cell membranes, and reduce formation of inflammatory eicosonoids. High dose oral magnesium appears to be effective in migraine prophylaxis. In a multi-centre placebo-controlled, double-blind randomized study (Peikert et al 1996) 600 mg (24 mmol) was used daily for 12 weeks. Migraine frequency was reduced by 41.6% in the magnesium group compared to 15.8% in the placebo group.

Toxic overload

Patients usually present to integrative doctors when conventional treatments have been exhausted. Commonly, these patients would have been thoroughly investigated with no specific cause found for the headache or migraine. For the rest of this chapter it is assumed that the migraine or headache has been thoroughly investigated and no cause has been found. The

---

Box 18.3

Therapeutic actions of magnesium and fish oil in migraine (Toth 2003).

Magnesium
Inhibition of platelet aggregation
Counteract vasospasm
Stabilize cell membranes
Reduce formation of inflammatory eicosonoids
Fish oil
Platelet stabilization
Antivasospastic action

focus then is to identify any toxic overload on the body. Chronic and multiple agent overload is more common than single agent or acute toxicity.

Medication- or substance-induced headache is probably an under-recognized condition with multiple etiologies. These include prescribed medication (including medication for the headache), over-the-counter medication, illicit drugs, anesthetic agents, inhaled substances, and substances used in diagnostic procedures (Toth 2003).

Proposed mechanisms by which toxicity can cause or contribute to headaches and migraine include interference with digestion, nutrient absorption, cellular transport, oxidative damage, enzyme interference and mimicking of hormones. Those relating to the gut and to the liver are discussed further.

The gut connection

The gut is another major source of toxicity. Poorly digested foods, by-products of digestion, altered gut bacterial populations caused by exogenous hormones, and antibiotics can all interfere with normal physiology.

The gastrointestinal tract (GIT) is a critical barrier between the internal and external environment. The normal intestinal epithelium is a semi-permeable (selective) barrier which prevents toxic, antigenic molecules or microorganisms and their by-products from entering the blood stream. The GIT is home to trillions of commensal bacteria. A state of controlled physiologic inflammation and contact with these bacteria are considered to be essential conditions for the proper development of the immune system, with over 50% of the immune system thought to be contained within the digestive tract (Fiocchi et al 1994). It is likely that cross-talk between the immune system and normal flora helps induce oral tolerance.

A key feature of the mucosal immune system is its ability to remain tolerant to these antigens while retaining the capacity to repel pathogens effectively.

GIT infections, excess intake of alcohol, NSAID use, stress, broad spectrum antibiotics, corticosteroid hormones, and chemical contamination of food are some of the factors that can adversely affect the barrier function of the GIT resulting in increased permeability. This change in permeability can stimulate hypersensitivity responses to foods (DeMeo et al 2002) and to components of the normal gut flora. Bacterial endotoxins, cell wall polymers, and dietary gluten may cause non-specific activation of inflammatory pathways mediated by complement and cytokines (Walker 1975). In susceptible individuals this can increase toxic load on the liver (Aldersley & Howdle 1999). Decarboxylation of amino acids by gut bacteria yields vasoactive and neurotoxic amines, particularly histamine, octopamine, tyramine, and tryptamine which are absorbed and transported to the liver to be deaminated. In severe cirrhosis, these amines enter the systemic circulation and contribute to encephalopathy and hypotension of hepatic failure (Brown 1977). Bacterial beta-glucuronidase deconjugates estrogens, increases enterohepatic recirculation of these steroids and decreases their rates of clearance from the body, effectively raising blood estrogen levels and the risk of breast cancer (Goldin 1986).

Testing for increased intestinal permeability involves the measurement of passive permeability of two sugars, mannitol and lactulose. This protocol was developed to measure intestinal hyperpermeability that could lead to food sensitivity (Andre 1986). The test measures the ability of these non-metabolized sugar molecules to permeate the intestinal mucosa. Since they are not metabolized any absorbed sugar is fully excreted in the urine within 6 hours. Urine is collected and the concentrations of the two sugars measured. Mannitol, a monosaccharide, is absorbed passively through the intestinal mucosa. In contrast, lactulose, a disaccharide, is normally not absorbed unless the mucosal barrier is compromised. Treatment of increased intestinal permeability involves a diet eliminating alcohol, possible food allergens and treatment with nutrients including L-glutamine, an amino acid that is a primary nutrient for coloncytes.

The liver connection

The liver is one of the most complex organs in the body with numerous functions. In addition to coordinating metabolic processes to ensure energy homeostasis and synthesis of plasma proteins and clotting factors, hepatocytes are active in biochemical biotransformation of many endogenous and exogenous substances (Corless & Middleton 1983).

One of the primary functions of the liver is toxin management and removal, known as detoxification. Toxins are chemical agents that produce adverse reactions in living things. More than 200 000 manufactured environmental chemicals (xenobiotics) exist. Most of these chemicals are subject to metabolism in the human body with the liver being the main organ involved in this detoxification. At least 30 different enzymes catalyse reactions involved in xenobiotic metabolism (Murray et al 2000).

Liver function can be assessed by administering an exogenous substance to quantify changes in hepatic blood flow, uptake, biotransformation and excretion. Characterization of drug half-life, clearance, and product formation rates are possible methods for measuring hepatic efficiency (Barstow & Small 1990). A test called a Functional Liver Detoxification Profile (Box 18.4) involves ingesting low doses of aspirin, paracetamol, and caffeine. (This test is available from specialist laboratories.)

Collected urine and saliva is tested and this gives information that determines the treatment to improve liver function. It is important to understand that the standard pathology liver function test does not provide any information on liver detoxification.

Repeated exposure to food-borne toxic chemicals, environmental pollutants, endotoxins produced by bowel bacteria, prescription and other drugs can increase the detoxification burden. This overload can lead to a greater production of free radicals and subsequent damage to various body systems. It is the author's clinical observation that headaches and migraines can be reduced by addressing the body burden of toxins.

Toxic compounds can accumulate and damage various enzyme systems. Common symptoms are fatigue, headache, nausea, poor concentration, hormonal imbalances, and multiple chemical sensitivities. People working as hair dressers, nail technicians, dry-cleaners commonly present with headache and fatigue, presumably caused by exposure to the chemicals used in those industries. Chronic pain patients with long term ingestion of analgesics are another common group where the liver is faced with an excessive toxic burden.

Phase 1 and 2 enzymes need to be in balance for efficient detoxification. If patients present with induced Phase 1 activity and normal or reduced Phase 2 activity, toxic substances from Phase 1 metabolism will increase. This will increase the risk of hepatotoxicity and the possibility of chronic disease including headache or migraine. Treatment will need to be directed at stimulating Phase 2 and reducing Phase 1 (Box 18.5).

In addition to the treatment of unbalanced Phase 1 or 2 activities, the liver can also be treated with *Silybum marianum* (also called milk thistle), as a general hepatoprotective agent (Rainone 2005). One of its active

Box 18.4

The functional liver detoxification profile.

The liver converts substances that are lipid soluble and toxic through a series of chemical reactions (called Phase 1 and Phase 2 reactions) to make them more water soluble and non-toxic.

The ability of the liver to clear a challenge dose of caffeine is an indicator of the detoxification capacity of the Phase 1 pathway. The enzyme system called microsomal P450 mixed-function oxidase is used to oxidize such compounds to prepare them for removal. Its activity towards all such molecules is reflected by how fast caffeine is removed from the body after a challenge dose. Saliva samples are taken at intervals of two and eight hours and analyzed for caffeine, the concentration of which closely parallels that in blood (Zylber-Katz et al 1984).

A high value indicates that the P450 system in the liver is actively working to remove toxins. When this activity is elevated it would be beneficial to reduce exposure to environmental toxins such as car exhausts and pesticides since the P450 enzymes can convert such substances to procarcinogenic compounds (Bralley & Lord 2005a). As the exposure decreases the enzyme activity should decline. A higher caffeine clearance will be seen in smokers and those on high protein diet as there would be a continuous induction of this enzyme. Gut microbes are another potential source of toxins that are detoxified by this pathway.

A low value of the caffeine clearance can indicate loss of liver function, e.g. alcoholic cirrhosis

(Wahllander et al 1990), and that the processing and degradation of foreign compounds is slower than normal. However, as the P450 enzyme system is an inducible, on-demand detoxification system, a low exposure to environmental inducers may result in a low caffeine clearance and not indicate a health problem. Clinical correlation can be useful in these circumstances.

Phase 2 is tested by ingesting a test dose of paracetamol and salicylic acid in the evening. These products are converted to various conjugation products overnight and the levels in the overnight urine reflect the activities of conjugation enzyme activities. The conjugation molecules are acted upon by specific enzymes to catalyze the reaction step. Molecules used by the liver for this purpose include glutathione, sulphate, glycine, acetate, cysteine, and glucuronic acid. Adequate amounts of these molecules are necessary for proper detoxification ability. There is also individual variation in the control mechanisms for Phase 1 and 2 processes depending on inherited or genetic strengths or weaknesses and ethnicity (Critchley et al 1986, Cupp & Tracy 1998, Patel et al 1992).

Phase 2 reactions are affected by numerous drugs and are susceptible to nutrient insufficiencies, obesity (Abernethy et al 1983), and cigarette smoking (Scavone et al 1990) and must be taken into account in the interpretation of results.

Box 18.5

Balancing Phase 1 and Phase 2 enzymes.

Herbs and nutrients that inhibit Phase 1 activity:
    Tumeric (Sugiyama et al 2006)
    Watercress (Hecht 1996)
    Garlic (Davenport & Wargovich 2005,
        Bhuvansewari et al 2005)
Herbs and nutrients that induce Phase 2 activity:
    Turmeric (Pfeiffer et al 2007)
    Rosemary (Offord et al 1997)
    Green tea (Maliakal et al 2001)
    Antioxidants – Vitamins A, C, E
    Lipoic acid (Flier et al 2002)
    Selenium (Bralley 2005b)

ingredients is silymarin (Pradhan & Girish 2006). The detoxification pathways need a number of B group vitamins, minerals, amino acids and other nutrients for efficient functioning (Flier et al 2002). Decreased hepatic clearance of estrogens can occur with these deficiencies which could occur from long term overload in the detoxification pathways and therefore a greater demand on these and other nutrients. Hormones have to compete with all the other substances for detoxification. So the total load on the liver needs to be considered if the patient is taking multiple medications.

A wide variety of substances induce liver enzymes and can potentially overload these systems. Some of these are alcohol, exhaust fumes, acetate, barbiturates, barbequed meats, dioxin, high protein diets, organophosphorus pesticides, and paint fumes.

The following case study illustrates how assessment of the functional liver detoxification profile and appropriate treatment can assist in the management of a patient's headache.

Case study

DY was a 42-year-old man who grew up in an orchard and had since taken over the family orchard business. About 3 years prior to attending he started to feel nausea and left-sided headaches. This lasted for a few days and cleared. A week later the symptoms recurred. He then noticed that every time he was exposed to spraying of the orchards his symptoms recurred. He then started to develop severe fatigue. He reported that the fruit is sprayed fortnightly from early September till April. The land is also sprayed regularly to control the weeds. After picking, the fruit is sprayed with a fungicide.

He had had blood tests at the nearest regional centre but was told that there was nothing abnormal found. He was apparently tested for various chemicals and told that nothing abnormal was discovered. He saw a neurologist and after investigation was given low dose amitriptyline. This did not help. He then saw another neurologist who treated him with another antidepressant which also did not help his symptoms.

Functional liver detoxification profile showed that his Phase 2 activity was slowed. Treatment involved the use of antioxidants, a herbal combination consisting of turmeric and rosemary, vitamin and mineral supplement. His headaches decreased considerably in intensity on this regime but did not clear as he was still living at the orchard and continuing to be exposed to the sprays.

Discussion

It is interesting that none of his family members living in the orchard had similar problems. A possible answer could emerge from the new field of pharmcogenomics or pharmacogenetics – the genetic tendency toward fast, slow, or normal metabolism of specific molecules due to genetic differences in the detoxification Phase 1 and Phase 2 systems (Critchley et al 1986). People with recurrent adverse effects from various chemicals including medications may have unique polymorphisms of the detoxification enzyme systems that make them more sensitive to these substances.

Conclusion

Effective assessment and treatment of headache or migraine depends on a good history, including a dietary history where food allergy or sensitivity is suspected. Identification of dietary triggers enables the practitioner to formulate an appropriate treatment plan. Specific nutrients have also been shown to help in the treatment of migraine. Finally, the core processes of gut and liver function may need to be investigated and treated if no other causes of the headache have been found.

References

Abernethy DR, Greenblatt DJ, Divoll M et al 1983 Enhanced glucuronide conjugation of drugs in obesity; studies of lorazepan, oxazepam and acetaminophen. J Lab Clin Med 101:873-880.

Aldersley MA, Howdle PD 1999 Intestinal permeability and liver disease. Eur J Gastroenterol Hepatol 11:401-403.

Andre C 1986 Food allergy. Objective diagnosis and test of therapeutic efficacy by measuring intestinal permeability. Presse Med 15:105-108.

Barstow L, Small RE 1990 Liver function assessment by drug metabolism. Pharmacotherapy 10:280-288.

Bhuvansewari V, Abraham SK, Nagini S 2005 Combinatorial antigenotoxic and anticarcinogenic effects of tomato and garlic through modulation of xenobiotic-metabolizing enzymes during hamster buccal pouch carcinogenesis. Nutrition 21:726-731.

Blumenthal HJ, Vance DA 1997 Chewing gum headaches. Headache 379:665-666.

Bralley JA, Lord RS 2005a Laboratory evaluations in molecular medicine. The Institute of Advances in Molecular Medicine, Norcross (GA) p 277.

Bralley JA, Lord RS 2005b Laboratory evaluations in molecular medicine. The Institute of Advances in Molecular Medicine, Norcross (GA) p 283.

Brown JP 1977 Role of gut bacterial flora in nutrition and health: a review of recent advances in bacteriological techniques, metabolism and factors affecting flora composition. CRC Crit Rev Food Sci Nutr 8:229-336.

Corless JK, Middleton HM 1983 Normal liver function. Arch Intern Med 143:2291-2294.

Critchley JA, Nimmo GR, Gregson CA et al 1986 Inter-subject and ethnic difference in paracetamol metabolism. Br J Clin Pharmacol 22:649-657.

Cupp MJ, Tracy TS 1998 Cytochrome P450: new nomenclature and clinical implications. Am Family Physician 57:107-116.

Davenport DM, Wargovich MJ 2005 Modulation of cytochrome P450 enzymes by organosulfur compounds from garlic. Food Chem Toxicol 43:1753-1762.

DeMeo MT, Mutlu EA, Keshavarzian A et al 2002 Intestinal Permeation and Gastrointestinal Disease. J Clin Gastroent 34:385-396.

Egger J, Carter CM, Wilson J et al 1983 Is migraine food allergy? A double-blind controlled trial of oligoantigenic diet treatment. Lancet 2:865-869.

Finelli PF, McEntee WJ, Ambler M et al 1980 Adult celiac disease presenting as cerebellar syndrome. Neurology 30:245-249.

Fiocchi C, Binion DG, Katz JA 1994 Cytokine production in the human gastrointestinal tract during inflammation. Curr Op Gastro 2:639-644.

Flier J, Van Muiswinkel FL, Jongenelen CA et al 2002 The neuroprotective antioxidant alpha-lipoic acid induces detoxication enzymes in cultured astroglial cells. Free Radic Res 36:695-699.

Gabrielli M, Cremonini F, Fiore G et al 2003 Association between migraine and Celiac disease: results from a preliminary case-control and therapeutic study. Am J Gastroenterol 98:625-629.

Goldin BR 1986 The metabolism of the intestinal microflora and its relationship to dietary fat, colon and breast cancer. In: Ip C, Birt DF, Rogers AE, Mettlin C (eds) Dietary fat and cancer. Alan R Liss, New York.

Hadjivassiliou M, Grunewald RA, Davies-Jones GAB 2002 Gluten sensitivity as a neurological illness. J Neur Neurosurg and Psychiatry 72:560-563.

Harel Z, Gascon G, Riggs S et al 2002 Supplementation with omega-3 polyunsaturated fatty acids in the management of recurrent migraines in adolescents. J Adolesc Health 31:154-161.

Hecht SS 1996 Chemoprevention of lung cancer by isothiocyanates. Adv Exp Biol 401:1-11.

Herskey AD, Powers SW, Vockell AL et al 2007 Coenzyme Q10 deficiency and response to supplementation in pediatric and adolescent migraine. Headache 47:73-80.

Jacome DE 2001 Hypoglycemia rebound migraine. Headache 41:895-898.

Jarisch R, Wantke F 1996 Wine and headache. Int Arch Allergy Immunol 110:7-12.

Koehler SM, Glaros A 1988 The effect of aspartame on migraine headache. Headache 28:10-14.

Lipton RB, Newman LC, Cohen JS et al 1989 Aspartame as a dietary trigger of headache. Headache 29:90-92.

Maliakal PP, Coville PF, Wanwimolruk S 2001 Tea consumption modulates hepatic drug metabolizing enzymes in Wistar rats. J Pharm Pharmacol 53:567-577.

Mansfield LE, Vaughan TR, Waller SF et al 1985 Food allergy and adult migraine: double blind and mediator confirmation of an allergic etiology. Ann Allergy 55:126-129.

Martin VT, Behbehani MM 2001 Headache: Toward a rational understanding of migraine trigger factors. Medical Clinics of North America 85:1-20.

Millichap JG 2001 The role of diet in migraine headaches. Pediatric Neurology Briefs 15:89.

Montagna P, Cortelli P, Brabiroli B 1994 Magenetic resonance spectroscopy studies in migraine. Cephalalgia 14:184-193.

Murray RK, Granner DK, Mayes PA (eds) 2000 Harpers Biochemistry, 25th edn. Appleton & Lange.

Newman LC, Lipton RB 2001 Migraine MLT-down: an unusual presentation of migraine in patients with aspartame-triggered headaches. Headache 41:899-901.

Offord ES, Mace K, Avanti O et al 1997 Mechanisms involved in the chemoprotective effects of rosemary extract studied in human liver and bronchial cells. Cancer Lett 114:275-281.

Patel M, Tang BK, Kalow W 1992 Variability of acetaminophen metabolism in Caucasians and Orientals. Pharmacogenetics 2:38-45.

Peikert A, Willizig C, Kohne-Volland R 1996 Prophylaxis of migraine with oral magnesium: results from a prospective, multi-center, placebo-controlled and double-blind randomized study. Cephalagia 16:257-263.

Pengiran Tengah DSNA, Wills A, Holmes GKT 2002 Neurological complications of coeliac disease. Postgrad Med J 78:393-398.

Pfeiffer E, Hoehle SI, Walsh SG et al 2007 Curcuminoids form reactive glucuronides in vitro. J Agric Food Chem 55:538-544.

Pizzorno J 2003 Lessons on integration from the White House Commission on Complementary and Alternative Medicine Policy. Integrative Med 2:10-11.

Pradhan SC, Girish C 2006 Hepatoprotective herbal drug, silymarin from experimental pharmacology to clinical medicine. Indian J Med Res 124:491-504.

Rainone F 2005 Milk thistle. Am Fam Physician 72:1285-1288.

Roche Herrero MC, Arcas Martinez J, Maritinez-Bermejo A et al 2001 The prevalence of headache in a population of patients with coeliac disease. Rev Neurol 32:301-309.

Rozen TD, Oshinsky ML, Gebeline CA et al 2002 Open label trial of coenzyme Q10 as a migraine preventative. Cephalalgia 22:137-141.

Sandor PS, DiClemente L, Coppola G et al 2005 Efficacy of Coenzyme Q10 in migraine prophylaxis: a randomised controlled trial. Neurology 64:713-715.

Scavone JM, Greenblatt DJ, LeDuc BW et al 1990 Differential effect of cigarette smoking on antipyrine oxidation versus acetaminophen conjugation. Pharmacology 40:77-84.

Scher AI, Stewart WF, Lipton RB 2004 Caffeine as a risk factor for chronic daily headache: a population based study. Neurology 63:2022-2027.

Schiffman SS, Buckley CE, Sampson HA et al 1987 Aspartame and susceptibility to headache. N Engl J Med 317:1181-1185.

Sugiyama T, Nagata J, Yamagishi A et al 2006 Selective protection of curcumin against carbon tetrachloride-induced inactivation of hepatic cytochrome P450 isoenzymes in rats. Life Sci 78:2188-2193.

Toth C 2003 Medications and substances as a cause of headache: a systematic review of the literature. Clin Neuropharmacol 26:122-136.

Wahllander A, Mohr S, Paumgartner G 1990 Assesment of hepatic function. Comparison of caffeine clearance in serum and saliva during the day and night. J Hepatol 10:129-137.

Walker WA 1975 Antigen absorption from the small intestine and gastrointestinal disease. Pediatr Clin North Am 22:731-746.

Zylber-Katz E, Granit L, Levy M 1984 Relationship between caffeine concentrations in plasma and saliva. Clin Pharmacol Ther 36:133-137.

19

Management of temporomandibular and cervical components of headache

Peter Selvaratnam, Stephen Friedmann, Jack Gershman
and Maria Zuluaga

Overlap between temporomandibular and cervical contributions to headache is common in many patients. In this chapter the authors, two musculoskeletal physiotherapists and two dentists, address the identification and management of these components with emphasis on temporomandibular and dental aspects.

Severe acute and chronic headache can cause substantial physical, social and financial distress due to the intensity, frequency, and duration of pain (Jull et al 2004, Rasmussen 2001, Rasmussen et al 1991). Epidemiologists estimate that direct costs for migraine per annum in USA was over US$1 billion in the late 1990s, and the indirect costs due to absenteeism and reduced effectiveness at work was US$13 billion (Hu et al 1999). In an Australian study of 1717 patients it was reported that 87% had experienced a form of headache in the previous year. Of these, 47% sought help from medical practitioners, pharmacists, dentists, physiotherapists, chiropractors, ophthalmologists, optometrists or masseurs, and 99% took medication (Heywood et al 1998).

The International Headache Society (IHS) has classified headache as either primary or secondary (Olesen et al 2004). Primary headaches are not associated with or caused by other diseases. Migraine, tension headache and cluster headache are examples of primary headache. Secondary headaches are caused by a medical condition or a disease process that may be minor, serious or life threatening (Biondi 2001, Olesen et al 2004). Headache arising from cervical or temporomandibular disorders (TMD) are examples of secondary headache. A detailed discussion of primary and secondary causes of headaches can be found in Chapter 2.

The incidence of cervicogenic headache in the general population is estimated to be 16–18% (Greenbaum 2006, Jull et al 2004, Nilsson 1995, Pfaffenrath et al 1990, Zito et al 2006). In comparison it is estimated that 25–33% of those with TMD may have pain or headache (Dworkin et al 1990, Gremillion et al 2000). Structures in both regions can cause referred pain to the temporal region of the head. The mechanism of such referral is considered to be through functional overlap of cervical afferent nerves with the spinal tract of the trigeminal nerve (Bogduk 1985, Govind et al 2005, Lance et al 2004). The biomechanical relationship between the head and neck could also be a contributory factor in such headache referral (Kraus 2007, Rocabado et al 1991, Santander et al 2000,

Watson et al 1993, Zito 2007). Clinicians therefore are faced with the task of differentiating TMD from cervical disorders likely to cause headache (Zito 2007, Zito et al 2008).

This chapter discusses the clinical assessment, differential diagnosis, and management of patients whose headache may be associated with or triggered by TMD or cervical disorders.

TMD and headache

Temporomandibular disorders (TMD) is a collective term for different musculoskeletal conditions involving the temporomandibular joints (TMJs) and/or masticatory muscle disorders (Nitzan et al, 2008) and is described in Chapter 7. Headache can be triggered by TMD due to TMJ or masticatory muscle involvement (Balasubramaniam et al 2008, Benoliel et al 2008a, Zito 2007) and this is referred to as 'TMD-related headache'. As well, headache can be associated with referred myofascial pain from the cervical region, tension type headache, migraine, fibromyalgia or bruxism and may refer pain to the TMJ and masticatory muscles resulting in 'secondary TMD' (Balasubramaniam et al 2008, Benoliel et al 2008a). Hence, TMD-related headache may need to be distinguished from other conditions that may contribute to TMD.

Bruxism

Bruxism may also play an important role in TMD and can occur while asleep or awake (Kato et al 2003). Sleep bruxism is defined as an oromotor movement disorder (Thorpy 2005) that can lead to tooth contact and result in activation of masticatory muscles (Lavigne 2005). However, it has been observed that rhythmic masticatory muscle activity can occur in the absence of tooth contact in 60% of normal controls and in those with rapid eye

movement, sleep disorders and somnambulism (sleep walking) (Kato et al 2003, Lavigne, 2005). Awake bruxism can be associated with habitual tooth clenching (Kato et al 2003). Jaw bracing, nail biting and tongue edge biting are also considered associated signs of bruxism (Kato et al 2003, Okeson 2005).

Bruxism is estimated to occur in approximately 6–20% of the population (Glaros, 1981, Goulet et al 1993, 1995, Lavigne 2005) with 17–20% of all bruxers complaining of TMJ pain and disability (Goulet et al 1993, Piekartz von et al 2001, Piekartz von 2007). The prevalence of sleep bruxism in a Canadian study was estimated to be approximately 8% of the adult population (Lavigne, 2005). Sleep studies indicate that tooth grinding occurs in 80% of young adults during Stages 1 and 2 of sleep and in about 5–10% during rapid eye movement (REM) (Kato et al 2003; Lavigne 2005). Laboratory studies also demonstrate that a large number of sleep bruxism episodes occur in the supine position similar to obstructive sleep apnea (Lavigne 2005, Lavigne et al 2006).

Bruxism has been described as either primary (idiopathic) or secondary (iatrogenic) (Kato et al 2003). Primary bruxism may be induced by the central nervous system (CNS) in the absence of an underlying medical pathology resulting in day time tooth clenching or sleep bruxism. Triggers of primary bruxism could be acute or prolonged anxiety and periods of prolonged stress. Psychological or psychiatric conditions can also trigger primary bruxism. Secondary bruxism may occur due to neurological conditions, sleep dysfunction or medication (Kato et al, 2003) such as selective serotonin reuptake inhibitors, anti-psychotic drugs or due to drug withdrawal (Lavigne 2005, Winocur et al 2003).

Bruxism was initially considered due to gnashing and grinding of teeth provoked by psychological factors. However, the evidence from the literature does not support this hypothesis (Kato et al 2003, Lavigne 2005, Raphael et al 2008). Laboratory studies demonstrate that cardiac autonomic activity and CNS mediated cortical function play an important role in initiating sleep micro-arousals during sleep bruxism (Kato et al 2001, 2003, Lavigne 2005, Lavigne et al 2006, Lobbezoo et al 2001, Macaluso et al 1998, Terzano et al 2002). These investigations show that there is an increase in autonomic cardiac activity 4 to 8 minutes prior to tooth grinding or phasic jaw muscle activity. Cortical activity then heightens followed by increased heart rate just prior to contraction of suprahyoid muscles. Following this, tooth contact occurs as the end result of a series of physiological episodes (Lavigne 2005, Lavigne et al 2006). Bruxism is therefore now considered to be mediated by cardiac autonomic and cortical activity.

Researchers and clinicians debate whether bruxism can trigger TMD. However, the relationship is very complex and not clearly understood (Lobbezoo et al 1997, Manfredini et al 2003). Review of the literature by Lobbezoo et al (1997) observed that 'a commonly held concept is that bruxism leads to signs and symptoms characteristic to one or more of the sub-diagnoses of TMD, while another hypothesis suggests that bruxism is a TMD itself and sometimes co-exists with other forms of TMD'. Their review indicated that the causal relationship between bruxism and TMD was unclear. Subsequently a prospective study by Manfredini et al (2003) demonstrated that there was a significant association between bruxism and TMD. They examined 212 patients with different research diagnostic criteria for TMD-related diagnoses, and compared them with 77 sex- and age-matched asymptomatic subjects. The highest incidence of bruxism was found in those with myofascial pain and disc displacement (87.5%), followed by myofascial pain, disc displacement, and

other joint conditions (73.3%), and then those with myofascial pain (68.9%). The investigators reported that there was a stronger association between bruxism and muscle disorders than with disc displacement and TMJ pathologies. Further studies need to be conducted in different populations to evaluate the relationship between bruxism and TMD

Some clinicians claim that bruxism contributes to headache. Cross-sectional studies addressing the prevalence of headache in bruxers indicate that 66–87% experience headaches (Hamada et al 1982, Molina et al 1997). Yustin et al (1993) screened 353 patients of whom 86 were identified as bruxers. They found that 60% of bruxers develop headache and neck pain. However, there have been only a few large scale double-blind randomized clinical trials or cohort studies that have evaluated the contribution of bruxism to headache and the level of available evidence is low (Dao et al 1994, Jennum 2002, Kampe et al 1997, Lobbezoo et al 2008, Macfarlane et al 2001, Rugh & Harlan 1988). These authors infer that while bruxism may trigger headache it may not always be associated with TMD.

Cervicogenic headache

Researchers have demonstrated that cervical structures can trigger headache in the temporal, frontal and orbital regions (Bogduk 1985, 2001, Jull et al 1988, 2002, Sjaastad et al 1983, Zito 2007, Zito et al 2006). Provocative stimulation of the occipital condyles, C1 dorsal root, C3 dorsal ramus and upper cervical zygapophyseal joints has been shown to refer pain to the cranium (Bogduk 1985, 2001, Campbell & Parsons 1944, Jull et al 1988). Local anesthetic blocks to the C3 dorsal ramus or radiofrequency neuromyotomy have also been demonstrated to relieve headache (Bogduk 1985, Govind et al 2005).

Myofascial trigger points (MTPs) in the sternocleidomastoid (SCM), splenius capitis, trapezius (Simons et al 1999) and sub-occipital muscles (Fernandez de las Penas et al 2006, 2008) have also been reported to refer pain to the head. Injecting these MTPs with local anesthetic (Okeson 2005, Simons et al 1999) or dry needling (Baldry 2005) have been described to relieve headache. The MTPs in the trapezius have also been shown to evoke pain in the face, the temple, the angle of the mandible, retro-orbital region and behind the ear (Okeson 1996, Simons et al 1999, Travell 1960). The MTPs in the SCM have also been known to refer pain to the temporal region, the anterior aspect of the face over the zygoma, and masseters (Kellgren 1949, Simons et al 1999).

These investigations demonstrate that upper cervical disorders can refer pain to the head. The neuroanatomical connection between the upper cervical region and head and the possible mechanism of referred pain to the head is described in Chapter 9. The characteristics of cervicogenic headache are described in Chapter 8.

Assessment

A detailed clinical history is important in the process of differential diagnosis of headache since patients with similar headache presentation may have a different etiology. In order to differentiate primary from secondary headache it is important to establish the history of onset of the headache and related symptoms, intensity, frequency and duration of the headache, any change in headache pattern and development of any new headache. The process may also be assisted by asking questions about factors that trigger and ease the headache, the presence of headache while sleeping and on waking, general health, past history of headache, previous and current interventions including medication and their effectiveness. Psychosocial factors (Chs 21

and 22) and food sensitivities (Ch. 18) may co-exist with chronic headache. Validated psychometric measures such as the Beck Depression Inventory may assist in evaluating depression (Dworkin et al 2005).

It is important to establish whether the TMD-related headache is due to musculoskeletal factors or associated with other rare joint related conditions that may present as TMJ pain. Conditions such as ear disorders, dental conditions, neurovascular conditions such as hemicrania continua, cardiac conditions, autoimmune disorders, infections, and benign or malignant tumors can refer pain to the TMJ and need to be differentially diagnosed (Nitzan et al 2008).

Similarly it is necessary to establish whether the cervicogenic headache is due to musculoskeletal factors or other causes. In rare instances, a dissecting vertebral artery or internal carotid artery may contribute to headache (Jull et al 2004). The authors recall seeing two patients with unusual signs that might have suggested cervical headache, who were later found to have a pituitary tumor and an upper cervical meningioma respectively. While these cases are uncommon, it is important to be aware of sinister underlying pathology as a possible differential diagnosis particularly with unusual clinical presentations or when there is poor response to musculoskeletal interventions.

Hence red flags such as the 'first or worst' headache need to be considered (Ch. 2). In a retrospective study of 111 patients with headache presenting for neuroimaging, it was found that paralysis, reduced conscious levels, and papilledema were statistically significant red flag features in predicting abnormal neuroimaging (Sobri et al 2003). Other red flag features included onset of new or different headache, nausea or vomiting, worst headache ever experienced, progressive visual or neurological changes, weakness, ataxia, or loss of coordination, drowsiness, confusion, memory impairment, onset of headache after age of 50 years, stiff neck, onset of headache with exertion, sexual activity or coughing, systemic illness, numbness, asymmetry of pupillary response, sensory loss and signs of meningeal irritation (Sobri et al 2003).

Some patients may have a combination of cervical disorders and TMD contributing to their headache. In these patients, the cervical region may need to be treated and signs and symptoms in both regions re-assessed to make a working diagnosis. If the condition is unaltered, the temporomandibular region needs to be treated and the signs and symptoms re-evaluated. Some patients may need both regions treated to evaluate the outcome. However, it is important to refer the patient to the medical practitioner for further investigation when a headache does not improve in the 'prescribed time' based on its severity, irritability and nature (Jull et al 2004, Niere & Selvaratnam 1995).

The visual analogue scale (VAS) can also be used to evaluate the intensity of headache on a 'good day' and a 'bad day' (where 0 is no pain, 1 mild pain, 5 moderate pain, and 10 the most severe imaginable pain). A pain diary can be used to assess the intensity, frequency and duration of the headache over a four week period to monitor the effects of treatment. Under experimental conditions females have been found to have a lower pain threshold during certain stages of their menstrual cycle (see Ch. 9). Lowered pain threshold was also observed in a study among women taking oral contraceptives (Fillingim et al 2000). Hence, it is important to consider these factors when assessing women with headache.

Guidelines for differential diagnosis

The following subjective and objective assessment provides further guidelines in differentiating a TMD-related headache from a cervicogenic

headache. These guidelines are based on findings in the literature (Jull et al 2004, Lavigne 2005, Lavigne et al 2006, Okeson 2005, Zito et al 2006), clinical findings of expert physiotherapists and musculoskeletal physiotherapists (Zito 2007), and the authors' clinical findings in patients with headache. Table 19.1 provides a summary of guidelines for differentiating patients with TMD-related headache from those with a cervicogenic headache.

Subjective assessment

Pain distribution

Pain caused by TMD-related headache can be unilateral or bilateral in the temporal and/or frontal regions (Lavigne et al 2006, Zito 2007). It is frequently associated with pain in the pre-auricular region, the muscles of mastication, in the distribution of the branches of the trigeminal nerve and as a feeling of fullness in the ear (Pettengill 1999, Zito 2007). Pain is rarely referred to the cervical region or trunk unless associated with fibromyalgia (Nitzan et al 2008).

Cervicogenic headache is usually referred from the upper cervical region to the fronto-temporal and orbital regions in the distribution of the ophthalmic nerve (Sjaastad et al 1983, 1998, Zito 2007). The headache is often associated with pain in the sub-occipital region, occipital region, or lower cervical region (Zito 2007). Cervicogenic headache is most often unilateral but at times can be bilateral (Jull et al 2004, Sjaastad et al 1983, Zito 2007).

Aggravating factors

Patients with TMD usually have difficulty with jaw functions, such as biting or chewing on foods such as apples, carrots and bread rolls, which may provoke headache. Those with

Table 19.1 Guidelines for differentiation of patients with TMD-related and cervicogenic headache.

Characteristics	TMD-related headache	Cervicogenic headache	Other causes
Subjective assessment			
Area of symptoms	Unilateral or bilateral temporal headache +/− TMJ and masticatory muscle pain Pain may radiate anteriorly from the pre-auricular region or superiorly	Unilateral fronto-temporal, or orbital headache but can occur bilaterally Pain may radiate superiorly from the cervical region to the cranium	TMJ pain in rare instances may be associated with ear disorder, dental conditions, neurovascular conditions such as hemicrania continua, cardiac conditions, autoimmune disorders, infections and benign or malignant tumors
Associated symptoms	Mandibular pain Fullness in the ear Sensitive teeth or periodontal structures	Pain in the occipital or sub-occipital region or in the upper trapezius muscle	
Aggravating factors	Jaw function exacerbates TMD-related pain or headache	Neck movements or sustained neck postures trigger headache	
Sleep pattern	Woken during sleep or on awakening with headache, mandibular, teeth or periodontal symptoms Patient or partner complains of snoring	Headache on waking associated with cervical pain or restriction Not associated with snoring	Waking in the early hours of morning could signify a red flag such as a brain tumor, or benign intracranial hypertension
Awake signs and symptoms	Headache associated with masseter or temporalis muscle tightness May be associated with a forward head posture while sitting	Headache may be associated with a forward head posture or while sitting and working in a slumped posture with cervical flexion	
Physical assessment			
Active movements	Active TMJ movements may be restricted and may reproduce headache	Active cervical movements may be restricted and reproduce or ease headache	
Spatula test	Placing spatula between premolars may reduce the patient's constant headache or TMJ pain. Examining cervical movements (with the spatula between premolars) reduces or alleviates headache compared to examining without a spatula	Headache is unaltered by placing spatula between premolars and on re-examining cervical movements	

Table 19.1 Guidelines for differentiation of patients with TMD-related and cervicogenic headache—Cont'd

Characteristics	TMD-related headache	Cervicogenic headache	Other causes
Muscles	Hypertrophied masseters	Hypertrophy of masseters is not associated with cervical disorder	Fibromyalgia, orofascial tumors, and blockages of the parotid duct need to be considered when masseters are hypertrophied
Palpatory examination	Palpation of the TMJ reproduces symptoms Presence of MTPs in masticatory muscles may reproduce headache or orofacial pain Some patients may have MTPs in cervical muscles which may trigger orofacial pain	Palpation of upper cervical motion segments reproduces headache Sustained pressure of the cervical motion segments for 30 to 60 sec may reproduce the headache or alleviate it Palpation of cervical MTPs reproduces or eases headaches	Red flags: dissecting vertebral artery or internal carotid artery
Slump test	Slump test negative	Slump test may reproduce headaches	
Odontogenic factors	Wear facets of the dentition Cracked tooth syndrome Tongue crenations and linea alba	Dental signs are not associated with cervicogenic headache	

TMJ = temporomandibular joint. MTPs = myofascial trigger points.

cervicogenic headache may attribute their headache to cervical movements, prolonged cervical postures while performing manual work, or sitting with a forward head posture. The forward head posture could impact upper cervical structures and contribute to headache (McKenzie 1983). This posture may also predispose to tooth clenching and contribute to awake bruxism-related headache (Okeson 2005). The relationship between the forward head posture and headache needs to be identified in the physical assessment.

Waking with headache. Patients who experience sleep bruxism/TMD may wake with a headache during sleep or on awakening (Kato et al 2003). This phenomenon could be due to rhythmic masticatory muscle activity or tooth grinding/clenching during Stages 1 and 2 or the REM sleep cycle. In others insomnia can cause morning headache (Lavigne 2005, Lavigne et al 2006).

Researchers infer from sleep studies that the most predictive indicator of sleep bruxism is whether a patient snores (Lavigne 2005, Lavigne et al 2006). Information about snoring should be obtained during the patient interview. If there is uncertainty, then the partner or those sharing the same dwelling should be questioned about whether the patient snores or makes jaw sounds (Lavigne 2005).

In the authors' experience most patients are either unaware of or deny snoring. Thus, if the patient or their partner is unable to shed further light then the diagnosis of sleep bruxism based on snoring is very limited. Symptoms associated with bruxism such as jaw muscle tightness, fatigue and pain and other odontogenic factors described in this chapter needs to be considered. Assessment for sleep apnea may be conducted at a sleep disorder clinic.

The patient's cervical region could also contribute to headache while sleeping and on waking (Jull et al 2004). The cervical sleep posture in different functional positions needs to be assessed to identify the contribution of the cervical region to headache. Changing the cervical posture or the number of pillows may assist in identifying whether it is a causative factor. In some patients wearing a cervical collar while sleeping may assist in identifying the cervical contribution to headaches. The collar may provide support to and relieve strain on cervical structures thereby easing headache.

Raised intracranial pressure can also cause individuals to awake with headache (Lance et al 2004). Those with a suspected raised intracranial pressure should be referred immediately to an emergency department for further evaluation (see Ch. 2).

Sensitive teeth or gums. Patients with TMD due to sleep bruxism may complain of a recent episode of sensitive teeth and/or gums on awaking or during functional activities while awake (Okeson 2005). Tooth sensitivity could be due to stimulation of nociceptive afferents of the maxillary and mandibular branches of the trigeminal nerve. Sensitivity of teeth to cold liquids may also be reported. The dentist may find that there is no odontogenic cause to their pain and bruxism may be suspected. Persistent pain may lead to hypertonicity of masticatory muscles and contribute to TMD-related headache (Okeson 2005).

Intermittent tooth pain. Patients who brux may complain of intermittent tooth pain lasting for two to three days on waking or at the end of a busy day (Okeson 2005). In contrast, the pain for patients with dental conditions may be variable (i.e., improving or worsening) or constant pain.

Clinical studies have also demonstrated that pain can be referred to the teeth from the temporalis and masseter muscles (Simons et al 1999), the SCM and trapezius muscles (Okeson 2005). Thus, in the absence of odontogenic causes, pain referral from the cervical and masticatory muscles should be considered (Okeson 2005).

Abscess. Clinicians need to be aware that dental abscess may also cause masticatory muscle co-contraction and TMD-related headache. Patients with a dental abscess may be incorrectly diagnosed with TMD. The pain in the affected tooth can be intense or throbbing and can occur quite suddenly and gradually worsen over a few hours or days. Red flags such as constant unremitting tooth pain associated with pain spreading to the ear, jaw and neck on the same side as the affected tooth should guide clinicians to promptly refer the patient to a dentist for further evaluation. Other symptoms of a dental abscess could include tenderness of the tooth and surrounding area to touch and pressure from biting, unpleasant taste in the mouth, sensitivity to food and drink that is very cold or hot, fever, a general feeling of being unwell, difficulty swallowing or opening the mouth and disturbed sleep (Benoliel et al 2008b, Doss et al 1999, Sharav et al 2008).

Physical assessment

The physical assessment needs to include the patient's posture, examination of the cervical and temporomandibular regions. The headache intensity during active and passive movement examination can be assessed with the verbal pain rating scale (which is an analogue to the VAS) where 0 is no pain, 1 is mild pain, 5 moderate pain and 10 is severe pain (Selvaratnam et al 1994). Dental pathology, secondary occlusal dysfunction such as missing teeth and open bites needs to be assessed by a dentist (Nitzan et al 2008).

Postural considerations

The patient's cervical posture (Braun et al 1989, McKenzie 1983, Mayoux-Benhamou et al 1994, Rocabado et al 1991, Watson et al 1993) as well as thoracic, lumbar and pelvic postures need to be assessed (Ch. 17) in the standing and sitting positions as part of the comprehensive headache examination (Gibbons et al 2006). Previous clinical studies did not support the effect of the forward head posture on the stomatognathic system (Braun et al 1991) in contributing to headache (Haughie et al 1995, Refshauge 1995, Treleaven et al 1994) or TMD (Olivo et al 2006, Sonnesen et al 2001). However, the clinical investigation by Fernandez de las Penas et al (2006) observed a relationship between forward head posture and unilateral migraine sufferers. They compared 20 unilateral migraineurs without side-shift and 20 matched controls. The craniovertebral angle was measured with side-view photographs in the sitting and standing positions. Neck mobility was measured with a goniometer. Migraine sufferers demonstrated a smaller cranio-cervical angle than controls ($p < 0.001$), and thereby presenting with a greater forward head posture in both positions. There was also a positive correlation between the craniovertebral angle and reduced cervical extension in migraineurs. This preliminary study lends support to the hypothesis that the forward head posture can be associated with headache sufferers.

A subsequent blinded pilot study also evaluated the effect of forward head posture in 15 episodic tension tension-type headache patients and 15 matched asymptomatic controls. (Fernandez de las Penas et al 2007). The study evaluated the differences in each group for the presence of forward head posture, active and latent MTPs in upper trapezius, sternocleidomastoid, temporalis, and neck mobility. Side-view photographs were taken in the sitting and standing positions to assess the craniovertebral angle. A goniometer was used to measure neck mobility.

The investigation identified that the patient group demonstrated a greater forward head posture than controls in both positions ($p < 0.05$). The patients with active MTPs in the analyzed muscles demonstrated a greater forward head posture than those with latent MTPs. They also had reduced neck mobility when compared with the asymptomatic patients. This study further demonstrates the importance of assessing the contribution of forward head posture in headache sufferers.

Correcting the forward head posture from upper cervical extension (Fig. 19.1a) to upper cervical flexion (Fig. 19.1b) in the sitting/standing positions and sustaining this position for 30 seconds may assist in evaluating the cervical component to headache. This sustained movement may need to be repeated 3 to 5 times due to long term adaptation of soft tissues. If the headache is unchanged, the patient is requested to place the tongue on the floor of the mouth to reduce masticatory muscle activity and jaw clenching (Carlson et al 1997). Any change in headache intensity may indicate a TMD-awake bruxism component. The effect of the tongue position may also be evaluated in different cervical positions. While these postural changes may infer a cervical/TMD component, the diagnosis can only be made following a comprehensive cervical and temporomandibular assessment.

Some patients may experience headache while seated in a slumped position with the cervical and thoracic spine in flexion. The slump test may assist in identifying the potential postural or spinal dural components of headache (Butler 2000). Anecdotal evidence suggests that changing a patient's sitting posture from a slumped position to a more erect sitting posture may reduce headache intensity and assist in diagnosing the spinal postural component to headache. Applying postural taping from the C7 to the T9 level (Fig. 19.2) to correct posture and improve postural awareness

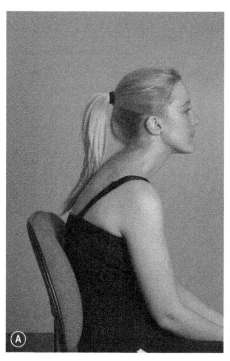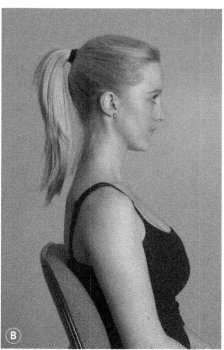

Figure 19.1 • The upper cervical spine in (A) extension and (B) flexion.

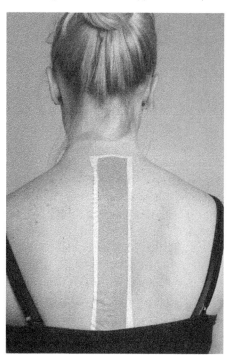

Figure 19.2 • Postural taping from the C7 to the T9 level.

may also assist in evaluating the postural component to headache.

It is also the authors' experience that attending to postural variations in some patients with a protracted scapula, a lumbosacral tilt, or an apparent leg length discrepancy has reduced their headache intensity or TMD-related pain due to biomechanical or neural effects. Thus, each patient's presenting condition and their postural variations need to be addressed carefully to evaluate whether postural changes alter the intensity or nature of the headache both within the session and over the long term. Patient-specific functional scales (Cleland et al 2006, Sterling 2007) would assist in evaluating the efficacy of postural changes.

Despite the paucity of large scale randomized clinical studies to support this empirical evidence, the benefit of postural correction and awareness in headache patients has support from the physiotherapy and dental professions.

Proponents of evidence informed medicine recommend that the patient's report on treatment outcomes and physician's experience must be considered in addition to systematic research findings (Sackett et al 1997). However, further clinical research is required to test these theories.

Cervical examination

Cervical diagnostic blocks are considered the gold standard in diagnosing cervicogenic headaches (Bogduk 2001, Govind et al 2005). These diagnostic blocks are not office procedures and cannot realistically be offered to each patient. However, diagnostic blocks assist in the diagnosis and indicate potential treatment options for patients with refractory cervicogenic headache and are described in Chapter 5. In most cases the diagnosis of cervicogenic headache can be made after a careful interview and physical examination of the cervical region (Jull et al 2004, Zito et al 2006).

Active movements of the cervical spine of flexion, extension, rotation, lateral flexion, and upper cervical flexion and extension (Niere & Selvaratnam 1995) may reproduce or ease a patient's headache (Jull et al 2002). Repeated movement of upper cervical flexion in the standing, sitting or supine positions (10 repetitions) may assist in evaluating changes in the intensity, quality, and directional preference (such as centralizing or peripheralizing) of the headache (Kent et al 2009, Long et al 2004, McKenzie 1983). Repeated movements can also be performed with other cervical movements to evaluate the behavior of the headache.

In addition, careful palpation of the cervical muscles, and passive physiological and accessory movements of the cervical motion segments will further assist in evaluating the cervical component (Brontfort et al 2004, Gibbons et al 2006, Jull et al 2002, Niere & Selvaratnam 1995). Reproducing or easing the patient's headache

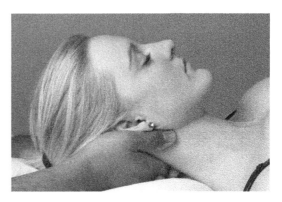

Figure 19.3 ● Application of manual upper cervical distraction.

by manual cervical distraction (Fig. 19.3) or posteroanterior palpation of the cervical region may assist in identifying the cervical contribution. If the headache is not reproduced, sustained palpation of the cervical region for 30 to 60 seconds may assist in reproducing or easing their headache. Treatment of the cervical region with passive physiological or accessory movements (Niere & Selvaratnam 1995), and re-examining active neck movements, functional activity and patient specific functional scales (Cleland et al 2006) will further assist in evaluating the cervical component.

Temporomandibular evaluation

Active opening and closure of the mouth, protrusion, retrusion, and lateral movement of the TMJ in the sitting or supine positions will assist in assessing TMD and/or related headache (Trott 1985, Zito 2007). The TMJ can be palpated laterally over the pre-auricular region or posteriorly via the external auditory meatus. The presence of TMJ clicking and/or crepitus during opening and closing may be assessed digitally over the lateral and posterior aspect of the TMJ. A stethoscope over the TMJs would assist in evaluating joint sounds since they can be present continuously or at a particular point of joint motion (Nitzan et al 2008).

The click usually occurs for a brief moment during opening and closing of the mouth. When it occurs during both directions it is referred to as a reciprocal click. In contrast, crepitus may occur throughout the joint motion (Nitzan et al 2008).

The normal range of inter-incisor opening in women is 35–45 mm and in men 45–54 mm; it can be assessed with a millimetre ruler or a measuring tape. The inter-incisor opening needs to be observed carefully to evaluate deviation or deflection of the mandible (Fig. 19.4) and whether correction to the deviation occurs. Persistent deviation to the side of the TMD is considered to be due to ipsilateral joint dysfunction or disc derangement without reduction. Deviation on opening which corrects itself is considered due to ipsilateral disc displacement with reduction (Nitzan et al 2008). However, deviation away from the TMD can also be due to muscle imbalance of the contralateral medial or lateral pterygoid and/or the unilateral temporalis (Okeson 2005). Headache in the presence of abnormal or restricted TMJ movement may suggest the possibility of TMD (Zito 2007) but needs to be taken in context with the total assessment of the patient.

Hypertrophied masseters may be observed in patients who brux or have TMD. However, fibromyalgia, orofascial tumors, and blockages of the parotid duct are diagnoses that should also be considered (Lavigne 2005). Palpation of the masseter, temporalis, medial pterygoid, SCM, trapezius, sub-occipital muscles and splenius capitis for the presence of MTPs will further assist in evaluating their contribution to headache related to TMD or cervical disorders (Simons et al 1999). The MTP examination of these muscles is described in Chapter 23.

Accessory movements of the TMJ such as postero-anterior gliding lateral movement and longitudinal gliding may also assist in the diagnosis of TMD (Trott 1985, Zito 2007) though their reliability has yet to be assessed.

Dental wear facets. Clinicians need to assess for dental wear facets as part of the examination. Prolonged teeth grinding may result in excessive dental wear facets (Fig. 19.5) that in some instances may appear as a diamond shaped

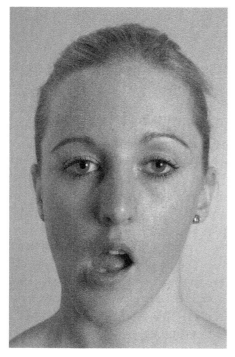

Figure 19.4 • Deviation of the mandible to the right.

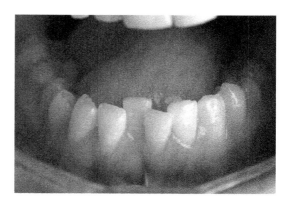

Figure 19.5 • Dental wear facets.

facet. However, the presence of dental wear does not provide an indication as to when it may have occurred. Dental wear may have occurred over many years and may not be an indication of bruxism that is ongoing. Attrition of dental facets could also be accelerated by an acidic diet and therefore may have no bearing on a patient's recent episode of tooth pain or TMD-related bruxism/headache.

Cracked tooth syndrome. Chronic bruxism could result in teeth cracking or overtly fracturing. Occlusal trauma or mastication of hard food can lead to a similar outcome. Dental wear facets and fractures may lead to an altered bite (Okeson 2005, Sharav et al 2008). An acute bite change may result in development of MTPs in masticatory muscles (Rocabado et al 1991, Simons et al 1999). Clinicians therefore need to be aware that while a cracked tooth could contribute to TMD-related headache it may not always be associated with a recent episode of headache.

Tongue indentation. The presence of indentations in the lateral aspects of the tongue (crenations) (Fig. 19.6) and cheek (linea alba) should

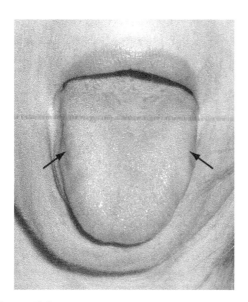

Figure 19.6 ● Indentations in the lateral aspect of the tongue (crenations).

be assessed as it could occur with bruxism or a tongue thrusting and/or chewing habit (Piquero et al 1999).

Spatula test

The spatula test is performed to identify if cervical disorders or TMD are contributing to the symptoms (Piekartz von et al 2001). Currently there is limited evidence on the discriminative validity and reliability of the spatula test despite its clinical utility. The spatula is placed between the points of most contact (for example, the pre-molars) in the sitting position (Piekartz von et al 2001, Piekartz von 2007) (Fig. 19.7a). The spatula reduces tooth contact between the upper and lower molars and is considered to lower peripheral neural receptor activity between the molars, and thereby reduce CNS input and/or activation of masticatory muscles (Piekartz von 2007).

Though clenching of the teeth is not the only means of determining TMD, a reduction of symptoms with application of the spatula at rest or in combination with cervical movements may indicate that it may be due to TMD or central sensitization. For example, when a patient presents with unilateral right temporal headache, active cervical movements are initially examined in the sitting position to determine whether they reproduce the patient's headache. If the patient's headache is reproduced at 60° of right cervical rotation, the neck is returned to the neutral position. A spatula is then placed between the points of most contact. Right cervical rotation is then re-assessed (Fig 19.7b). If the headache is eased, this change may be inferred due to TMD or central sensitization (Piekartz von et al 2001). If the headache is unaltered it is possibly due to cervical involvement. The cervical component can be further assessed by palpating the upper cervical zygapophyseal joints or cervical muscles with the cervical spine rotated. Reproduction of the headache further confirms the

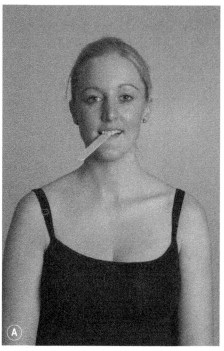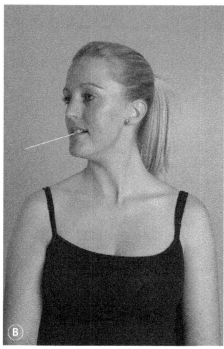

Figure 19.7 • Spatula positioned between the points of most contact (e.g., the pre-molars) in A. neutral cervical position and B. with the cervical spine rotated.

cervical contribution. Other cervical movements such as upper cervical flexion or cervical flexion could be examined with the spatula, particularly when forward head posture or cervical flexion causes headaches.

The spatula test may give rise to false-positives and false-negatives. However, it provides clinicians with an assessment tool to evaluate the contribution of cervical or TMD to headache in the absence of expensive laboratory tests to examine sleep apnea or injection studies to the cervical region.

Investigations

Appropriate investigations and imaging need to be conducted when suspecting catastrophic or sinister headaches (Ch. 2). Blood tests or lumbar puncture may be indicated. A CT scan or MRI of the brain will be required to rule out some sinister or catastrophic causes of headache. Cervical

X-rays or MRI may be required for cervical disorders. Panoramic radiographs of the TMJ are usually taken for routine assessment (Nitzan et al 2008). Cone beam CT scans have replaced panoramic radiographs and other plain films as a routine examination for the TMJ and other bone pathology. MRI would be useful for more detail investigation of the articular disc and soft tissues (Nitzan et al, 2008).

Clinical decision making and management

Effective management of headache will depend on the practitioner's clinical decision making and diagnosis. To this end it can be useful to sub-group patients on the basis of subjective and physical assessment findings rather than 'clumping' them and treating them in a prescriptive manner (Kent et al 2004). This approach seems to be supported by the results of a survey of 650 participants in two Australian low back pain meetings, where it was found that physiotherapists, medical practitioners, specialist physicians, musculoskeletal physicians, chiropractors, and osteopaths are more likely to sub-group patients according to their physical impairments (signs and symptoms) rather than the pathoanatomy (Kent et al 2009).

Sub-grouping patients by physical impairments may assist in identifying those headache patients who require immediate medical attention (Ch. 2), referral for management of anxiety/depression (Chs 21 and 22), food sensitivity (Ch. 18), or hormonal dysfunction (Ch. 9). Sub-grouping may also assist in identifying patients with other medical conditions that can cause TMJ pain (Table 19.2) or who have a musculoskeletal headache due to TMD or cervical disorders.

Musculoskeletal headache may be further classified as acute or chronic. As well it is useful to evaluate irritability, which is the degree to which the headache is provoked by functional movements (Niere & Selvaratnam 1995). Aggravating factors are likely to implicate specific cervical or mandibular functional movements/postures that could contribute to headache and may suggest possible management strategies which will vary in each patient.

The TMD may be sub-grouped according to TMJ or masticatory muscle involvement (Table 19.3). The TMJ component may be further subdivided into joint locking, hypermobility, internal disc derangement with or without reduction and deviations of the mandible. Treatment selection will depend on the condition being managed. Likewise, masticatory muscle involvement may be sub-grouped according to the muscles that cause the disorder, their action, particularly when these muscles contribute to mandibular deviation.

Table 19.2 Sub-grouping of patients for diagnosis and management.

Diagnosis	Management
Catastrophic or sinister headache (Ch. 2)	Referral to Emergency Department/medical practitioner/neurologist
Anxiety/depression	Cognitive strategies/referral to psychiatrist/psychologist/psychoanalyst (Chs 21 and 22)
Food sensitivity	Referral to integrative medical practitioner (Ch. 18)
Hormonal headache (Ch. 9)	Referral to medical practitioner/endocrinologist/integrative medical practitioner
Temporomandibular disorders(TMD) A. TMD-related headache B. Entities that may in rare occasions be associated with TMJ pain; e.g. ear (Ch. 10), dental, neurovascular conditions such as hemicrania continua, cardiac, auto-immune and malignant condition	See Table 19.3 Referral to medical/dental practitioner
Cervicogenic headache A. Non-musculoskeletal; e.g., vertebral artery/internal carotid artery dissection, cervical meningioma, pituitary tumor mimicking as cervicogenic headache B. Musculoskeletal	Referral to medical practitioner See Table 19.4

Table 19.3 Sub-grouping of TMD-related headache for diagnosis and management.

Diagnosis	Management

Muscles
Assess function of masticatory and cervical agonist and antagonist.
Assess MTPs in the cervical and temporomandibular regions (Ch. 23)
	• Improve coordination of masticatory agonist and antagonist
	
	• Deactivate MTPs with:
	  a. MTP therapy (Ch. 23)
	  b. Dry needling (Ch. 24)
	• Pain management:
	  a. Medication
	  b. Cognitive therapy (Chs 21 and 22)
	  c. Progressive muscle relaxation
	  d. Breathing relaxation
	  e. Feldenkrais therapy (Ch. 25)
	• Exercise:
	  a. CCFP, upper cervical flexion in sitting, mandibular exercises (Ch. 20)

Joint Locking, hypermobile, clicking, crepitus, internal disc derangement with or without reduction	• Eat soft foods/soup • Reduce mouth opening • Support mandible with fist while-yawning • Apply moist heat • Mandibular stabilizing exercises • Medication • Stabilizing occlusal splint • Referral to orofacial surgeon
Posture Evaluation of postural biomechanics	• Ergonomic recommendations for work and home environment • Evaluate effect of changing forward head posture
Bruxism Sleep/awake bruxism	• Pain management • Referral to dental specialist for medication/stabilizing occlusal splints • Evaluation of sleep/awake posture • Sleep clinic
Neural Pain referral in the trigeminal nerve distribution	• Medication • Pain management • Dry needling • Counseling
Referred from cervical region	Treatment of: a. Cervical MTPs b. Zygapophyseal joint c. Postural changes
TMD-related headache associated with temporalis muscle, myofascial pain, migraine and tension headache	Assess for: a. primary or secondary TMD signs b. medical versus dental referral c. management of secondary masticatory muscle signs (Ch. 23)

CCFP = Craniocervical flexor program. MTP = Myofascial trigger point.

Similarly cervical disorders may be sub-grouped according to structures involved – the zygapophyseal joint, muscular or neural structures and the cervical segment contributing to the disorder (Table 19.4). Investigators have assessed patients with neurocompressive and

Table 19.4 Sub-grouping of cervicogenic headache for diagnosis and appropriate management.

Diagnosis	Management
Postural	• Ergonomic recommendations for work and home environment • Evaluate the effect of changing forward head posture or the slumped posture • Postural taping program

Muscles
Muscle function (e.g. altered endurance of cervical stabilizers (Ch. 14) or presence of MTPs (Ch. 23)
	• Exercise programs
	• CCFP (Ch. 15)
	• Perform CCFP and evaluate if craniocervical flexor endurance improves and/or MTP is deactivated
	• Isometric cervical extensor program
	• Upper cervical flexion in sitting
	• Lumbar core stability programs
	• MTP therapy (Ch. 23)
	• Dry needling (Ch. 24)
	• Pain management
	  a. Cognitive therapy (Chs 21 and 22)
	  b. Progressive muscle relaxation
	  c. Breathing relaxation
	  d. Feldenkrais therapy (Ch. 25)
	  e. Medication

Zygapophyseal joint	• Passive mobilization (Chs 15, 16 and 17) • Cervical stabilization with CCFP • Zygapophyseal joint block (Ch. 5)
Nerve	• Neural mobilization (e.g. manual cervical distraction, slump test, upper limb neurodynamic test) • Radiofrequency neurotomy (Ch. 5)

CCFP-Craniocervical flexor program. MTP-myofascial trigger point.

non-specific low back pain. They report that exercise prescription by manual therapists based on centralization/peripheralization was strongly predictive of the specific exercise that would assist patients (Kent et al 2009, Long et al 2004). Based on these findings, repeated cervical movements, for example, upper cervical flexion may further identify which movement eases the headache and exercises prescribed accordingly (McKenzie 1983).

Preliminary studies indicate that lumbar mobilization/manipulation and stabilization exercises can be used successfully in patients with physical impairments due to non-specific low back pain (Childs et al 2004, Flynn, 2002, Hicks et al 2005). From these findings, it is hypothesized that physical impairments may indicate whether manual cervical distraction, passive accessory cervical zygapophyseal joint or TMJ mobilization, cervical, or masticatory muscle interventions is the best approach for the patient. Impairments may indicate the need for zygapophyseal joint blocks, radiofrequency neurotomy, MTP injections, or dry needling. Similarly, impairments may suggest that a patient requires stabilization exercises for the cervical region (Ch. 15) and temporomandibular region compared to range of movement exercises or referral to a dentist for a stabilizing occlusal splint. Sub-grouping may also identify patients likely to benefit from postural re-training, postural taping intervention, or an ergonomic assessment at work or home.

As a group, headache patients can be complex. However, sub-grouping will assist informed decision making regarding physical management and identifying those patients who may benefit from a multi-disciplinary approach.

It is imperative that the management includes an explanation of the clinical findings so that the patient understands the nature of the condition and proposed plan of management. The explanation will assist patients to comply with the management plan. In this way, the patient is more likely to play an active role in management. In contrast, a hasty explanation may lead to confusion, reduce compliance, and compromise the outcome of intervention.

The following management strategies are a guide to clinicians and are neither prescriptive nor exhaustive. There is published evidence supporting some of these management strategies while other interventions are based on evidence-informed medicine (Sackett et al 1997) and have consensus within the medical, physiotherapy, and dental professions based on anatomical, biological, and biomechanical concepts. The outcome measures described in Chapter 13, the mandibular function impairment questionnaire (Stegenga et al 1993), and patient specific functional scales (Cleland et al 2006, Sterling 2007) may assist clinicians to plan and evaluate interventions. Some of these management strategies are described in the following section.

Pain management

Relaxation skills, behavior modification, time management, work-life balance, adequate sleep, and managing psychosocial stressors are all important in the management of people with headache. While clinicians are aware of stress management skills, some patients may require referral to a psychologist/psychiatrist to deal with specific mental health factors or stressors that may contribute to headache. Chapters 21 and 22 address psychological issues and management strategies. Pharmacotherapy for different conditions is discussed in Chapters 2, 3, 10, and 22.

Addressing lifestyle stressors is important since headache and orofacial patients may suffer from anxiety, depression, and distress (Nitzan et al 2008). Some patients may benefit from progressive muscle relaxation (Jacobsen 1929, Lance et al 2004), breathing techniques, visual imagery (Ricks 1994) and prayer (Benson 1996) in

managing their headache/TMD. Evidence-based outcome studies indicate that cognitive behavioral therapy benefits patients with tension-type headache, migraine, and TMD (Raphael & Ciccone 2008). A review of the literature disputes a psychogenic explanation to orofacial pain, though there is evidence that psychological factors can perpetuate ongoing pain and dysfunction (Raphael & Ciccone 2008). Thus behavioral therapy programs need to be prescribed judiciously and take into account the patient's condition and personality in order to provide the best management strategy.

Ergonomics and postural awareness

Postural considerations in relation to sleep position (described previously), work and home ergonomics are imperative in the individual's management. Applying taping to the cervicothoracic region to improve postural awareness (Fig. 19.8) will limit slumping while seated and reduce forward head posture. The tape can be worn for 2 days and then be removed for a day. If the patient is able to function without experiencing skin irritation, the tape can be trialed over one to three weeks. Patients need to be advised about potential skin irritation and also to remove the tape gently. The effect of posture and taping on the outcome of headache can be evaluated with a VAS scale or a pain diary. Taking pause breaks and changing one's work posture every 20 minutes, prioritizing work, and conflict resolution are also important tools to manage headache.

Spinal mobilization and exercise

Spinal mobilization (Gibbons et al 2006, Jull et al 2002, Niere & Selvaratnam 1995) and low load exercises focusing on the craniocervical flexor muscles have been shown to benefit those

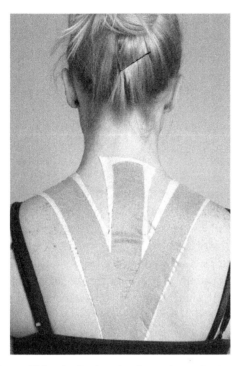

Figure 19.8 • Application of taping to the cervicothoracic region to improve postural awareness and reduce hypertonicity of the upper trapezeii. The skin is first prepared to reduce the risk of skin irritation followed by application of anti-allergenic tape and then adhesive tape.

with cervicogenic headache (Jull et al 2002). In a randomized clinical study in 200 patients with chronic unilateral cervicogenic headache, spinal manipulative therapy (SMT) performed by musculoskeletal physiotherapists, and combining SMT with a low load craniocervical flexor program significantly reduced the frequency and intensity of headache in a large majority of patients compared to controls on medication (Jull et al 2002). The investigation demonstrated that SMT or exercise with SMT is effective in the management of those with chronic cervicogenic headache and the effects maintained over a 12 month period. However, it is important while performing SMT or exercise therapy that the muscle and joint changes correlate with changes in headache pattern. If the

headache is alleviated for only a few hours, despite improved upper cervical joint and muscle signs, it is wise to refer them to an appropriate specialist (Jull et al 2004). More details on the cervical rehabilitation program can be found in Chapter 15.

Patients with TMD may also benefit from a rehabilitative exercise program to the temporomandibular region. Randomized clinical trials have been conducted in patients with TMD (de Wijer 2005, Michelotti et al 2004, van der Glas 2000). Exercise therapy was compared with occlusal splint therapy in 71 patients with 'myogenous temporomandibular dysfunction' (de Wijer 2005, van der Glas 2000). The findings of the study indicated that exercise therapy prescribed by physiotherapists to the temporomandibular region might be preferred to occlusal splint therapy due to lower costs, similar efficacy, and shorter treatment duration. In another study of 70 'myogenous TMD' patients, education about their condition was compared with a combination of education and a home exercise program (Michelotti et al 2004). The exercise involved gently opening the mouth to the point of pain onset and maintaining the stretch for one minute. This exercise was performed a total of six times. Co-ordination exercises were also performed by opening and closing the mouth 20 times. The home program included diaphragmatic breathing and self mobilization of the masseters and temporalis. After 3 months the success rate in the education only group was 57% and 77% in the combination therapy group. These findings support education and exercises in patients with TMD.

Clinicians need to take care when prescribing mandibular exercises. There is a risk of overstretching the TMJ, accentuating mandibular protrusion while performing mandibular exercises, and aggravating the condition. Hence, when prescribing these exercises, specific instructions must be provided to move within pain free limits. From clinical experience and based on the biomechanical relationship of the cervical and temporomandibular regions, it is recommended that patients commence cervical exercises prior to commencing an exercise program directed at the temporomandibular region. For example they can perform upper cervical flexion in the sitting position (see Fig. 19.1b), or craniocervical flexion in the supine position (see Fig. 15.1).

Masticatory muscle relaxation can be achieved by placing the tongue on the floor of the mouth (Carlson et al 1997) and quietly breathing in and out for 5 sec. This exercise can then be repeated 5 times. Orofacial exercises can also be performed by placing the tip of the tongue on the upper gums and moving the tongue over the upper gums and then over the lower gums. The tip of the tongue can then be placed on the cheek pouch and slow circular movements performed in the clockwise and counter clock-wise direction without causing excessive stretching of the TMJ. The exercise program described in Chapters 20 and 25 can also be performed within pain free limits.

Conclusion

Temporomandibular and cervical disorders can refer pain to the temporal regions of the head. Diagnosis can be a complex challenge requiring a comprehensive history and clinical examination to differentiate TMD-related from cervicogenic headache, and to assess the possible contribution of bruxism. Sub-grouping can be useful in differential diagnosis and management, and to identify the need for referral to other health professionals. High quality research into chronic cervicogenic headache supports the use of spinal mobilization therapy and craniocervical exercise to produce long term positive outcomes in the management of this patient group. Similarly, research supports education in conjunction with exercise programs conducted by physiotherapists for those with TMD. The evidence also supports the view that relaxation therapy and stress management skills can produce positive outcomes. However, other treatment approaches which have sound anatomical, biological, and biomechanical paradigms are based on convention, and need to be monitored with appropriate outcome measures to justify ongoing use in clinical practice.

References

Balasubramaniam R, Ram S 2008 Orofacial movement disorders. Oral maxillofacial surgery clinics of North America 20(2):273-285.

Baldry PE 2005 Acupuncture, Trigger points and musculoskeletal pain. Elsevier, Edinburgh.

Benoliel R, Sharav Y 2008a Masticatory myofascial pain, and tension-type and chronic daily headache. In: Sharav Y, Benoliel R (eds) Orofacial pain and headache. Elsevier, Edinburgh, p 109-148.

Benoliel R, Sharav Y 2008b The trigeminal autonomic cephalgias (TACs) In: Sharav Y, Benoliel R (eds) Orofacial pain and headache. Elsevier, Edinburgh, p 225-254.

Benson H 1996 Timeless healing. The power and biology of belief. Harvard Medical School and Mind Body Medical Institute. Hodder Headline, Australia.

Biondi D (2001) Headaches and their relationship to sleep. Dent Clin North Am 45:685-700.

Bogduk N 1985 Cervical causes of headache and dizziness. In: Grieve G (ed) Modern manual therapy of the vertebral column. Churchill Livingstone, Edinburgh, p 289-302.

Bogduk N 2001 Cervicogenic headache: anatomic basis and pathophysiologic mechanisms. Curr Pain Headache Rep 5:382-386 and J Craniomandib Disord 5:239-244.

Braun BL, Amundson LR (1989) Quantitative assessment of head and shoulder posture. Arch Phys Med Rehabil 70:322-329.

Braun B, Schiffman EL 1991 The validity and predictive value of four assessment instruments for evaluation of the cervical and stomatognathic systems. J Craniomand Disorder 5: 239-244.

Bronfort G, Haas M, Evans RL, Bouter LM 2004 Efficacy of spinal manipulation and mobilization for low back pain and neck pain: a systematic review and best evidence synthesis. Spine J 4:335-356.

Butler D 2000 The sensitive nervous system. Noigroup Publications, Adelaide, Australia.

Campbell DG, Parsons CM 1944 Referred head pain and its concomitants. J Nervous Mental Diseases 99:544-551.

Carlson CR, Sherman JJ, Studts JL et al 1997 The effects of tongue position on mandibular muscle activity. J Orofac Pain 11(4):291-297.

Childs JD, Fritz JM, Flynn W et al 2004 A clinical prediction rule to identify patients with low back pain most likely to benefit from spinal manipulation: a validation study. Annals Internal Medicine 141:920-928.

Cleland JA, Fritz JM, Whitman JM et al 2006 The reliability and construct validity of the neck disability index and patient specific functional scale in patients with cervical radiculopathy. Spine 31(5):598-602.

Dao TT, Lund JP, Lavigne GJ 1994 Comparison of pain and quality of life in bruxers and patients with myofascial pain of the masticatory muscles. J Orofac Pain 8:350-356.

de Wijer A 2005 Physiotherapy for TMD-the evidence base. (Abstract) The 4th International Conference on Orofacial Pain and Temporomandibular Disorders-the Scientific Basis of Clinical Decision Making (ed Kleinberg I) Sydney, Australia p 14-15.

Doss A, Taylor N, Down PF 1999 A rare complication of dental abscesses Postgrad Med J 75:749-750.

Dworkin SF, Huggins KH, Leresche L et al 1990 Epidemiology of signs and symptoms in temporomandibular disorders: clinical signs in cases and controls. Journal of the American Dental Association 120:273-281.

Dworkin RH, Turk DC, Farrar JT et al 2005 Core outcome measures for chronic pain clinical trials. IMMPACT recommendations. Pain 113(1-2):9-19.

Fernandez de las Penas C, Cuadrado ML, Pareja JA 2006 Myofascial trigger points, neck mobility and forward head posture in unilateral migraine. Cephalgia 26(9): 1061-1070.

Fernandez de las Penas C, Cuadrado ML, Pareja JA 2007 Myofascial trigger points, neck mobility and forward head posture in episodic tension-type headache. Headache 47(5):662-672.

Fernandez-de-Las-Penas C, Cuadrado ML, Arendt-Nielsen L et al 2008 Association of cross-sectional area of the rectus capitis posterior minor muscle with active trigger points in chronic tension-type headache: a pilot study. Am J Phys Med Rehabil 87(3):197-203.

Fillingim RB, Ness T J 2000 Sex-related hormonal influences on pain and analgesic responses. Neurosci Biobehav Rev 24 (4):485-501.

Flynn T, Fritz JM, Whitman M et al 2002 A clinical predictive rule for classifying patients with low back pain who demonstrate short-term improvement with spinal manipulation. Spine 27 (24):2835-2843.

Gibbons PT, Tehan P 2006 Manipulation of the spine thorax and pelvis. Churchill Livingstone/Elsevier, Edinburgh.

Glaros AG 1981 Incidence of diurnal and nocturnal bruxism J Prosthet Dent 45:545-549.

Goulet JP, Lund J, Montplaisir J et al 1993 Daily clenching, nocturnal bruxism, and stress and their association with CMD symptoms J Orofacial Pain 7:120-127.

Goulet JP, Lavigne GJ, Lund JP 1995 Jaw pain prevalence among French-speaking Canadians in Quebec and related symptoms of temporomandibular disorders. J Dent Res 74:1738-1744.

Govind J, King W, Giles P et al 2005 Headache and the cervical zygapophyseal joints (cervicogenic headache). (Orthopaedic Proceedings). J Bone Joint Surg 87B (suppl III):399-340.

Greenbaum T 2006 Thesis. The effectiveness of passive manual modalities versus acupuncture in the treatment of primary and cervicogenic headache. University of South Australia.

Gremillion HA, Mahan PE 2000 The prevalence and etiology of temporomandibular disorders and orofacial pain. Texas Dental Journal 117:30-39.

Hamada T, Kotani H, Kawazoe Y, Yamada S 1982 Effect of occlusal splints on the EMG activity of masseter and temporal muscles in bruxism with clinical symptoms. J Oral Rehabil 9:119-123.

Haughie LF, Fiebert IM, Roach KE 1995 Relationship of forward head posture and cervical backward bending to neck pain. Journal of Manual and Manipulative Therapy 3:91-97.

Heywood J, Colgan T, Coffey C 1998 (Abstract) Prevalence of headache and migraine in an Australian city. J Clin Neuroscience 5(4):485.

Hicks G E, Fritz J M, Delitto A et al 2005 Preliminary development of a clinical prediction rule for determining which patients with low back pain will respond to a stabilization program. Archives Physical Medicine Rehab 86 (9):1753-1762.

Hu X, Markson L, Lipton RB 1999 Disability and economic costs of migraine in the United States: A population-based approach Arch Intern Med 159:813-818.

Jacobsen E 1929 Progressive relaxation. University of Chicago Press, Illinois.

Jennum P, Jensen R 2002 Sleep and headache. Sleep Med Rev 6:471-479.

Jull G, Bogduk N, Marsland A 1988 The accuracy of manual diagnosis for cervical zygapophyseal joint pain syndromes. Med J Aust 148:233-236.

Jull G, Niere K 2004 The cervical spine and headache. In: Boyling G, Jull G (eds) Grieve's modern manual therapy. The vertebral column, 3rd edn. Elsevier, Edinburgh, p 291-309.

Jull G, Trott P, Potter H et al 2002 A randomized controlled trial of exercise and manipulative therapy for cervicogenic headache. Spine 27:1835-1843.

Kampe T, Tagdae T, Bader G et al 1997 Reported symptoms and clinical findings in a group of subjects with longstanding bruxing behaviour. J Oral Rehabil 24:581-587.

Kato T, Rompre P, Montplaisir JY et al 2001 Sleep bruxism: an oromotor activity secondary to micro-arousal. J Dent Res 80:1940-1944.

Kato T, Montplaisir JY, Guitard F et al 2003 Evidence that experimentally induced sleep bruxism is a consequence of transient arousal. J Dent Res 82:284-288.

Kellgren JH 1949 Deep pain sensibility. Lancet 1:943-949.

Kent PM, Keating J 2004 Do primary-care physicians think that non-specific low back pain is one condition? Spine 29:1022-1031.

Kent PM, Keating J, Buchbinder R 2009 Searching for a conceptual framework for non-specific low back pain. Manual Therapy (in press).

Kraus S 2007 Temporomandibular disorders, head and orofacial pain: cervical spine considerations. Dent Clin North Am 51:161-193.

Lance JW, Goadsby PJ 2004 Mechanism and management of headache. Butterworth Heinemann, Oxford.

Lavigne G 2005 Principles and practice of sleep medicine. Elsevier Saunders, Philadelphia.

Lavigne G, Morisson F, Khoury S et al 2006 Sleep-related pain complaints: morning headaches and tooth grinding. Insom 7:4-11.

Lobbezoo F, Lavigne G 1997 Do bruxism and temporomandibular disorders have a cause-and-effect relationship? J Orofac Pain 11(1): 15-23.

Lobbezoo F, Naeije M 2001 Bruxism is mainly regulated centrally not peripherally. J Oral Rehab 28:1085-1091.

Lobbezoo F, Van Der Zaag J, Van Selms M K A et al 2008 Principles for the management of bruxism. J Oral Rehab 35(7):509-523.

Long A, Donelson R, Fung T 2004 Does it matter which exercise? A randomized controlled trial of exercise for low back pain. Spine 29:2593-2602.

Macaluso GM, Guerra P, Di Giovanni G et al 1998 Sleep bruxism is a disorder related to periodic arousals during sleep. J Dent Res 77:565-573.

Macfarlane TV, Gray RJM, Kincey J, Worthington HV 2001 Factors associated with the temporomandibular disorder, pain dysfunction syndrome (PDS): Manchester case-control study. Oral Dis 7:321-330.

Manfredini D, Cantini E, Romagnoli M, Bosco M 2003 Prevalence of bruxism in patients with different research diagnostic criteria for temporomandibular disorders (RDC/TMD) diagnoses. Cranio 21 (4):279-285.

Mayoux-Benhamou M, Revel M, Vallee C et al 1994 Longus colli has a postural function on cervical curvature. Surgical & Radiologic Anatomy 16:367-371.

McKenzie R 1983 Treat your own neck. Spinal Publications. Waikanae, New Zealand.

Michelotti A, Steenks MH, Farella M et al 2004 The additional value of a home physical therapy regimen versus patient education only for the treatment of myofascial pain of the jaw muscles: short-term results of a randomized clinical trial. J Orofac Pain 18:114-125.

Molina OF, dos Santos J Jr, Nelson SJ, Grossman E 1997 Prevalence of modalities of headaches and bruxism among patients with craniomandibular disorder. Cranio 15:314-325.

Niere K, Selvaratnam PJ 1995 The cervical region. In: Zuluaga M et al (eds) Sports physiotherapy-applied science and practice. Churchill Livingstone, Edinburgh, p 325-341.

Nilsson N 1995 The prevalence of cervicogenic headache in a random population sample of 20-59 year olds. Spine 20:1884-1888.

Nitzan D, Benoliel R, Heir G et al 2008 Pain and dysfunction of the temporomandibular joint. In: Sharav Y, Benoliel R (eds) Orofacial pain and headache. Elsevier, Edinburgh, p 149-192.

Okeson J 1996 Orofacial pain: guidelines for assessment, diagnosis, and management. Quintessence Publishing Co. Inc., Chicago.

Okeson J 2005 Bell's Orofacial pain. The clinical management of orofacial pain. Quintessence Publishing Co. Inc., Chicago.

Olesen J, Bousser MG, Diener HC et al 2004 The international classification of headache disorders. The International Headache Society, 2nd edn. Cephalalgia 24(suppl 1):1-160.

Olivo SA, Bravo J, Magee DJ et al 2006 The association between head and cervical posture and temporomandibular disorders: a systematic review. J Orofac Pain 20:9-23.

Pettengill A 1999 A comparison of headache symptoms between two groups: a TMD group and a general dental practice group. Cranio 17:64-69.

Pfaffenrath V, Kaube H 1990 Diagnostics of cervicogenic headache. Funct Neurol 5:159-164.

Piekartz von H J M, Bryden L 2001 Craniofacial dysfunction and pain. Butterworth, Heinemann, Oxford.

Piekartz von H J M 2007 Management of craniomandibular region. Clinical patterns and management. Elsevier, Edinburgh.

Piquero K, Ando T, Sakurai K 1999 Buccal mucosa ridging and tongue indentation: incidence and associated factors. The Bulletin of Tokyo Dental College 40(2):71-78.

Raphael K G, Ciccone D S 2008 Psychological aspects of chronic orofacial pain. In: Sharav Y, Benoliel R (eds) Orofacial pain and headache. Elsevier, Edinburgh, p 57-74.

Rasmussen B K, Jensen R, Schroll M et al 1991 Epidemiology of headache in a general population – a prevalence study. Journal of Clinical Epidemiology 44:1147-1157.

Rasmussen B 2001 Epidemiology of headache. Cephalalgia 21:774-777.

Refshauge K 1995 Clinical reasoning in physiotherapy. Butterworth Heinemann, Oxford.

Ricks S 1994 Superworking. How to achieve peak performance without stress. Simon & Schuster, Sydney, Australia.

Rocabado M, Iglarsh ZA 1991 Musculoskeletal approach to maxillofacial pain. JB Lippincott Co., Philadelphia.

Rugh JD, Harlan J 1988 Nocturnal bruxism and temporomandibular disorders. Adv Neurol 49:329-341.

Sackett D, Richardson W 1997 Evidence-based medicine. How to practice & teach EBM. Churchill Livingstone, New York.

Santander H, Miralles R, Perez J et al 2000 Effects of head and neck inclination on bilateral sternocleidomastoid EMG activity in healthy subjects and in patients with myogenic cranio-cervical-mandibular dysfunction Cranio 18:181-191.

Selvaratnam PJ, Matyas TA, Glasgow EF 1994 Noninvasive discrimination of brachial plexus involvement in upper limb pain. Spine 19:26-33.

Sharav Y, Benoliel R 2008 Acute orofacial pain In: Sharav Y, Benoliel R (eds) Orofacial pain and headache. Elsevier, Edinburgh, p 75-90.

Simons D, Travell J, Simons LS 1999 Travell and Simons' myofascial pain and dysfunction: the trigger point manual. Upper half of the body. Lippincott Williams and Wilkins, Philadelphia.

Sjaastad O, Saunte C, Hovdahl H et al 1983 Cervicogenic headache. An hypothesi. Cephalalgia 3:249-256.

Sjaastad O, Fredriksen TA, Pfaffenrath V 1998 Cervicogenic headache: diagnostic criteria. The Cervicogenic Headache International Study Group. Headache. 38:442-445.

Sobri M, Lamont AC, Alias N A et al 2003 Red flags in patients presenting with headache: clinical indications for neuroimaging. Br J Radiology 76:532-535.

Sonnesen L, Bakke M, Solow B 2001 Temporomandibular disorders in relation to craniofacial dimensions, head posture and bite force in children selected for orthodontic treatment. Eur J Orthod 23:179-192.

Stegenga B, de Bont LGM, de Leeuw R, Boering G 1993 Assessment of mandibular function impairment associated with temporomandibular joint osteoarthrosis and internal derangement. Journal Orofacial Pain 7:183-195.

Sterling M 2007 Patient specific functional scale. Clinimetrics. Aust J Physio 53:65.

Terzano MG, Parrino L, Rosa A et al 2002 CAP and arousals in the structural development of sleep: an integrative perspective. Sleep Med 3:221-229.

Thorpy M 2005 Classification of sleep disorders. Elsevier Saunders, Philadelphia.

Travell J 1960 Temporomandibular joint pain referred from muscles of the head and neck. J Prosthetic Dent 10:745-763.

Treleaven J, Jull G, Atkinson L 1994 Cervical musculoskeletal dysfunction in post-concussional headache. Cephalalgia 14:273-279.

Trott P 1985 Examination of the temporomandibular joint. In: Grieve G (ed) Modern manual therapy of the vertebral column. Churchill Livingstone, Edinburgh, p 521-529.

van der Glas H 2000 Vergelijk tussen behandelingsvormen bij myogene emporomandibulaire dysfunctie. Ned Tijdsch Tandhk 107:505-512.

Watson DH, Trott PH 1993 Cervical headache: an investigation of natural head posture and upper cervical flexor muscle performance. Cephalalgia 13:272-284.

Winocur E, Gavish A, Voikovitch M et al 2003 Drugs and bruxism: a critical review. J Orofac Pain 17:99-111.

Yustin D, Neff P, Rieger MR, Hurst T 1993 Characterization of 86 bruxing patients with long-term study of their management with occlusal devices and other forms of therapy. J Orofac Pain 7:54-60.

Zito G 2007 Diagnostic criteria used by physiotherapists to differentiate cervicogenic headache from temporomandibular headache. Clinical doctoral thesis. Brownless library. The University of Melbourne, Melbourne. Parkville, Australia.

Zito G, Jull G, Story I 2006 Clinical tests of musculoskeletal dysfunction in the diagnosis of cervicogenic headache. Man Ther 11:118-129.

Zito G, Morris M, Selvaratnam PJ 2008 Characteristics of TMD headache – a systematic reviews. Physical Therapy Reviews 13(5):324-332.

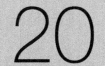

Chapter Twenty

Management of parafunctional activities and bruxism

Harry von Piekartz

There is some evidence of a relationship between parafunctional activities and orofacial pain. In this chapter the author, a musculoskeletal physiotherapist, outlines the clinical patterns and management of parafunctional activities and bruxism. These conditions are often managed by dentists, manual therapists, and psychologists.

Parafunctional activities (abnormal oral habits) are not always recognized by clinicians in patients with long term head and face pain. A possible reason for this is because parafunctional activities may not be directly associated with symptoms. However, there is some evidence of their contribution in patients with headache and orofacial pain (Glaros et al 2007, Lobezzoo 2006, Okeson 2005, Svensson et al 2001). This chapter discusses some aspects of neuromusculoskeletal therapy and behavioral re-education of patients with these conditions.

Bruxism, a form of parasomnia, was defined as 'continued or rhythmic contraction of the masticatory muscles combined with tooth contact' (Hathaway 1995a, McMillan & Blasberg 1994). Currently, bruxism is considered an oro-motor disorder (Lavigne et al 2005), but its effects mimic those of parafunctional activities. Bruxism may include abnormal orofacial behavior such as bracing and grinding while sleeping and/or awake (Lavigne et al 2008, Thorpy 1990).

The term bruxomania or diurnal bruxism is sometimes used when referring to bruxism that occurs during both day and night (Grozev & Michailov 1999, Marbach et al 1990, Marie & Pietkiewicz 1997). Bracing is defined as diurnal teeth pressing without vertical teeth movement (Kampe et al 1997, Kraus 1988).

Epidemiology

The prevalence of bruxism is estimated at 6–20% in studies conducted on students (Carlsson et al 2003, Glaros 1981) and the general population (Goulet et al 1993, Lavigne & Montplaisir 1995). Of these people, 10–20% are conscious that they brux (Carlsson & Magnusson 1999). The incidence decreases with age, especially beyond the age of 50 (Dao et al 1994). There is a positive correlation between bruxism, lip-cheek-nail-biting, and craniofacial dysfunctions and pain (Kieser & Groeneveld 1998, Widmalm et al 1995). However, parafunctional activities may not always cause symptoms. For example, 60% of healthy volunteers assessed in sleep laboratories show rhythmic masticatory muscle activities without having temporomandibular symptoms (Marklund & Wänman 2008). Furthermore, only 17–20% of patients with bruxism may suffer from pain and dysfunction (Goulet et al 1993).

Etiology

The etiology of bruxism is not clearly under-stood. Stress is frequently cited as a domi-nant factor producing increased muscle tension in masticatory muscles during normal orofacial activities (Flor et al 1991, Kapel et al 1989, Moss & Adams 1984, Rugh & Montgomery 1987). However, psychological stress and associated occlusal dysfunctions have not been found to correlate strongly with symptoms associated with bruxism (Clark 1985, Goulet et al 1993, Marie & Pietkiewicz 1997). The only direct correla-tion with sleep bruxism has been observed with sleep disorders. Sleep studies indicate that sleep bruxism occurs predominantly during Stages 1 and 2 of the sleep cycle and to a lesser extent during rapid eye movement (REM) sleep (Dao et al 1994, Kato et al 2003, Lobbezoo et al 1996).

Several pathophysiological mechanisms have been proposed. Current research indicates that sleep bruxism is centrally mediated involving subcortical structures. Affective and cognitive influences are considered to induce changes in autonomic and motor outputs, leading to peripheral changes in the masticatory muscles (Gastaldo et al 2006, Lobbezoo & Naeije 2001, Yu et al 1995).

Clinical examination

Areas of motor control that clinicians need to be aware of are listed in Box 20.1. Parafunctional activities are not easy to identify; however, there are often clinical patterns present that may assist in their recognition. Box 20.2 lists the common clinical characteristics of patients with long term parafunctional activities.

Box 20.3 lists the factors that need to be con-sidered when assessing a patient.

Box 20.1

Areas of motor control that may be affected by parafunctional activities.

Linguistic activities
  Speaking
  Singing
Social/sexual activities
  Kissing
  Nonverbal expression
Digestive activities
  Swallowing
  Sucking
Respiratory activities
  Inspiration and expiration

Box 20.2

Motor dysfunctions that may be clinically associated with parafunctions.

Oral habits
  Chewing, nail biting
Sensory overactivity
  Overactivity of the lips
  Tongue sucking, biting
Incoordination
  Insufficient timing with deep cervical muscles
  Dysphagia
Unpredictable motor patterns
  Bruxism/Bruxomania
  Bracing
  Trismus

Parafunctional activities may lead to hyper-trophy of the masticatory muscles, especially the masseters (Kiliaridis & Carlsson 1994) (Fig. 20.1A & B). This hypertrophy can lead to facial asymmetry which may affect the patient's social communication and cause emotional con-flict (Rhodes 2006). Parafunctions are often accompanied by other neuromusculoskeletal dysfunctions (Winocur et al 2001) such as craniocervical and shoulder pain, TMJ, and motor dysfunction. The study by Manfredini and co-workers (2003) on 289 subjects partially

Box 20.3

Essential components of the subjective and physical examination.

Subjective examination

History

- Recent history (in the last 6 months) of grinding the teeth, usually observed by partner or friends
- Recent history of temporomandibular disorder and or dental treatment

Behavior

The patient:

- Is conscious of teeth grinding and clenching during the day
- Perceives that the masticatory muscles are stiff and tense
- Wakes during the night because of the grinding sounds and/or their partner is aware of them grinding
- Is aware that the masseter muscle is 'tired' on awakening
- Experiences muscle tiredness during the day which is associated with jaw function
- Wakes with a locked jaw
- Wakes with soreness of the masseters and temporalis

- Experiences neck pain on waking, usually combined with one or more of the above mentioned symptoms
- Reports feeling physically tired due to disturbed sleep
- Reports experiencing toothache on waking.

Physical examination

On physical examination the following clinical patterns may be observed:

- Inadequate counter reaction of the mandible when gentle resistance is applied
- Hypertonicity and sensitivity of the masticatory muscles on palpation
- Mildly reduced active range of motion on opening of the mouth. The range may improve after passive examination
- Protective muscle guarding of the masticatory muscles during passive examination of the temporomandibular joint (TMJ).

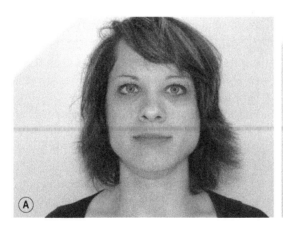 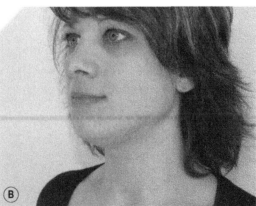

Figure 20.1 • Patient exhibiting hypertrophy of the left masseter. (A) Frontal view. (B) Left side view.

supports this concept; they observed that 212 subjects with bruxism had TMJ disorders (such as disc displacements and joint pathology) as classified by the Research Diagnostic Criteria of Temperomandibular Disorders (RCD/TMD). Motor dysfunctions such as impaired timing, speed and coordination may be present while talking, swallowing and singing (Castelo et al

2005, Corvo et al 2003) (see Box 20.2). Motor control of the masticatory muscles can be affected by many factors including mood, posture, the environment and sleep disorders (Glaros et al 2007). Longitudinal studies have shown that parafunctions in childhood predict increased anterior tooth wear 20 years later. This phenomenon suggests that oral parafunctions in children may be a persistent trait in the future that needs more attention (Lawrence & Samson 1988). However, current research suggests that tooth wear can be due to prolonged grinding or build up of acid and may not necessarily be causing the patient's current symptoms (Lobbezoo 2006).

Factors that may contribute to parafunctional activity include: occlusal dysfunctions which require dental assessment (Glaros et al 2005); abnormal craniocervical, facial, and mandibular morphology in the head, face, and neck regions (Piekartz von & Bryden 2001); and cognitive and emotional influences such as extreme stress, anxiety, discontentment and frustration. Patients may not relate these to parafunctional activities. A 24 hour diary monitoring symptoms and activities may assist the correlation between certain situations, environments and emotions (Dahlstrom et al 1982). Sleep disorders such as sleep apnea, insufficient or disturbed sleep may also be present (Tosun et al 2003).

A multifactorial model of the factors contributing to parafunctions is shown in Figure 20.2.

Management

The intervention for bruxism/bruxomania will vary in each patient due to multiple etiological factors. Some of the most common interventions include:

Night time occlusal splints: considered to influence parafunctional activities during the night (Clark 1985). However, while occlusal

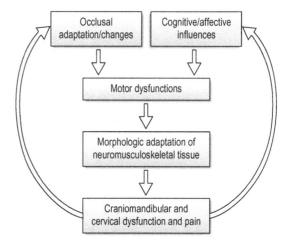

Figure 20.2 • Factors that could contribute to craniomandibular and cervical dysfunction.

splints were previously considered to reduce the effects of bruxism (Nagels et al 2001, Okeson 1996), the evidence supporting the use of splints is lacking (Nagels et al 2001).

Stress management: progressive muscle relaxation, hypnosis, and biofeedback applied to change the effects of stress and psychosocial problems (Hathaway 1995b, Heller & Forgione 1975, Kardachi & Clarke 1977). Stress management has been shown to provide short term improvement in patients with bruxism (Goulet et al 1993). However, the long term effects have not been investigated.

Physiotherapy intervention: craniofacial soft tissue and TMJ mobilization, education of motor control and behavior modification to influence the neuromusculoskeletal factors contributing to parafunctional activities.

Clinically, patients with parafunctions can be divided into three broad groups:

1. Patients who have a direct correlation between their symptoms and parafunctional activities based on subjective examination and symptom behavior (Lobbezoo & Naeije 1997, Piekartz von 2007). These patients may benefit from occlusal splint therapy, physiotherapy intervention, an educational approach, or a combination of these may reduce complaints.

2. Patients who do not have a direct correlation between their symptoms and parafunctional activities. This phenomenon may be due to a lack of conscious awareness of parafunctional activities. Clinicians can assess the possible correlation with trial treatments followed by reassessment of physical signs and patient specific outcome measures.

3. Patients who do not have craniofacial symptoms but present with clear parafunctional activities. The treatment approach will depend on the presentation of each patient's parafunction.

Treatment of tissue dysfunction

Craniofacial tissue mobilization

There is clinical evidence that passive mobilization can lead to the reduction of abnormal orofacial motor activity and may have a positive effect on parafunctional activities (Chaitow 2005, Piekartz von 2007). Assessment and treatment of craniofacial bone tissue is often underestimated by clinicians when managing patients with parafunctional activities. There are many models explaining how cranial manipulative interventions can change signs and symptoms (Chaitow 2005).

The techniques described below are based on a pragmatic functional approach related to clinical evidence from orthodontics and cranial plastic surgery (Oudhof 2001, Zöller et al 2005). Craniomandibular-facial dental dysfunctions such as malocclusion or TMJ disc displacements are considered to facilitate an abnormal interactive bone tension (stress-transducing). This phenomenon may facilitate (abnormal) craniofacial

growth which may influence the masticatory muscles leading to abnormal afferent input or nociception (Proffit & Fields 1993, Piekartz von 2007). For example, facial asymmetry caused by unilateral maxillary sinusitis may lead to an abnormal stress-transducer effect on facial and neurocranial bone tissue. This asymmetry can lead to abnormal bone growth and craniofacial morphology (Linder-Aronson & Woodside 2000). The patient may express these abnormal motor responses with an increase in muscle tone in both sternocleidomastoid and masseter muscles (Palazzi et al 1996).

Cranial accessory movements (passive movements between cranial bones which cannot be performed actively by the patient) described in the following examples have the potential to influence stress-transducer mechanisms of the craniofacial region (Piekartz von 2007). For an excellent overview of different theories of cranial manual therapy the reader is referred to the work of Chaitow (2005).

In the author's experience the following mobilization or movement strategies have been shown to be beneficial for patients with craniofacial symptoms due to parafunctional activities.

Temporal-zygomatic region

The temporal bone forms the lateral side of the neurocranium and is connected to the parietal, sphenoid and occipital bones of the neurocranium. Together with the facial skeleton it has a strong connection with the zygoma and provides the origin to the masseter muscle (Fig. 20.3A & B).

Starting position. The patient is instructed to lie comfortably in the supine position on a plinth. The clinician sits at the top end of the plinth facing the patient's head (Fig. 20.4). The clinician then positions the right hand on the posterolateral aspect of the patient's right temporal bone directly over the ear. The right mid finger is placed in the external auditory meatus. The right

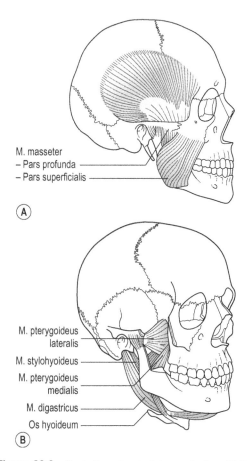

Figure 20.3 ● Illustration of a skull demonstrating: **(A)** the temporalis and masseter, and **(B)** the pterygoids, digastric and stylohyoid muscles. From Piekartz HJ (ed) 2007 Craniofacial pain. Neuromusculoskeletal assessment, treatment and management. Elsevier, Edinburgh.

M. masseter
– Pars profunda
– Pars superficialis

M. pterygoideus lateralis
M. stylohyoideus
M. pterygoideus medialis
M. digastricus
Os hyoideum

thumb is positioned on the superior aspect of the zygomatic process and the index finger is positioned on its inferior aspect (Fig. 20.4).

Following this, the clinician rotates the patient's head and neck to the left by 30°. The clinician then holds the right zygomatic bone between the left thumb and index finger. **Method.** From this position the clinician performs accessory movements of the temporal and/or zygomatic bone. Rotational movements around a transverse axis are performed by the clinician pronating and supinating the forearm. The movements can also be initiated by the clinician's trunk.

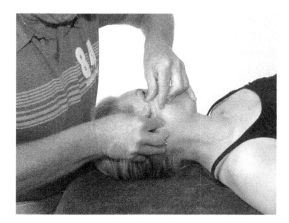

Figure 20.4 ● Craniofacial tissue mobilization of the temporo-zygomatic region.

When performing lateral transverse movement, the clinician needs to hook their right ring finger in the external auditory canal while the middle and index fingers squeeze the zygomatic process.

Temporal-parietal region

Starting position. The patient is instructed to lie comfortably in the supine position on a plinth with the head and neck rotated to the left by 30° (Fig. 20.5). The clinician sits at the right side of the patient's head and positions the right hypothenar eminence over the patient's right pars squamosa of the temporal bone with their fingers facing towards the face. The right thumb and index finger are positioned on the superior and inferior aspects of the zygomatic process of the temporal bone respectively. The right little finger is in contact with the mastoid process. The palm of the left hand is positioned on the top of the skull with the fingers placed on the parietal bone superior to the parietotemporal region.

Method. The clinician's trunk initiates parietal bone movement in the direction that they propose to treat. A slight counter pressure is applied in the opposite direction with the right hand on the temporal bone to emphasize the squeeze action of the pars squamosa (the temporoparietal region) (Fig. 20.5).

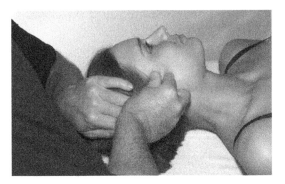

Figure 20.5 • Craniofacial tissue mobilization of the temporal-parietal region.

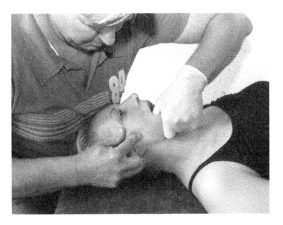

Figure 20.6 • Craniofacial tissue mobilization of the temporomandibular region.

Accessory movements of the temporal-parietal region can be performed such as longitudinal movements in caudad and cephalad directions applying compression and distraction. Rotational movements about the longitudinal, transverse and sagittal axes and anterior/posterior or posterior/anterior movements can also be performed.

Temporomandibular region

Starting position. The patient lies in the supine position on the plinth. The clinician's right hand is positioned in the similar starting position as the temporo-zygomatic technique. The clinician's left thumb is placed intra-orally on the right lower molars while the fingers grasp the mandible extra-orally (Fig. 20.6).

Method. From this starting position, accessory movements of the mandible, the temporal bone, and a combination of these movements can be performed. Muscular stretching techniques can also be performed from this position. Similarly myofascial trigger point treatment of the masseters, temporalis, lateral and medial pterygoid muscle can also be performed (Piekartz von 2007) (see Chapter 23). These manual techniques need to be integrated with patient education and behavioral interventions.

Patient education and behavioral interventions

Habitual reverse technique

The 'habitual reverse technique' is implemented to educate patients about their parafunctions, improve awareness of causative factors, the etiology, the precursors, the nature of their condition, and self management (Azin & Nunn 1973). As patients gain kinesthetic awareness of their parafunctional activity they can learn motor control to modify this activity. The technique involves the following steps:

Response description. Patient awareness using mirrors as well as education about the consequences of parafunctions, such as asymmetrical muscle atrophy and abrasion of teeth.

Early warning procedure. Kinesthetic awareness of early signs such as increased muscle tension in the cheek or increased pressure in the throat.

Awareness of aggravating factors. Identification of trigger factors in discussion with the patient. Such awareness may take several weeks and therefore a logbook may assist the process.

Habitual discomforts. A description of the unpleasant emotions, thoughts and consequences experienced by the patient. If the patient cannot spontaneously express their irrational thoughts, the clinician should specifically question them. For example, if the patient is aware that working in front of a computer increases their facial tension, they need to verbalize what they experience and of any discomfort.

Competing responses. Describes the exercise/s that patients need to perform when they experience the onset of parafunctions (early warning procedure). The exercise should have the following prerequisites:

– isometric exercise (with the teeth separated) that is opposite to the parafunction (Fig. 20.7)
– the exercise needs to be performed until the signs of oncoming parafunction wears off. This process generally may take up to a minute
– the exercise should be easy to perform and fit in with activities of daily living

Note. In order to prevent over stretching of the masticatory muscles, exercises need to be performed isometrically without associated movements of the jaw and neck, or in abnormal habitual postures.

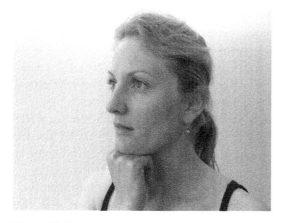

Figure 20.7 • Habitual reverse technique performing isometric mandibular depression exercise (with the teeth separated).

Tongue teeth breathing and swallowing (TTBS) exercise

The TTBS exercise promotes neuromuscular re-education (Damsté 1980). The TTBS exercise includes the components 'tongue-up', 'teeth apart' and 'breathing and swallowing' in order to gain control over diurnal parafunctions (Kraus 1995). The exercise aims to improve patient awareness of parafunctions and motor control during both rest and mandibular movements to eliminate parafunctional activity (Selms van et al 2004).

Correct posture of the head, neck and trunk is imperative for the TTBS exercise to be successful since it affects tongue movement, the tongue position against the teeth, as well as tension in the masticatory and cervical muscles. Either TTBS exercise or other habitual reverse technique must be integrated into the patient's daily activities in order to reprogram motor activity if parafunctional activity is triggered.

Starting position. The clinician needs to correct the patient's head, neck and trunk posture to minimize masticatory muscle activity (Rugh & Drago 1981). Electromyography tests may assist in the achievement of this position; however, its use may be time consuming.

TTBS, tongue-up exercise. Patients are not commonly aware of their teeth or tongue position. Assistance to achieve kinesthetic awareness is a fundamental aspect of the treatment process. The middle of the tongue should be in contact with the central palate and the tip of the tongue should contact the posterior aspect of the middle upper incisor teeth without producing increased pressure. This position promotes nose breathing and relaxes the mandibular elevator muscles (Derkay & Schlechter 1998). If this tongue posture cannot be achieved, the patient should be prescribed tongue coordination exercises. These exercises include rotating the tongue around the longitudinal and transverse axis to improve kinesthetic awareness of tongue position and tongue movement. The clinician may use a spatula to assess the tongue position by palpating it for the presence or absence of increased tension.

TTBS, teeth apart. This position improves awareness of teeth position, whereby the individual's teeth are not in contact. Separation of the upper and lower teeth may be confirmed by inserting a spatula between the upper and lower molars (Fig. 20.8).

TTBS, breathing. The advantage of nose breathing is that it filters dirt particles, warms the incoming air, and promotes diaphragmatic activity. Nasal breathing is associated with the normal resting position of the tongue as described in the tongue-up exercise and inhibits masticatory muscle tension (Damsté & Idema 1994, Jordaan & Piekartz von 2007, Lowe & Johnston 1979). Mouth breathing in contrast is associated with upper cervical extension, facilitates accessory respiratory muscle activity (Sharp et al 1976) and reduces diaphragmatic breathing (Ormeno et al 1999, Sharp et al 1976).

The clinician needs to facilitate nasal and diaphragmatic breathing in neutral position of the head, neck and trunk. During inspiration the clinician ensures that the:

* tongue pressure does not increase
* diameter of the nostrils does not increase
* correct neck posture is maintained (commonly the neck moves into extension)
* masticatory muscle tension does not increase
* teeth do not touch.

TTBS, swallowing. Normal swallowing (Box 20.4) involves movement of the tongue as well as maximal teeth contact (Butler & Stallard 2006). An adult swallows on average 1200 times a day with a total duration of about 6–10 minutes (Gupta et al 1996). Swallowing dysfunction can increase teeth contact and may change motor function of the masticatory system and the craniocervical region (Milidonis et al 1993).

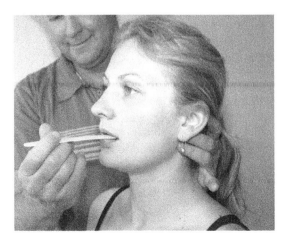

Figure 20.8 ● Tongue teeth breathing and swallowing (TTBS) exercise. Separation of the upper and lower teeth may be confirmed by inserting a spatula between the upper and lower molars.

Box 20.4

A summary of normal swallowing.

The requirements for normal swallowing occur in the following order:

The tongue is positioned behind the upper incisor teeth.

The tongue moves to the floor of the mouth once food or fluids enter the mouth.

To initiate swallowing the tongue moves to the palatinum but the pressure on the incisor teeth increases.

Intermediate phase: the tension in the dorsal two thirds of the tongue increases, while the activity in the tip of the tongue is reduced. The tongue performs a wave-like motion and the muscle activity occurs more posteriorly. This activity takes place with or without contact with the (pre-)molar teeth.

Final phase: the tongue moves back into its resting position and swallowing is completed.

Method. The clinician ensures that:

- the head and/neck maintains a neutral position throughout
- there is no molar contact thereby decreasing the risk of excessive masticatory muscle activity
- the tongue is returned to its rest position behind the upper incisors without any pressure of the mid-tongue against the palate.

The TTBS swallowing exercise is performed with the clinician seated at the same height as the patient to observe and correct muscle activity and compensatory movements. The patient is requested to swallow a sip of water several times while the clinician observes the function of their lips, the hyoid bone and the cervical region (Fig. 20.9). The patient will gain valuable feedback if they observe the swallowing function in a mirror.

The clinician then places the thumb and index finger of one hand on the sub-occipital region. The thumb and index fingers of the other hand are then placed gently around the hyoid. The head/neck position should be maintained in the neutral position, without the upper cervical spine moving into extension. The sub-occipital muscles can be palpated to detect any increase in tension. The hyoid bone should initially be move cephalad and then caudad while swallowing. It is difficult to quantify a 'normal range' of hyoid movement. However, if the hyoid does not move between the palpating fingers, its motion while swallowing is considered to be restricted.

Awareness phase. If the patient has difficulty with components of the exercise, more time should be spent with the swallowing phase of the movement. For instance, if the patient has difficulty relaxing the upper lip after the final phase of swallowing, lip exercises are indicated. Examples of lip exercises are: passive stretching of the upper lip, manually or with the aid of a small tampon; this stretch may be combined with proprioceptive stimulation of the facial muscles like: pouting the lips, spreading the lips, sucking the lips into the mouth cavity, whistling and stretching the lip with tongue movements (Piekartz von 2007).

The next treatment session should then include repetition of the complete TTBS swallowing exercise.

In the author's clinical experience combining passive stretching with lip coordination exercises can lead to a more 'normal' swallowing pattern.

Indicators of orofacial dysfunctions during swallowing

Lips: during the tongue resting phase the lips usually move slightly and then should relax again. Upper lip dysfunction is observed when it curls slightly upwards due to increased activity of the buccinator which connects to the superficial masseter and orbicularis oculi. When there is increased tension in both masseters and orbicularis oculi, the upper lip activity is increased and this results in the upper lip to curl slightly inwards.

Hyoid: in the intermediate phase of swallowing the hyoid can be palpated. The hyoid

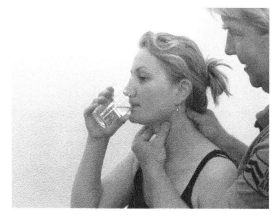

Figure 20.9 ● Tongue teeth breathing and swallowing (TTBS) exercise.

usually moves cephalad and returns to the normal position. Indicators for hyoid dysfunction are: the range of motion of the hyoid is smaller than usual; and on palpation the hyoid is positioned more cranially (i.e. above the C2–C3 level) or tilted forward/backward in the sagittal plane.

Treatment methods during bracing activities

Brace-relax technique

This technique involves small, oscillating, pain free passive or active movements of opening the mouth, performed with minimal muscle activity. A prerequisite for the success of the technique is the ability of the patient to consciously relax the mandible. The aim of the exercise is first explained to the patient, following which they are requested to concentrate in order to relax and 'let go' their mandible.

Starting position. The patient initially sits in a relaxed position in a chair. They are instructed to gently press the tip of their tongue against the hard palate. The clinician then stands on the right side of the patient and holds their head with the left hand.

Method. Following this, the clinician places the right hand on the patient's mandible (Fig. 20.10). In this position small amplitude oscillating movements of the mandible are performed, initially only into laterotrusion (sideway movement) to the right and then to the left side with an average frequency of two repetitions per second. The patient is requested to relax the mandible during the intervention. The following guided imagery suggestions may assist the patient to relax the mandible:

- 'Imagine your jaw is so heavy that it weighs more than 10 kilograms'.
- 'Imagine the bottom of your jaw is so big that it almost touches the floor'.

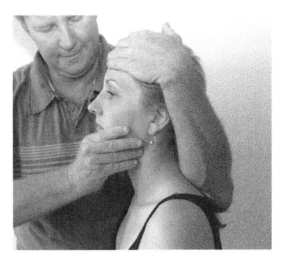

Figure 20.10 ● The brace-relax technique.

- 'Imagine that your jaw is so warm and heavy that it becomes impossible to shut your mouth'.

Often the patient is able to relax initially but tenses the masticatory muscles after a short period of time. The clinician should prompt the patient to be aware of masticatory muscle tension so that they can consciously relax.

Variations. Once the basic exercise is mastered, variations may be introduced. For example:

Frequency. The frequency of the oscillating movements may be increased to 4–8 repetitions per second.

Direction. Protrusion and retrusion of the mandible may be performed in the same position.

If the patient is able to relax the mandibular muscles, laterotrusion may be combined with other mandibular movements (e.g. laterotrusion with protraction).

Duration. The initial duration of the exercise is approximately 60–90 seconds. The duration may be extended as treatment is progressed. Clinical experience suggests that even when the patient performs the exercise well, some appear to experience difficulty with progressions of the exercise. Sometimes bracing re-occurs after 20–30 seconds of relaxation. In this case the exercise should be progressed gradually.

Position of the head. The position of the head may influence the masticatory muscles. Therefore a variation of positions may be used as a starting position. Variations add or reduce the grade of difficulty for the patient. In most cases the clinician will aim for the position that usually triggers the symptoms.

Mind imagery. Once the mandible is relaxed, the patient can be instructed to think of triggering a pain provoking situation. The clinician constantly assesses for motor reactions and provides feedback to the patient. The duration of this exercise depends on the outcome of mandibular muscle relaxation.

Combinations of the above may increase the difficulty of the exercise.

Wiggle technique

When the patient has learnt to experience a relaxed mandible they can be introduced to exercises such as the 'wiggle' technique into their daily activities.

Starting position and method. The patient sits in a relaxed position and places their left thumb and index finger on the mandible. Their right hand supports the occiput (Fig. 20.11). They then passively move the mandible between the fingers over a few millimeters. The technique is then progressed by moving the mandible towards the right and then the left side. It is important that the patient does not experience any symptoms during the exercise; overstretching of the mandible or compensatory movements are avoided.

Rapid opening and closing in mid-position

Starting position and method. The patient is instructed to press the tongue gently against the hard palate so that the mouth is opened no more

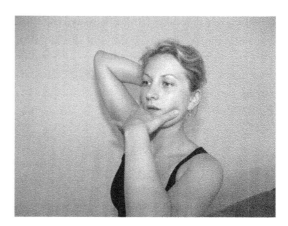

Figure 20.11 ● The wiggle technique.

than 20–25 mm. The clinician then places the index and middle fingers of both their hands on the angle of each mandible to add proprioceptive input. During opening and closing of the mouth:

- both index and middle fingers palpate and guide the physiological opening and closing via the rami of the mandible
- no neck movement should occur
- the exercise should be pain free
- the movement should not be perceived to be unpleasant.

The exercise is ceased at the earliest signs of fatigue.

Once the patient is able to perform the exercise with ease, the degree of difficulty can be increased by removing the contact on the angle of the mandible.

Conclusion

This chapter has described the clinical assessment of patients with orofacial pain. It provides a detailed description of the neuromusculoskeletal management of the most common parafunctional activities and bruxism. Neuromusculoskeletal treatment of cranial tissue dysfunction integrating educational and behavioral interventions is discussed.

References

Azin N, Nunn R 1973 Habit reversal: A method of eliminating nervous habits and tics. Behav Res Therapy 11: 619-623.

Butler JH, Stallard R 2006 Physiologic stress and tooth contact. J Periodontal Research 4(2):152-158 (published online 30 June 2006).

Carlsson GE, Magnusson T 1999 Management of temporomandibular disorders in the general dental practice. Quintessence Publishing, Chicago, p 41-42.

Carlsson GE, Egermark I, Magnusson T 2003 Predictors of bruxism, other oral parafunctions, and tooth wear over a 20-year follow-up J Orofac Pain 17(1):50-57.

Castelo PM, Gaviao MB, Pereira LJ, Bonjardim LR 2005 Relationship between oral parafunctional/nutritive sucking habits and temporo-mandibular joint dysfunction in primary dentition. Int J Paediatr Dent 15(1):29-36.

Chaitow L 2005 A brief historical perspective in cranial manipulation, therapy and practice, 2nd edn. Elsevier, Edinburgh, p 1-13.

Clark G 1985 Kieferfunktionen, Diagnostik und Therapie. Quintessenz, Berlin, p 145-157.

Corvo G, Tartaro G, Giudice A, Diomajuta A 2003 Distribution of craniomandibular disorders, occlusal factors and oral parafunctions in a paediatric population. Eur J Paediatr Dent 4(2):84-88.

Dahlstrom L, Carlsson GE, Carlsson SG 1982 Comparison of effect of electromyographic biofeedback and occlusal splint therapy on mandibular dysfunction. Scand J Dent Res 90:151-156.

Damsté PH 1980 Tongue function in the rehabilitation of speech disorders, faulty breathing habits and deglutition disorders. Acta Otorhinolaryngol Belg 34 (6):630-645.

Damsté P, Idema N 1994 Habitueel mondademen. Houten/Zaventem: Bohn Stafleu Van Loghum, p 12-34.

Dao TT, Lund JP, Lavigne GJ 1994 Comparison of pain and quality of life in bruxers and patients with myofascial pain of the masticatory muscles. J Orofac Pain 8(4):350-356.

Derkay C, Schlechter G 1998 Anatomy and physiology of pediatric swallowing disorders, dysphagia in children. Adults and Geriatrics 31-38.

Flor H, Birbaumer N, Schulte W et al 1991 Stress-related EMG responses in patients with chronic temporomandibular pain. Pain 46:145-153.

Gastaldo E, Quatrale R, Graziani A et al 2006 The excitability of the trigeminal motor system in sleep bruxism: A transcranial magnetic stimulation and brainstem reflex study. J Orofacial Pain 20:145-155.

Glaros AG 1981 Incidence of diurnal and nocturnal bruxism. J Prosthet Dent 45:545-551.

Glaros AG, Williams K, Lausten L, Friesen L 2005 Tooth contact in patients with temporomandibular disorders. Cranio 136:188-193.

Glaros AG, Owais Z, Lausten L 2007 Reduction in parafunctional activity: a potential mechanism for the effectiveness of splint therapy. Oral Rehab 34:97-104.

Goulet J, Lund J, Montplaisir J et al 1993 Daily clenching, nocturnal bruxism, and stress and their association with CMD symptoms. J Orofacial Pain 7:120-127.

Grozev L, Michailov T 1999 Treatment of bruxism and bruxomania (clinically tested). Folia Med (Plovdiv) 41(1):147-148.

Gupta V, Reddy N, Canilang E 1996 Surface EMG Measurements at the throat during dry and wet swallowing. Dysphagia 11:173-179.

Hathaway K 1995a Bruxism: Definition, measurement and treatment. In: Fricton J, Dubner R (eds) Orofacial pain and temporomandibular disorders. Raven Press, New York, p 375-380.

Hathaway K 1995b Bruxism: definition, measurement and treatment. In:

Fricton J, Dubner R (eds) Orofacial pain and temporomandibular disorders. Raven Press, New York, p 375-387.

Heller RF, Forgione AG 1975 An evaluation of bruxism control: massed negative practice and automated relaxation training. J Dent Res 54(6):1120-1123.

Jordaan R, von Piekartz H 2007 Management of craniofacial and cervical postural changes in the child with altered breathing patterns in craniomandibular, head-en craniocervical region. Neuromusceloskeletal assessment – treatment and management (von Piekartz (ed)). Elsevier, Edinburgh, p 637-654.

Kampe T, Edman G, Bader G et al 1997 Personality traits in a group of subjects with longstanding bruxing behaviour. J Oral Rehabil 24 (8):588-593.

Kapel L, Giaros A, McGlynn F 1989 Psychophysiological responses to stress in patients with myofascial pain-dysfunction syndrome. J Behav Med 12:397-403.

Kardachi B, Clarke N 1977 The use of biofeedback to control bruxism. J Periodontol 48:639-645.

Kato T, Thie NM, Huynh N et al 2003 Topical review: sleep bruxism and the role of peripheral sensory influences. 191-213.

Kieser JA, Groeneveld HT 1998 Relationship between juvenile bruxing and craniomandibular dysfunction. J Oral Rehabil 25 (9):662-665.

Kiliaridis S, Carlsson GE 1994 Bruxing and growth, angle. Orthod 64 (4):244-245.

Kraus SL 1988 Cervical spine influence on the craniomandibular region. In: Kraus SL (ed) TMJ disorders management of the craniomandibular complex. Churchill Livingstone, New York, p 367-404.

Kraus SL 1995 Cervical influences on management of temperomandibualr disorders. In: Kraus SL (ed) TMJ Disorders management of the craniomandibular complex. Churchill Livingstone, New York, p 325-412.

Lavigne G, Montplaisir J 1995 Bruxism: epidemiology, diagnosis, pathophysiology and pharmacology. Adv Pain Res Therapy 21:387-392.

Lavigne G, Woda A, Truelove E et al 2005 Mechanisms associated with unusual orofacial pain. J Orofac Pain 19(1):9-21.

Lavigne GJ, Khoury S, Abe S et al 2008 Bruxism physiology and pathology: an overview for clinicians. J Oral Rehabil 35(7):476-494.

Lawrence E, Samson G 1988 Growth development influences on the craniomandibular region. In: Kraus S (ed) TMJ Disorders: management of the craniomandibular complex. Churchill Livingstone, New York, p 241-274.

Linder-Aronson S, Woodside D 2000 Excess face height malocclusion. Etiology 1-35.

Lobezzoo F 2006 Bruxism: its multiple causes and its effects on dental implants-an updated review. J Oral Rehabil 33(4):293-300.

Lobbezoo F, Naeije M 1997 Bruxisme en myofasciale pijn van kauwspieren. De relatie kritisch bekeken. Ned T Fysiother 107:70.

Lobbezoo F, Naeije M 2001 Bruxism is mainly regulated centrally, not peripherally. J Oral Rehabil 28 (12):1085-1091.

Lobbezoo F, Montplaisir J, Lavigne G 1996 Bruxism: a factor associated with temporomandibular disorders and orofacial pain. J Back Musculoskeletal Rehab 6:165-201.

Lowe AA, Johnston WD 1979 Tongue and jaw muscle activity in response to mandibular rotations in a sample of normal and anterior open-bite subjects. Am J Orthod 76(5):565-576.

Manfredini D, Landi N, Romagnoli M et al 2003 Etiopathogenesis of parafunctional habits of the stomatognathic system. Minerva Stomatol 52(7-8):339-345, 345-349.

Marbach J, Raphael K, Dohrenwend B et al 1990 The validity of tooth grinding measures: Aetiology of pain dysfunction syndrome revisited. J Am Dent Assoc 120:327-324.

Marie H, Pietkiewicz K 1997 La bruxomanie: Mémoires originaux. Rev Stomatol 14:107-111.

Marklund S, Wänman A 2008 Incidence and prevalence of myofascial pain in the jaw-face region. A one-year prospective study on dental students. Acta Odontol Scand 66(2):113-121.

McMillan A, Blasberg B 1994 Pain-pressure threshold in painful jaw muscles following trigger point injection. J Orofacial Pain 8:384-391.

Milidonis M, Kraus S, Segal R, Widmer C 1993 Genioglossi muscle activity in response to changes in anterior/neutral head posture. Am J Orthod Dentofac Orthop 103:39-44.

Moss R, Adams H 1984 Physiological reactions to stress in subjects with and without myofascial pain dysfunction symptoms. J Oral Rehabil 219-224.

Nagels G, Okkerse W, Braem M et al 2001 Decreased amount of slow wave sleep in nocturnal bruxism is not improved by dental splint therapy. Acta Neurol Belg 101(3):152-159.

Okeson J 1996 Orofacial pain. Guidelines for assessment, diagnosis, and management. Quintessence Books, Chicago, p 68-69.

Okeson J 2005 The clinical management of orofacial pain. Bell's orofacial pain. Quintessence Publishing Co. Inc., Chicago.

Ormeno G, Miralles R, Loyola R et al 1999 Body position effects on EMG activity of the temporal and suprahyoid muscles in healthy subjects and in patients with myogenic cranio-cervical-mandibular dysfunction. J Craniomandibular Practice 17(2):132-142.

Oudhof H 2001 Skull growth in relation with mechanical stimulation, Craniofacial Dysfunction 1-22.

Palazzi C, Miralles R, Soto M et al 1996 Body position effects on EMG activity of sternocleidomastoid and masseter muscle in patients with myogenic craniocervical-mandibular Dysfunction. Cranio 14:200-207.

Piekartz von HJM 2007 Management of craniomandibular region. Clinical patterns and management. In: von Piekartz (ed) Craniofacial pain.

Neuromusculoskeletal assessment, treatment and management. Elsevier, Edinburgh, p 214-243.

Piekartz von HJM, Bryden L 2001 Craniofacial dysfunction and pain. Butterworth Heinemann, Oxford.

Proffit W, Fields H 1993 Contemporary orthodontics, 2nd edn. Mosby Year Book section II. p 18-34.

Rhodes G 2006 The evolutionary psychology of facial beauty. Annu Rev Psychol 57:199-226.

Rugh JD, Drago CJ 1981 Vertical dimension: a study of clinical rest position and jaw muscle activity. J Prosthet Dent 45(6):670-675.

Rugh JD, Montgomery GT 1987 Physiological reactions of patients with TM disorders vs symptom-free controls on a physical stress task. J Craniomandib Disord 1 (4):243-250.

Selms van MK, Lobbezoo F, Wicks DJ et al 2004 Craniomandibular pain, oral parafunctions, and psychological stress in a longitudinal case study. J Oral Rehabil 31(8):738-745.

Sharp J, Druz W, Danon J et al 1976 Respiratory muscle function and the use of respiratory muscle electromyography in the evaluation of respiratory regulation. Chest 70 (suppl):150-156.

Svensson P, Graven-Nielsen T 2001 Craniofacial muscle pain: review of mechanisms and clinical manifestations. J Orofacial Pain 15:117-145.

Thorpy M 1990 Parasomnias. In: Thorpy MJ (ed) International classification of sleep disorders: Diagnostic and coding manual. American Sleep Disorders Association. Allen Press, Rochester MN, p 142-149.

Tosun T, Karabuda C, Cuhadaroglu C 2003 Evaluation of sleep bruxism by polysomnographic analysis in patients with dental implants. Int J Oral Maxillofac Implants 18(2):286-292.

Widmalm SE, Christiansen RL, Gunn SM 1995 Oral parafunctions as temporomandibular disorder risk factors in children. Cranio 13(4):242-246.

Winocur E, Gavish A, Volfin G et al 2001 Oral motor parafunctions among heavy drug addicts and their effects on signs and symptoms of temporomandibular disorders. J Orofac Pain 56-63.

Yu XM, Sessle BJ, Vernon H, Hu JW 1995 Effects of inflammatory irritant

application to the rat temporo-mandibular joint on jaw and neck muscle-activity. Pain 60:143-149.

Zöller JE, Küber AC, Lorber WD, Mühling JFH 2005

Kraniosynosthosen in Kraniofaziale Chirurgie. Diagnostik und therapie kraniofazialer Fehlbildung. Thieme, Stuttgart p 3-25.

21

Psychological management

Paul R Martin

Individuals suffering from chronic headache are rarely referred to psychologists, which is unfortunate as they have much to offer. While headache may arise from central and peripheral mechanisms, psychosocial issues can trigger headache and influence the headache experience. In this chapter the author, a clinical psychologist, presents a functional model of headache, the psychological assessment of patients with headache, and reviews the approaches used in the treatment of patients with headache.

Most individuals have experienced a headache at one time or another but the event is less than overwhelming and passes quickly. On the other hand, a significant proportion of the population experience headaches and associated symptoms of such intensity that they are quite debilitating; and a significant proportion of the population experience headaches with high frequency or even continuously. Some individuals have suffered from headaches for most of their lives. Headaches lead to lost work days and impact on families.

The contribution of psychologists stems from a range of factors including the following. First, by definition, headaches are 'pain in the head' and whilst the pain may arise from various central and peripheral mechanisms, the experience of pain is influenced by cognitive and emotional processes, such as whether attention is focused on the pain or elsewhere, and the anxiety level of the headache sufferer. Second, the most common trigger of headaches is stress and negative emotions such as anxiety, anger and depression. Third, headaches arise out of an interaction between the person and her/his environment, that is, behaviour and lifestyle provide the psychosocial context in which headaches unfold. Finally, maladaptive reactions to a headache occurring, by the sufferer and sometimes significant others, can aggravate headaches in the short-term and contribute to the development of a chronic disorder in the long-term.

This chapter presents a functional model of chronic headaches which seeks to explain the variance in headache activity, that is, why headaches occur at one time rather than another, why the person is getting headaches at this stage of her/his life rather than at other stages, why the headache problem began when it did, and why the person is vulnerable to developing a headache disorder. This model is then used as a framework for reviewing briefly what we know about headache from a psychological perspective, and how headache should be assessed and treated.

The functional model of chronic headache

When psychologists seek to answer the 'why' questions posed above, they typically resort to functional models that analyse disorders in terms of their antecedents and consequences. Figure 21.1 presents a schematic outline of a functional model of chronic headaches.

In the centre of the model, labelled as 'headache phenomena', are headaches and associated symptoms, and the underlying central and peripheral mechanisms. It is important to remember that headaches are often preceded by, and accompanied by, a variety of other symptoms, such as aura, nausea and vomiting, photophobia and phonophobia, and vertigo and tinnitus. These symptoms are sometimes perceived as more distressing than the head pain itself. The central and peripheral mechanisms are complicated and still not fully understood as evidenced by the fact that in the 'bible' of the field, there are 16 chapters devoted to the mechanisms of just one headache type – migraine (Olesen et al 2006).

To the left of the model are the antecedents of headaches arranged along a temporal continuum. The immediate antecedents are the triggers or precipitating factors. Most headache sufferers report multiple triggers with Kelman (2007) finding that the mean number reported per patient was 6.7. The most commonly reported triggers are stress and negative emotions, hormonal factors for females, sensory stimuli (flicker, glare, eyestrain, noise, odors), hunger, eating certain foods (e.g., chocolate, cheese, oranges), alcohol consumption, lack of or excess of sleep, and certain weather conditions (e.g., changes in weather, heat, humidity) (Martin & MacLeod, 2008). Some of these triggers have been validated experimentally including stress (Martin & Seneviratne, 1997), visual disturbance (Martin & Teoh 1999), noise (Martin et al 2005), and hunger (Martin & Seneviratne 1997).

'Setting factors' refers to the psychosocial context in which headaches occur. Once triggers have been identified, it is important to understand how they arise in the lifestyle of the patient. For example, if stress is a trigger of headaches, what are the main sources of stress for that person (e.g. marital relationship, work)? Also, stress is moderated by variables such as coping skills and social support so that an understanding of headaches triggered by stress needs to take into account the strategies the individual uses for coping with stress and her/his social support network. As emotional states are a common trigger of headaches, emotional disorders are obvious setting factors for recurrent headaches. Research has shown that chronic headaches are associated with anxiety disorders (particularly panic and phobia) and major depression (Radat & Swendsen 2004, Sheftell & Atlas 2002). If headaches are associated with hunger, eating, and drinking, then an analysis of their dietary patterns is needed to document the relevant behaviors and explanatory factors for the behaviors (e.g. why does a person sometimes go for long periods without eating?).

'Onset factors' refer to events associated with the headaches beginning when they did or becoming significantly worse when they did. The most common onset factor is periods of high stress. For women, events associated with hormonal factors are often linked to headache onset such as menarche, use of oral contraceptives and pregnancy (see Ch. 9). Onset factors are not always important from a management perspective, as the factors that are responsible for a problem beginning are not always the same as the factors responsible for a problem continuing, but sometimes they are. For example, one type of stressful event that has been identified as an

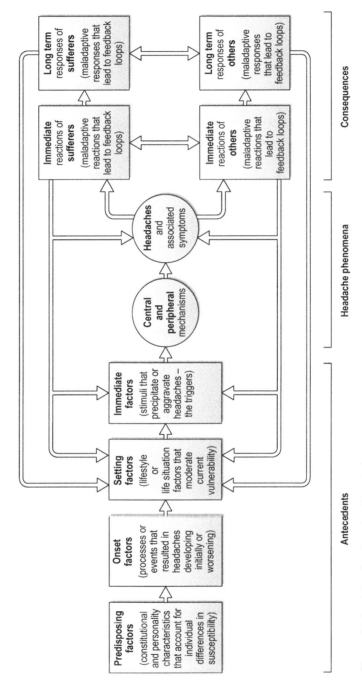

Figure 21.1 • A functional mode of headaches. (Adapted from Martin: Psychological Management of Chronic Headaches, 1993.)

onset factor for headaches is physical and sexual abuse. If such abuse has not been resolved, then it is likely to need attention.

With respect to 'predisposing factors', headaches run in families and have a genetic predisposition, but genes explain only 20% to 50% of the variance (Russell & Olesen 1995). From a psychological perspective, it can be asked whether particular personality types are more vulnerable to developing a chronic headache disorder. There is a long tradition of describing the 'migraine personality' or 'headache personality' using terms such as 'tense', 'sensitive', 'obsessional', 'perfectionist' and 'inflexible'. Many studies have failed to find support for such hypotheses, however, particularly the better controlled studies that have investigated the relationship in community rather than clinic samples (e.g. Philips 1976). This does not mean that personality is not a vulnerability factor for headaches, however, only that the relationship is complicated and therefore difficult to pin down in research studies. Put simply, there are many different routes to becoming a chronic headache sufferer, and a variety of different personality traits or combinations of traits may make individuals vulnerable. Any characteristics that result in individuals reacting excessively to 'stressful' situations are likely to make people vulnerable, for example.

The consequences of headaches are divided into immediate and long-term reactions, for headache sufferers and for significant others. The significance of these reactions is that they are often maladaptive because they lead to vicious cycles whereby the reaction feeds back to the headaches or antecedent factors. An individual may react to a headache by becoming (more) anxious, as a consequence of, for example, worrying about the cause or impact of the headache. As anxiety exacerbates the experience of pain, a loop is created between the affective reaction and headache. Alternatively, if the headache trigger was anxiety and the reaction is

anxiety, then a loop is created between the reaction and the immediate antecedent of the headache. If the trigger was stress, and the main source of stress was a dysfunctional marriage, then if the headache sufferer reacted to the headache by feeling tense and irritable leading to conflict with the spouse, this could create a loop whereby the reaction exacerbated the setting factor of marital discord. Responding to headaches by trying to avoid the triggers of headaches may result in decreased tolerance for the triggers thereby increasing the probability of headaches in the future. Excessive consumption of medication in response to headaches can result in 'medication-overuse headache'.

Partners can react in a number of ways that are maladaptive. If the complaint of headache is always followed by positive reinforcement (e.g., attention, sympathy) and negative reinforcement (e.g., avoiding unappealing tasks), then there is a danger of headache complaints increasing. Alternatively, if the partner responds in ways that are experienced as aversive by the headache sufferer (e.g., reacting against having to take over unappealing tasks), then this can complete loops whereby stress leads to headaches and the reaction of the partner causes more stress.

Long-term consequences that can prove maladaptive include withdrawing from leisure and recreational activities after such activities have been spoiled on a number of occasions by the development of headaches. This can have a number of adverse consequences such as a reduction in the size of a person's social network, thus resulting in less social support with consequent implications for increased stress response. This is an example of a long-term response feeding back to the setting factor of inadequate social support. Withdrawal can lead to reduced positive reinforcement, pleasure and activities that engender a sense of achievement, all changes that increase the likelihood of depressed mood, a potential trigger or aggravating factor for headaches.

Psychological assessment of headache

Three methodologies are used to collect information in the psychological assessment of headache: interviewing, self-monitoring, and questionnaires/inventories. Before discussing each methodology, the role of diagnosis in assessment is reviewed briefly.

Functional analysis v. diagnosis

The critical starting point in assessing headaches is to make a diagnosis (Headache Classification Subcommittee of IHS 2004), because if the headache is a secondary headache caused by, for example, an intracranial neoplasm, ischemic stroke, intracranial infection or intracerebral hemorrhage, the diagnosis will determine management. Psychologists are not qualified to make such a diagnosis which is why they should always work collaboratively with medical practitioners. However, the vast majority of individuals suffering from recurrent headaches have headaches that would be diagnosed as migraine or tension-type headache.

It is argued here, that once it is clear that headaches fall into the migraine or tension-type headache categories, there is limited value in pursuing from a psychological perspective, the type of headache, let alone the subtype. This statement is somewhat counter to traditional practice, but where psychological treatments have been administered to both migraine and tension-type headache sufferers in the same study, there has been no differential response as a function of diagnosis (e.g. Martin et al 2007, Williamson et al 1984). It is argued here that functional analysis is complementary to diagnosis, and provides more relevant information for the psychological management of primary headache.

Interviewing

The questions to be asked at interview in completing a headache assessment from a psychological perspective have been listed in Martin (1993). A starting point is to take a personal and social history as this provides the developmental and psychosocial context for understanding headaches. In assessing headaches, it is important to begin by ascertaining whether the individual can identify one or more than one type of headache. It is common for individuals to suffer from both migraine and tension-type headache, and if this is not identified at the beginning of the assessment, a very confused history can evolve as individuals respond to some questions on the basis of one type of headache and other questions on the basis of the other type of headache.

The headache assessment needs to include a description of the headaches and associated symptoms, and of the history of the assessment and treatment of the headaches. A functional analysis of the headaches should follow that assesses the triggers of headaches, setting, onset and predisposing factors. Questioning can begin with open-ended questions but checklists often help people to remember. For example, patients recall more headache triggers when they are shown a list of potential triggers than without such a list (Kelman 2007). A list of common stressful events can assist people recall onset factors. The reactions of the headache sufferer and significant others in the short and long-term should also be assessed with the objective of identifying maladaptive responses. Such an assessment usually takes two sessions but varies according to factors such as whether there are one or two types of headaches, and the length and complexity of the headache history.

There are advantages to involving partners in assessments as they can provide information and insights that help the formulation, and it provides a vehicle for eliciting their support in managing the headache disorder. However, there is a danger of 'disseminating responsibility' whereby the patient assumes that the partner will take responsibility for solving the headache problem. This is counter to the principle of empowering patients and increasing their confidence in their ability to learn the skills and make the lifestyle changes necessary for overcoming their headache disorder.

Self-monitoring

Patients keeping records of their headaches and related factors is an important component of psychological assessment. Many different types of 'diaries' have been advocated. The most commonly used system is 'time-sampling', for which patients are requested to rate their headache intensity at regular intervals (usually hourly) throughout the waking day, and to record the ratings by placing crosses on a graph at the intersection of the rating and the time of day. If patients experience two types of headaches, both can be monitored in the same diaries by using crosses for one type of headache and circles for the other. Patients are also asked to record in these diaries medication consumed. The information yielded by this system aids the assessment by revealing frequency, duration and severity of headaches, as well as patterns in headache activity such as whether the headaches are worse at some times of the day than others, worse some days of the week than others, and worse at certain times of the month. They also show the impact on the headaches of taking medication. By self-monitoring before, during and after treatment, the records allow evaluation of treatment efficacy. Some researchers/clinicians have advocated recording other types of information in the diaries such as pain location, associated symptoms and triggers.

Another type of self-monitoring is 'event-sampling', whereby recording is triggered by an 'event' rather than a time interval. For example,

Martin (1993) advocated completing 'change' cards whenever a headache begins or gets worse, or ends or improves. These cards involve recording feelings, thoughts and activities, before and after the change occurred. Hence, they have the advantage of focusing on the time of most interest to assessment – the period associated with change.

Diaries have traditionally been kept on cards or forms but electronic recording systems have been developed. Patients are given instructions on how to complete the records verbally and in writing. Experience shows that headache sufferers have a great capacity for keeping records, and research shows that it results in minimal change to headaches (i.e. no appreciable increase or decrease in headaches). The records generate very detailed information, and information relatively free of memory distortions, unlike interviews.

Questionnaires/inventories

Questionnaires can be useful particularly for assessing setting factors. Headaches are so often associated with anxiety and depression that a case can be made for routinely administering inventories such as the Beck Depression Inventory and State-Trait Anxiety Inventory. Measures of stress such as the Perceived Stress Scale may be valuable. If inadequate social support is suspected as a setting factor, administration of scales measuring support such as the Interpersonal Support Evaluation List can provide detailed information in this domain. Questionnaires can also be useful for assessing potential predisposing factors such as low self-esteem and Type A behavior pattern ('hurry sickness').

A number of questionnaires have been developed for measuring disability and quality of life in headache sufferers such as the Migraine Disability Assessment, Headache Impact Test, and Headache Disability Inventory (Andrasik et al 2005).

Treatment of headache

There are three main categories of psychological treatment for headaches although there are significant variations within the categories and overlap between the categories. The categories are biofeedback training, relaxation training and cognitive behavior therapy. There are psychological approaches to headaches that arguably do not fit into these three categories, such as transcendental meditation and hypnosis, but these will not be discussed here as there is relatively little evidence pertaining to their efficacy. A more detailed account of psychological treatment of headache can be found in Borkum (2007).

Biofeedback training

Biofeedback training involves helping patients learn to control biological processes by providing real-time feedback with respect to the process. This is accomplished by attaching electrodes or transducers to patients to monitor the process, and providing feedback to the patient in an auditory (e.g. tone varying in frequency) or visual form (e.g. line varying in length). Patients are sometimes provided with home trainers to practice at home between office visits.

Biofeedback training as a treatment for headaches has been based on traditional (outdated) beliefs with respect to peripheral physiological mechanisms for headaches, that is, the mechanism of migraine is vascular and the mechanism of tension-type headache is muscular. The most common forms of biofeedback training for headaches are EMG biofeedback training and thermal biofeedback training, with the former tending to be used for tension-type headache and the latter tending to be used for migraine, but both types of biofeedback have been used with both types of headache. Other forms of biofeedback training have been used such as feedback of temporal pulse amplitude, EEG biofeedback and skin conductance biofeedback, but they have been evaluated less fully. Biofeedback training is usually combined with relaxation training, including instructions to practice at home.

EMG biofeedback training usually provides feedback from the frontalis muscle (forehead), although other pericranial muscle sites are sometimes used such as the temporalis and trapezius muscles, and the task is for the patient to learn to reduce muscle tension. Thermal biofeedback training usually involves placing a thermisistor on the third finger of the dominant hand, and the task is for patients to learn to warm their hands, which is accomplished by increasing blood flow to their hands.

Relaxation training

The most commonly used forms of relaxation training with headache patients are progressive relaxation and autogenic training, particularly the former. The goal of progressive relaxation training is to help the patient learn to recognize and control tension as it arises in the course of daily activities. It proceeds by the patient sequentially tensing and then releasing specific groups of muscles throughout the body, and noticing how tension feels relative to relaxation. It usually begins with 16 muscle groups, and then combines muscle groups to form 7 groups, finally combining muscle groups to form 4 muscle groups. Autogenic training has foundations in hypnosis and uses autosuggestion. It involves six standard exercises that use self-instructions of warmth and heaviness to promote a state of deep relaxation (e.g. 'my right arm is heavy'). All forms of relaxation training include instructions to practice at home, usually assisted by an audiotape or CD.

Cognitive behavior therapy

Cognitive behavior therapy (CBT) takes on a number of different forms with some authors advocating a 'standard package' of cognitive and behavioral techniques (e.g. Holroyd 2002), and others advocating a broader more individualized approach based on the results of a functional analysis (Martin 1993). The defining technique of this approach is identifying and challenging maladaptive thoughts and beliefs related to headaches. These thoughts and beliefs pertain to the antecedents and consequences of headaches. For example, as stress and negative affect are the most common triggers of headaches, cognitive techniques can be used to modify the thoughts that give rise to stress and negative emotions, and the beliefs that underlie the thoughts. Also, headaches are perceived as stressful and give rise to negative emotions that feedback to aggravate the headaches, and cognitive techniques can be used to break this vicious cycle. Other components of CBT include education, pain management strategies such as imagery training and attention-diversion training, and relaxation training.

The results of a functional analysis suggest a variety of ways of intervening. One level is to consider behavioral management of triggers. The traditional wisdom is to advise that the best way to prevent headaches is to avoid the triggers (e.g. World Health Organization (2006)), but we have argued that avoidance can result in sensitization to triggers in the same way that avoidance of situations that can elicit anxiety results in an increased capacity for those situations to elicit anxiety in the future (Martin & MacLeod 2008). We have provided some evidence to support this position (e.g. Martin 2001), and that repeated, prolonged exposure to triggers can desensitize patients to triggers (Martin 2000). Hence, we advocate a 'coping' approach to triggers that involves controlled exposure for some triggers to promote desensitization to the

trigger, and avoidance of triggers when exposure would clearly be inappropriate.

Other types of intervention suggested by a functional analysis include intervening in the domain of setting factors, for example, targeting the main source of stress such as marital dysfunction, or social support if support is considered inadequate. Predisposing factors such as low self-esteem can be part of a treatment plan. Maladaptive reactions to headaches are potential targets. For example, some headache sufferers respond to a headache beginning by rushing to complete activities that they would not be able to do when a headache has fully developed, thus guaranteeing that the headache will be worse than if they had adopted a strategy designed to minimize headache development. Partners who respond to headaches with reinforcement need to be trained to maintain the level of reinforcement but to reduce the link between reporting headaches and receiving reinforcement.

How effective are psychological treatments?

Borgards and ter Kuile (1994) completed a meta-analysis of psychological treatment for tension-type headache and concluded that EMG biofeedback training, either when administered alone or with relaxation training, and CBT, are associated with at least a 50% reduction in headaches. Improvements reported with these three treatments and with relaxation alone were significantly larger than improvements reported with placebo control treatments or untreated controls. The four treatments did not differ significantly in effectiveness. Goslin et al (1999) reported a meta-analysis of relaxation training, thermal biofeedback, thermal biofeedback plus relaxation training, EMG biofeedback, and CBT plus thermal biofeedback, as treatment for migraine. These psychological interventions yielded 32% to 49% reductions in migraine versus 5% reduction for no-treatment controls. The effect size estimates indicated that relaxation training, thermal biofeedback combined with relaxation training, EMG biofeedback training and CBT were all statistically more effective than waiting-list control.

Rains, Penzien, McCrory and Gray (2005) recently summarized the results of four meta-analytic reviews for psychological treatment of tension-type headache (EMG biofeedback, relaxation training and CBT) published between 1980 and 2001, and concluded that average improvements ranged between 35% and 55%, compared with 2% for no-treatment controls. These authors also summarized the results of five meta-analyses for psychological treatment of migraine (thermal biofeedback, EMG biofeedback, relaxation training and CBT) published between 1980 and 1999, and concluded that average improvement ranged from 33% to 55%, compared with 5% for no-treatment controls. In the most recent review of biofeedback training for headache disorders, Nestoriuc et al (2008) reported medium-to-large mean effect sizes for biofeedback in migraine and tension-type headache patients.

Individual studies have reported superior results. For example, Martin et al (2007) evaluated CBT using an individualized approach based on the results of functional analysis on a mixed sample of tension-type headache and migraine, and reported an average decrease in headaches of 68% post-treatment, which had extended to 77% at 12-month follow-up.

In addition to reducing headaches, psychological treatments lead to many other positive changes (Martin 1993). Treatment is associated with decreased consumption of medication, and decreases in negative moods such as depression and anxiety. It is also associated with various cognitive changes including a shift toward a more internal locus of control, enhanced self-efficacy to cope with headaches, and alterations in cognitive reactions to stress, such as changes in appraisal and coping processes. Reduced neuroticism, hysteria, somatisation, psychosomatic symptoms, and enhanced quality of life, have been reported in treatment studies.

How long do improvements last?

In a review of 10 prospective follow-ups of at least 12 months duration, Blanchard (1987) concluded as follows. Headache reductions achieved with EMG biofeedback for tension headache and thermal biofeedback for migraine, were maintained to 12 months, but deteriorated progressively at 2 and 3 years post-treatment. With relaxation training, a similar pattern of deterioration after 12 months was reported for migraine, but effects were well maintained for tension headache for at least 4 years. Benefits from CBT for tension headache were maintained at 2-year follow-up. Since this review, some studies have produced findings suggesting that treatment effects last longer than 12 months. For example, Lisspers and Ost (1990) reported benefits derived from thermal biofeedback training for migraine persisting for 6 years after treatment, and in fact slightly increasing during the follow-up period. Sorbi, Tellegen and Du Long (1989) reported benefits from relaxation training and CBT for migraine lasting for 3 years after treatment. Blanchard et al (1997) found that 91% of migraine headache patients remained significantly improved 5 years after completing psychological treatment.

Predictors of response to psychological treatment

Excessive use of analgesics limits the benefits associated with psychological treatment (and prophylactic pharmacotherapy). Michultka et al (1989) reported that less than one third of 'high medication users' showed a 50% or greater reduction in headache activity following psychological treatment, whereas more than half of 'low medication users' showed this level of improvement.

Depressive symptoms prior to treatment have been shown to be associated with a poor prognosis (e.g. Jacob et al 1983, Martin et al 1988). It seems likely that patients with co-morbid psychiatric disorders would be less likely to respond to psychological treatment, although controlled studies evaluating this possibility are unavailable.

Patients with near continuous headaches appear less responsive to relaxation training or biofeedback training than do patients with more delimited headache episodes (Blanchard et al 1989). However, studies have shown that it is possible to get positive results in this group. For example, Holroyd et al (2001) compared CBT, antidepressant medication, and the combination of the two approaches, for chronic tension-type headache. They found that all three approaches produced modest but clinically significant improvements in headaches.

In the 1980s, it was thought that relaxation and EMG biofeedback training might be ineffective for patients over the age of 50 years (e.g. Holroyd & Penzien 1986). However, subsequent research showed that relatively simple adjustments in the treatment procedures yielded positive outcomes. For example, treating patients who ranged in age from 60 to 78 years (mean 68 years), Mosley et al (1995) found CBT to be more effective than relaxation training alone, with 64% of patients showing clinically significant improvement.

Can treatment be administered cost-effectively?

Psychological treatment has typically involved about 10 individual sessions, and from the 1980s researchers have investigated ways of delivering treatment in more cost-effective ways. One approach has been to use minimal contact approaches in which skills training is introduced in the clinic but training primarily takes place in the home with the patient guided by printed materials and audiotapes or CDs. This approach reduces the number of clinic sessions to three or four. Three meta-analytic reviews have demonstrated that minimal contact interventions for headache can be as effective as clinic-based approaches (e.g. Rowan & Andrasik 1996).

Another approach has been to deliver treatment in a group format. Penzien, Rains and Holroyd (1992) completed a meta-analytic review and reported a 53% improvement associated with the group format, a similar figure to that achieved with individual sessions.

Treatment interventions have been developed that utilize the internet. Initial efforts indicate that some individuals are able to effectively learn headache management skills via the internet, but have been plagued by high dropout rates (e.g. Anderson et al 2003, Strom et al 2000).

Should treatments be combined?

Given the hundreds of trials of psychological treatments and the thousands of trials of pharmacological treatments, it is surprising that only a few studies have compared the two approaches or integrated them. Meta-analyses comparing propranolol, flunarizine and combined relaxation and biofeedback training, in migraineurs, show greater than a 50% improvement in headache for each of these approaches compared to 12% improvement with a placebo pill (e.g. Holroyd et al 1992). Combined propranolol plus relaxation training and thermal biofeedback training have proven highly effective in controlling migraine in two studies yielding more than a 70% reduction in headache activity (e.g. Holroyd et al 1995).

Holroyd et al (1991) compared CBT administered in minimal contact format and amitriptyline HCL to patients with tension-type headache. Each treatment yielded significant reductions in headaches with a 56% reduction for CBT and a 27% reduction for amitriptyline HCL. Holroyd et al (2001) compared amitriptyline HCL, matched placebo, CBT administered in minimal contact format plus placebo, and combined CBT and amitriptyline HCL for tension-type headache. The three active treatments produced similar improvements in headaches and quality of life.

Holroyd et al (1998) proposed algorithms to guide the integration of drug and psychological treatments. They suggest for tension-type headache that integrated treatment be considered if tension-type headaches are unremitting or a co-morbid mood or anxiety disorder is present. If neither condition is present, psychological treatment may be the intervention of choice. However, more intensive psychological interventions also deserve consideration when headaches are unremitting, and CBT interventions with proven effectiveness in treating mood and anxiety disorders deserve consideration when mood and anxiety disorders are present.

Holroyd, Martin and Nash (2006) have suggested that pharmacological and psychological treatments have different effect profiles. For example, psychological treatments compared to pharmacological treatments have been observed to produce improvements more slowly, to yield fewer side effects, to require more time and effort to complete, and to produce more psychological benefits.

Conclusion

Psychologists have much to offer patients with chronic headache. The functional model of chronic headache provides a rational approach to the assessment and treatment of this patient group. There is strong evidence to support the use of contemporary psychological interventions such as biofeedback, relaxation therapy, and CBT. These interventions may help to reduce headache and prevent its recurrence.

References

Anderson G, Lunstom P, Strom LA 2003 A controlled trial of self-help treatment for recurrent headache conducted via the Internet. Headache 43:353-361.

Andrasik F, Lipchik GL, McCrory DC, Wittrock DA 2005 Outcome parameters in behavioral headache research: Headache parameters and psychosocial outcomes. Headache 45:429-437.

Blanchard EB 1987 Long-term effects of behavioral treatment of chronic headache. Behavior Therapy 18:375-385.

Blanchard EB, Appelbaum KA, Radnitz CL et al 1989 The refractory headache patient: I. Chronic, daily, high-intensity headache. Behaviour Research and Therapy 27:403-410.

Blanchard EB, Appelbaum KA, Guarnier P et al 1997 Five year prospective follow-up on the treatment of chronic headache with biofeedback and/or relaxation. Headache 27:580-583.

Borgards MC, ter Kuile MM 1994 Treatment of recurrent tension-type headache: A meta-analytic review. Clinical Journal of Pain 10:174-190.

Borkum JM 2007 Chronic headaches: Biology, psychology and behavioral treatment. Lawrence Erlbaum Associates, Mahwah, NJ.

Goslin RE, Gray RN, McCrory DC 1999 Behavioral and physical treatments for migraine headache (Technical Review 2.2). Prepared for the Agency for Health Care Policy and Research under Contract No. 290-94-2025. Available from the National Technical Information Service; NTIS Accession No. 127946.

Headache Classification Subcommittee of the International Headache Society (2004). The International Classification of Headache Disorders, 2nd ed. Cephalalgia (suppl 1);24:1-151.

Holroyd KA 2002 Assessment and psychological treatment of recurrent headache disorders. Journal of Consulting and Clinical Psychology 70:656-677.

Holroyd KA, Penzien DB 1986 Client variables in the behavioral treatment of recurrent tension headache: A meta-analytic review. Journal of Behavioral Medicine 9:515-536.

Holroyd KA, Nash JM, Pingel JD et al 1991 A comparison of pharmacological (amitriptyline HCL) and nonpharmacological (cognitive-behavioral) therapies for chronic tension headaches. Journal of Consulting and Clinical Psychology 59:387-393.

Holroyd KA, Penzien DB, Rokicki LA et al 1992 Flunarizine vs. propanolol: A meta-analysis of clinical trials. Headache 32:256.

Holroyd KA, France JL, Cordingley GE et al 1995 Enhancing the effectiveness of relaxation-thermal biofeedback training with propanolol hydrochloride. Journal of Consulting and Clinical Psychology 63:327-330.

Holroyd KA, Lipchik GL, Penzien DB 1998 Psychological management of recurrent headache disorders: Empirical basis for clinical practice. In: K.S. Dobson KS, Craig KD (eds) Best practice: Developing and promoting empirically supported interventions. Sage, Newbury Park CA, p 193-212.

Holroyd KA, O'Donnell FJ, Stensland M et al 2001 Management of chronic tension-type headache with tricyclic antidepressant medication, stress-management therapy, and their combination: A randomized controlled trial. Journal of the American Medical Association 285:2208-2215.

Holroyd KA, Martin PR, Nash JM 2006 Psychological treatments of tension-type headaches. In: Olesen J et al (eds) The headaches, 3rd edn. Lippincott Williams & Wilkins, Philadelphia, p 711-719.

Jacob RG, Turner SM, Szekely BC, Eidelman BH 1983 Predicting outcome of relaxation therapy in headaches: The role of 'depression'. Behavior therapy 14:457-465.

Kelman L 2007 The triggers or precipitants of the acute migraine attack. Cephalalgia 27:394-402.

Lisspers J, Ost L 1990 Long-term follow-up of migraine treatment: Do the effects remain up to six years? Behaviour Research and Therapy 28:313-322.

Martin PR 1993 Psychological management of chronic headaches. Guilford Press, New York.

Martin PR 2000 Headache triggers: To avoid or not to avoid, that is the question. Psychology and Health 15:801-809.

Martin PR 2001 How do trigger factors acquire the capacity to precipitate headaches? Behaviour Research and Therapy 39:545-554.

Martin PR, MacLeod C 2008 Behavioral management of headache triggers: Avoidance of triggers is an inadequate strategy. (Manuscript submitted for publication.)

Martin PR, Seneviratne HM 1997 Effects of food deprivation and a stressor on head pain. Health Psychology 16:1-9.

Martin PR, Teoh H-J 1999 Effects of visual stimuli and a stressor on head pain. Headache 39:705-715.

Martin PR, Nathan PR, Milech D, van Keppel M 1988 The relationship between headaches and mood. Behaviour Research and Therapy 26:353-356.

Martin PR, Todd J, Reece J 2005 Effects of noise and a stressor on head pain. Headache 45:1353-1364.

Martin PR, Forsyth MR, Reece J 2007 Cognitive-behavioral therapy versus temporal pulse amplitude feedback training for recurrent headache. Behavior Therapy 38:350-363.

Michultka DM, Blanchard EB, Appelbaum KA et al 1989 The refractory headache patient: II. High medication consumption (analgesic rebound) headache. Behaviour Research and Therapy 27:411-420.

Mosley TH, Grotheus CA, Meeks WM 1995 Treatment of tension headache in the elderly: A controlled evaluation of relaxation training and relaxation combined with cognitive-behavior therapy. Journal of Clinical Geropsychology 1:175-188.

Nestoriuc Y, Martin A, Rief W, Andrasik F 2008 Biofeedback treatment for headache disorders: A comprehensive efficacy review. Applied Psychophysiology and Biofeedback 33:125-140.

Olesen J, Goadsby PJ, Ramadan NM et al (eds) 2006 The headaches, 3rd edn. Lippincott Williams & Wilkins, Philadelphia.

Penzien DB, Rains JC, Holroyd KA 1992 A review of alternative behavioral treatments for headache. The Mississipi Psychologist 17:8-9.

Philips HC 1976 Headache and personality. Journal of Psychosomatic Research 20:535-542.

Radat F, Swendsen J 2004 Psychiatric comorbidity in migraine: a review. Cephalalgia 25:165-178.

Rains JC, Penzien DB, McCrory DC, Gray RN 2005 Behavioral headache treatment: History, review of empirical literature, and methodological critique. Headache 45(suppl 2):S92-S109.

Rowan AB, Andrasik F 1996 Efficacy and cost-effectiveness of minimal therapist contact treatments for chronic headache: A review. Behavior Therapy 27:207-234.

Russell MB, Olesen J 1995 Increased familial risk and evidence of genetic factor in migraine. British Medical Journal 311:541-544.

Sheftell FD, Atlas SJ 2002 Migraine and psychiatric comorbidity: from theory and hypothesis to clinical application. Headache 42:934-944.

Sorbi M, Tellegen B, Du Long A 1989 Long-term effects of training in relaxation and stress-coping in patients with migraine: A 3-year follow-up. Headache 29:111-121.

Strom L, Peterson R, Anderson G 2000 A controlled trial of self-help treatment of recurrent headache conducted via the internet. Journal of Consulting and Clinical Psychology 68:722-727.

Williamson DA, Monguillot JE, Jarrel HP et al 1984 Relaxation for the treatment of headache: Controlled evaluation of two group programs. Behavior Modification 8:407-424.

World Health Organization 2006 Neurological disorders: Public health challenges. Switzerland: WHO.

$$22$$

Psychiatric management

P Rajan Thomas

Headache and psychiatric disorders frequently co-exist. The psychiatrist plays a pivotal role in assisting health professionals with the difficult task of evaluating and managing this group of patients. In this chapter the author, a psychiatrist, addresses the association between headache, migraine, and psychiatric disorders, and presents an approach to patient management.

Psychiatric factors often influence the onset and severity of headache yet these may not be acknowledged. Patients who experience headache as part of a psychiatric disorder may symbolically express their psychological conflict through pain. They are likely to state that 'nothing helps'. They are often very distressed by the pain and may have a history of multiple medical consultations; they also use various pain killers and some become dependent on opiates. They are preoccupied with the pain and cite it as the main source of their misery, but they do not fake the pain. They may have multiple headache complaints and when one disappears a new one will appear. The patient is keen to convince the clinician of the pain and describes the pain as unique. Anxiety about an attack itself may lead to continuation of headache. Individuals with chronic daily headache often present with a sense of emptiness and sadness that may be visible on their facial expression.

Patients may also have underlying depression. Breslau et al (1991, 2003) found that, compared to a control group, migraine sufferers are four to five times more likely to suffer from affective disorders including dysthymic disorder, major depression, and bipolar disorder. Stewart et al (2001) examined the role of stress in chronic daily headache. Specific stressful events such as bereavement, divorce, separation and problems with children were associated with chronic daily headache. In addition De Fidio et al (2000) showed that patients with chronic daily headache had high profiles of hypochondria, depression, and hysteria scales in the revised version of the Minnesota Multiphasic Personality Inventory (MMPI-2).

Patients living with chronic pain experience negative cognitive, emotional and behavioral changes which can lead to a depressive illness. In individuals who have a biochemical predisposition to major depression or dysthymic disorder, chronic headache can act as a stressor and precipitate the psychiatric condition.

Headache and psychiatric conditions

According to the diagnostic criteria of the Diagnostic and Statistical Manual IV (American Psychiatric Association 1994) (DSM IV), headache can be a somatic symptom of major depression as well as a manifestation of anxiety and panic disorders. It could be a delusional pain in schizophrenia and other psychotic conditions. It can also occur as an adverse effect of psychotropic medication. Individuals with, for example, histrionic, borderline, dependent, and avoidant personality disorders can have headache as a co-morbid condition.

Psychogenic headache is a term collectively used to describe a headache unexplained by any pathophysiological process. A headache can occur as a symptom of somatoform disorder. Somatoform disorder is characterized by symptoms that mimic disease or injury for which there is no identifiable physical cause. There may be depression, or physical symptoms such as pain, nausea, and dizziness. However, no general medical condition, other mental disorder, or substance is adequately diagnosed as a cause. The complaints are serious enough to cause significant emotional distress and impairment of social and/or occupational function.

Psychiatric assessment

A psychiatric assessment focuses on the reason for referral, understanding of the psychological and medical factors associated with the condition, the disability caused by the headache, the purpose served by the headache, and the social factors which contributed to the onset and maintenance of the condition. It also addresses whether the pain is driven by nociceptive stimuli or maladaptive changes within the central nervous system, whether it is a complaint of depression, or whether it is a delusional pain.

Interview

Although the interview considers the above questions, rigid adherence to a structured format may not elicit all the information. The clinician

Box 22.1

Elements of a psychiatric interview.

Headache
- Anticipatory symptoms and behaviors
- Precipitating factors
- Frequency, severity, duration, distribution
- Behaviors and factors that increase or decrease the pain
- Impact on function and quality of life
- Past treatment

Psychiatric factors
- Past history of depression, anxiety and other psychiatric conditions
- Family background, personal history including childhood trauma and experiences, work history and relationship history
- Alcohol and drug history
- Personality traits and coping abilities
- Mental state examination
- General appearance, behavior, speech, mood, thought content, perceptions, and cognitive function
- Attitude to psychiatric assessment

Other factors
- Appetite, sleep, weight, sexual functioning

should have empathy and genuine concern about the impact of the condition. The patient is given time to describe the problem and associated difficulties. Development of a therapeutic relationship forms the cornerstone of correct diagnosis and management. The interview should cover the items contained in Box 22.1.

Depression and other mood disorders

The patient is questioned about whether they have been feeling low in mood, pessimistic about the future, unable to enjoy activities previously enjoyed (anhedonia), socially isolated and withdrawn from others, tearful, hopeless, or experiencing suicidal thoughts. The depressed patient may also have poor concentration, be forgetful due to lack of concentration, and may experience loss of appetite, loss of weight, poor sleep with early morning awakening and diurnal mood variation. Depression can also be associated with other mood disorders like bipolar affective disorder. In this condition, the patient has a history of manic or hypomanic episodes in addition to depressive episodes.

Anxiety disorder

Features of anxiety may manifest as physiological and psychological symptoms, and spasm of scalp and neck muscles can lead to tension-type headache. Other features of anxiety include fine tremors, sweating, tightness of chest, and shortness of breath. Patients may have heaviness in the chest, fear of doom, or may feel restless and sometimes there may be a feeling of hot and cold. Those with panic attacks have an accentuation of the above symptoms as well as severe palpitations, sweating, fear of collapse and fear of a heart attack or stroke. They may present with sweaty palms and fine tremors. A severe headache can also occur at this time. Those who have migraine may develop anticipatory anxiety due to fear of another attack of migraine. This is likely to cause further headaches.

Substance abuse

Individuals with chronic headache may also abuse multiple prescribed and illicit substances. Commonly abused among prescribed drugs are opiate pain killers and benzodiazepines. Substances abused include alcohol, cannabis, heroin and amphetamines. These substances are initially used as a means to control the headache, but soon control is lost and dependence develops. Due to the development of tolerance and the need to avoid withdrawal symptoms, higher doses of the medication or substances are used. Often analgesics are used as an excuse of preventing a headache.

Excessive use of analgesics is recognized as one of the frequent causes of chronic headache. The family physician should recognize this and take steps to identify and treat the underlying causes.

Schizophrenia and other psychoses

Headache can occur as part of delusional symptoms in schizophrenia and delusional disorder. Patients with paranoid psychosis may have delusions of being poisoned which may cause headache. The patient may have an abnormal belief of being controlled by external forces. In addition to the delusions they have thought disorder and hallucinations. They may have a blunted facial expression. The other psychotic conditions are delusional disorder, brief psychotic illness and psychosis secondary to a medical condition.

Side effects of medication

Headache can also be a side effect of some psychotropic medication, most often with serotonin specific reuptake inhibitors (SSRI anti-depressants). Sumatriptan, a migraine medication and other triptans can interact with SSRIs. Triptans mimic serotonin effect and SSRIs increase the availability of serotonin in synaptic spaces. This can potentially cause a serotonin syndrome. Serotonin syndrome manifests as headache, agitation, confusion, hallucinations, myoclonus, tremors, hyper-reflexia, sweating, shivering and coma. An early symptom of this condition is headache. This has to be differentiated from other types of headache. Opiates, too, when misused can cause headache.

Personality disorders

Undiagnosed personality disorders are common in those with chronic headaches. Common personality disorders and personality traits

291

observed are Cluster B personality disorders (borderline personality, histrionic personality, anti social personality and narcissistic personality) and Cluster C personality disorders (dependent personality, avoidant personality and obsessive-compulsive personality). Patients with Cluster B and C personality disorders are more prone to have co-morbid headache. These individuals develop maladaptive behavioral patterns to cope with day to day stressors. Those who have a history of childhood physical or sexual abuse have difficulty trusting others and have strained relationships. Such abuse can manifest as anger and some exhibit self harming behavior when under stress. They are also prone to mood swings. Among the Cluster C group, anxiety related symptoms predominate. Free floating anxiety and their reaction to stress are seen with headache. The personality disorder group generally shows changes in the manifestations of symptoms according to the environment.

Hypochondriasis

Patients with chronic headache can fulfill the criteria for hypochondriasis. They are likely to be preoccupied with headache and their life may be greatly influenced by headache. They may visit the doctor frequently and may undergo multiple investigations. Hypochondriasis could be present as part of a major depressive illness. Patients with hypochondriasis believe that they have a serious illness and attribute their symptoms to an undiagnosed illness. The patient experiences these symptoms and abnormal beliefs for at least six months. Multiple doctors are consulted for investigation and explanation. In spite of negative findings in the neurological examination and investigations, the patient is not convinced that they do not have a serious illness. Those with a headache believe that they suffer from a brain tumor or meningitis. The intensity

of the beliefs may not reach delusional proportions but persist in spite of reassurances. The distress caused affects their day to day life.

Conversion disorder

Headache can manifest as a symptom of conversion disorder. Conversion disorder is not a diagnosis of exclusion, but is made on specific criteria. The patient presents with headache and reports that it affects day to day functioning. The description of headache may vary and tends to be dramatic. It may not conform to any recognizable pattern of headache or anatomical site. These patients may not show the distress of the headache as shown by the pain disorder patients. The patients with conversion disorder usually have primary and secondary gain. The primary gain is the control of anxiety symptom. The secondary gain is the attention they obtain due to the symptom. Psychological factors usually initiate and exacerbate the symptoms. This condition was previously called hysteria.

Somatization disorder

Headache can be a symptom of somatization disorder, which is recognized by the presence of multiple bodily complaints. This disorder is differentiated from other somatoform disorders by the following criteria. The somatic symptoms develop before the age of 30 years and gradually continue to develop into various symptoms. The somatic symptoms are headache, shortness of breath, burning sensation in genitals, menstrual complaints, chest pain, a lump in the throat, and vomiting. DSM IV diagnostic criteria list the clusters of the symptoms. The neurological symptoms are headache, amnesia, tremors and weakness; individuals seek excessive medical treatment. Patients also have personality disorder traits, most frequently Cluster B group of personality characteristics.

Factitious disorder

Headache is a symptom that cannot be measured objectively. This makes it easy for someone to fake the condition leading to a diagnosis of factitious disorder. There may also be a conscious exaggeration of the symptom. In conversion disorder, secondary gain is usually identified and the symptom usually serves a purpose for the patient, although they often avoid painful diagnostic procedures. In comparison patients with factitious disorder cannot fake their symptoms all through the day. They also have differential pain manifestation in different settings. Individuals usually admit to faking symptoms when they are found out. The information the patient provides about the headache may be verified with a relative to check the validity of the symptoms. Patients may have associated antisocial or histrionic personality or borderline personality traits.

Management

Often, patients with headache are referred for psychiatric management fairly late in the management process. Health professional education tends to focus on treatment of conditions with organic causes and they are thus ill-equipped to manage the co-morbid psychiatric aspects of care. If there are significant issues, it is important to refer patients to psychiatrists for assessment to diagnose the psychiatric condition associated with headache.

The first principle in management is to understand that the patient is suffering and to develop a concerned therapeutic relationship. The pain of headache may seem exaggerated but it is a subjective experience. It is not helpful to say 'It is all in your mind'. This comment often breaks the therapeutic relationship and the patient can become overtly hostile. The best approach is to recognize and acknowledge the suffering of the patient. The physician should ensure that all relevant investigations have been carried out. It is also useful to provide an acceptable explanation for the headache. The focus is therefore changed to how this person can cope with the headache and function.

Some patients may also develop an abnormal illness behavior where they consult different medical practitioners seeking investigations and treatment. These patients are preoccupied with the headache and this alters their life style. The physician can be drawn into this maladaptive pattern of behavior and respond to the patient's demands by prescribing different pain killers and arranging further investigations. Patients can become angry and hostile if their needs are not met.

Every patient who has chronic headache is also likely to suffer psychological consequences. They should have an individual treatment plan which should address the following issues:

1. Patient's commitment to treatment plan
2. Goal of treatment
3. Physical treatments
4. Psychological treatments
5. Focus on improving quality of life.

Pharmacological approaches

Psychiatric treatment includes managing the co-morbid psychiatric conditions as mentioned above. Depression is the most frequent psychiatric condition that exists with chronic headache and antidepressant medications have been most helpful in managing the depression and dysthymia associated with headaches. Previous studies have suggested amitryptiline as the antidepressant of choice. It is still very effective, but new selective serotonin reuptake inhibitors (SSRI) and selective noradrenalin reuptake inhibitors (SNRI) can be used initially before amitryptiline is prescribed. They include: duloxetine (60 mg), venlafaxine (75 to 225 mg), mirtazapine (15 to 45 mg), citalopram (20 to 40 mg), escitalopram (10 to 20 mg), sertraline (50 to 200 mg), fluoxetine (20 to 40 mg) and paroxetine (20 to 40 mg). The side effect profile of SSRI is well tolerated compared to amitriptyline. Amitriptyline (50 to 150 mg) has been found useful as adjunctive in pain management. Other tricyclic antidepressants such as imipramine (50 to 150 mg), dothiepin (75 to 150 mg) are also useful. Tricyclic antidepressants are superior to SSRI in pain management, even where there is no depression.

Anticonvulsants have also been used in management of headache. Sodium valproate, gabapentin, and topiramate have been found to be useful. Carbamazapine has also been used for the treatment of trigeminal neuralgia and other facial pain. Anticonvulsants also have mood stabilizing and antidepressant effects.

Benzodiazipines are also used in treating anxiety related symptoms. This group of medication is addictive and should not be used for a prolonged duration. Among the benzodiazepines, Diazepam is still the most frequently used drug. It has a very long half life, up to 72 hours. Other shorter acting benzodiazepines are oxazepam and lorazepam, whose half life is about 12 hours. These drugs should not be used on their own for the treatment of anxiety. Antidepressants (SSRI) are effective in treatment of anxiety, especially sedating antidepressants, but they take two to three weeks for the full effect to be observed. Benzodiazepines may be used in this period to control the symptoms.

Non-pharmacological approaches

Non-pharmacological treatments that have been found useful in managing headache and co-morbid depression have been cognitive behavioral therapy, relaxation therapy, biofeedback therapy. Other approaches include stress management, group therapy, hypnosis, and dry needling (see Ch. 24) or acupuncture.

Cognitive behavioral therapy

Cognitive behavioral therapy (CBT) for pain is based on the patients' beliefs about their pain and can influence adjustment to the pain experience. Jenson and Karoly (1991) found that patients who ignored their pain, those who used self statements to cope with pain, and those who increased their daily activities, had better psychological functioning than those who did not engage in these behaviors. Acceptance of pain has been associated with lower reports of pain intensity, less anxiety related to pain, decreased avoidance behaviour and depression. These individuals experienced decreased disability and improved work status. Turk and Rudy (1988) provide some assumptions for the foundation of cognitive-behavioral interventions. Cognitions interact with emotions, physiological sensations, and behavior. Altering one of these components can alter other components. Effective intervention must address the cognitive emotional and behavioral aspects of the presenting problem. Some studies have shown that chronic headache responds to cognitive therapy. Johnson and Thorn (1989) demonstrated that cognitive behavior therapy (CBT), individually administered, and group CBT were superior to no psychological treatment for chronic headache. Holroyd and Stensland (2005) found that antidepressant medication, CBT, and stress management therapy were equally effective in tension type headache. They observed that CBT and stress management therapy had better psychosocial outcome measures.

In understanding CBT for depression, the depressed mood is the outcome of depressive cognition. Negative cognitions lead to depressed mood; e.g. viewing pain as the worst thing in the world and believing that it will never get better.

These thoughts are challenged and changed to positive thoughts leading to improvement. The individual must participate actively in the treatment and learn more adaptive ways to deal with their problem. Other behavioral procedures follow operant methods. The patient responds to pain behaviors with neutral attitudes (extinction) and non-pain behaviors are rewarded positively. Reinforcement of non-pain behaviors such as a special meal, recreation and attention from significant others may be beneficial.

Relaxation and biofeedback therapy

Relaxation therapy involves helping the patient to relax using one of the relaxation techniques, e.g. progressive muscular relaxation, deep breathing, or visualizing technique. Relaxation therapy uses techniques such as calming music and other relaxation methods to reduce excessive stimulation. Biofeedback uses thermal (hand warming) and electromyographic (EMG) techniques. Both treatments have been shown to reduce the headache index (measure of frequency and severity) by 40% (Dowson 2003).

Case studies

Three case vignettes are given below which illustrate some of the presentations of headache where psychiatric factors are prominent.

Case study 1

A 42-year-old divorced woman with four children presented to the hospital after a serious attempt to kill herself with methadone tablets. She had experienced severe migraine for the past 25 years. Previously she had presented with a throbbing headache, photophobia, and nausea lasting up to 48 hours. She was prescribed various medications for migraine, including nonsteroidal antiinflammatories, benzodiazepines, and opiates. Other medications prescribed were diazepam tablets (up to 40 mg daily), methadone tablets (40 mg daily) and morphine injections (30 mg, one to two injections daily). These medications had been taken for more than 10 years with no beneficial effect. She commenced using methadone tablets and morphine injections to prevent attacks but was still experiencing severe headaches. She was depressed because of constant headache. Prior to the overdose, she visited the family doctor and asked to discuss how she was feeling, but he gave her another prescription. She took an overdose of methadone tablets with alcohol and had a serious intention to die.

The woman had been sexually abused by a neighbor at the age of 16 and her headache commenced from that time. She had multiple relationship problems and could not trust any one. She had been divorced three times.

Psychiatric assessment showed that she was severely depressed. The sexual abuse had started the maladaptive pattern of behavior. She could not discuss the abuse and developed headache. The personality difficulties of dependence and mistrust developed. She needed someone to cling to, and was using medication to drown her anxiety. Her diagnosis was major depressive illness, dependent personality traits, and opiate and benzodiazepine dependence.

In managing her problem, initially a therapeutic relationship was established, by listening to her regarding the headache and psychosocial problems. She was commenced on an SSRI. The opiates and benzodiazepines were gradually reduced. Initial problems with trust were overcome and she was able to engage in treatment. She discussed the abuse and the problems in her life. As her depression improved, she was able to use cognitive therapy to overcome the headache. Interpersonal psychotherapy and antidepressants were used to prevent further episodes of depression.

This case illustrates that patients with severe depression, dependence on drugs, and childhood trauma can present with headache.

Case study 2

Mrs J was a 36-year-old woman who had been experiencing severe headache for two years which was not responding to analgesic medication. Her headache was usually experienced in the mornings which prevented her from attending work. In the afternoons she felt better and was able to perform housework. She was not anxious about not attending to work. Mrs J experienced episodes of spasm in her hand when she was 12 years old which stopped her from attending school. Later it was revealed that she was bullied at school. Once the bullying ceased she recovered.

In exploring her current situation, Mrs J revealed the difficulties she was experiencing at work. She was bullied by her supervisor and the way Mrs J was bullied reminded her of her school days. The psychiatric diagnosis was conversion disorder. In managing her situation, first a therapeutic relationship was established. The headache was fully investigated by her family physician and she was reassured that there was no organic problem causing the headache. A full psychiatric history was taken. During the sessions, Mrs J revealed the bullying by her supervisor and at school. She was able to understand the link between the bullying at school and work. The maladaptive way in which she responded in both situations was also identified. The primary gain was reduction of anxiety and the secondary gain was not going to work. She was persuaded to go to work and deal with the stress in an appropriate way. She responded to the treatment and the headache subsided. There was no indication for any medication.

This case illustrates how headache can arise secondary to conversion disorder, and with appropriate psychiatric intervention the patient can be helped.

Case study 3

Ms R was a 27-year-old single woman who was experiencing severe headaches which were diagnosed as migraines. She was prescribed medication for the migraines.

As a teenager, she was sexually abused by a family member and her personality was affected by it. She was getting depressed and suicidal. She was also cutting her wrists frequently and having frequent mood swings. She had developed features of major depression with persistent low mood, feeling hopeless, recurrent suicidal thoughts, loss of appetite, loss of weight, lack of energy, early morning wakening and diurnal mood variation. The depression had been present during the past year.

Her psychiatric diagnosis was major depression and borderline personality disorder. Her treatment was complicated by the fact that SSRI antidepressant medication can interact with sumatriptan and other similar migraine treatments, potentially leading to serotonin syndrome. She had SNRI (mirtazapine) for the depression, which was used in small doses and with psychotherapy she gradually improved. With the improvement of depression, her migraine attacks also reduced.

This case illustrates that migraine can co-exist with major depression and borderline personality disorder; intervention to treat the psychiatric disorders can assist the resolution of the physical pain.

These case vignettes illustrate the link between psychiatric issues and headache. In many cases, more than one psychiatric factor comes into play. Most frequent is depression.

Conclusion

Headache may be part of the constellation of symptoms of psychiatric disorders. Patients with a psychiatric diagnosis may experience concurrent headache. This chapter has explored the association between headache and psychiatric conditions including depression and anxiety disorders. Practitioners are given guidelines to assess affective conditions in patients presenting with headache. The importance of an individualized treatment plan involving both medication and non-pharmacological approaches is emphasized.

References

American Psychiatric Association 1994 Diagnostic and statistical manual of mental disorders, fourth edition, Washington, DC.

Breslau N, Davis GC, Andreski P 1991 Migraine, psychiatric disorders and suicide attempts: an epidemiologic study of young adults. Psychiatry Res 37(1):11-23.

Breslau N, Lipton RB, Stewart WF et al 2003 Comorbidity of migraine and depression: investigating potential etiology and prognosis. Neurology 60(8):1308-1312.

De Fidio D, Libro G, Prudenzano MP et al 2000 Stress and chronic headache, Journal of Headache and Pain 1(suppl 1):S49-S52.

Dowson AJ 2003 Your questions answered: Migraine and other headaches. Churchill Livingstone, Edinburgh, p 90-94.

Holroyd K, Stensland M 2005 Separate and combined effect of CBT and Drug Therapy; psychosocial outcomes in the treatment of chronic tension type headache. Journal of pain 2005; Vol 6. Online. Available: http://www.headachedrugs.com. archives2/cbt.html September 2005.

Jenson MP, Karoly P 1991 Control beliefs, coping efforts and adjustment to chronic pain. J Consult Psychol 59:431.

Johnson PR, Thorn BE 1989 Headache 29(6):358-365. Cognitive behavioral treatment of chronic headache: group versus individual treatment format.

Stewart WF, Scher AL, Lipton RB 2001 Stressful life events and risk of chronic daily headache: results from the frequent headache epidemiology study. Cepalalgia 21:279.

Turk DC, Rudy TE 1988 A cognitive-behavioral perspective on chronic pain: Beyond the scalpel and syringe. Handbook of chronic pain management. William and Wilkins, Baltimore.

Section **Three**

Treatment

23

Myofascial trigger point treatment for headache and TMD

Kerrie Bolton and Peter Selvaratnam

Cervical and temporomandibular disorders may contribute to the production of headache. In this chapter the authors, a myotherapist and a musculoskeletal physiotherapist-anatomist, identify muscles that can refer pain to the head and describe clinically effective hands-on management and treatment strategies.

Headache and temporomandibular disorders (TMD) can cause significant suffering to many patients including anxiety, disability, and catastrophizing with regard to pain (Jerjes et al 2007). The contribution of cervical muscles (Fernandez de las Penas et al 2006a & b, 2007, Kellgren 1938a,1938b, Jull et al 2002, Jull et al 2004, Zito et al 2006) and the muscles of mastication (Benoliel et al 2008, Fernandez de las Penas et al 2006a & b, Okeson 2005, Simons et al 1999, Zito 2007, Zito et al 2008) to headache has been reported. Similarly, the contribution of masticatory muscle disorders to TMD has also been well described (Okeson 2005, Simons et al 1999) and is discussed in Chapter 7.

Myofascial trigger points (MTPs) can contribute to headache and TMD (Benoliel et al 2008, Brukner et al 2006, Okeson 2005, Simons et al 1999). Similarly, reduced endurance of the deep neck flexors and reduced extensibility of the cervical and axio-scapular muscles can contribute

to headache by eliciting symptoms created by muscle imbalance, faulty posture, and movement (Janda 1985, Jull et al 2002). Myofascial tightness, muscle hypertonicity, local muscle tenderness, superficial soft tissue tightness, and skin tightness are also common in patients with musculoskeletal disorders (Janda 1985, Magarey 2007 personal communication). Clinical experience indicates that attention to these factors can be as effective as passive cervical mobilization in patient outcomes despite the limited rigor of current evidence.

This chapter addresses the examination and treatment of MTPs as part of the musculoskeletal evaluation and management of patients with headache and TMD.

Myofascial trigger points

Pioneering work in myofascial trigger point management was conducted during the late 1920s and early 1930s by Sir Thomas Lewis (Lewis 1938). Subsequently, Kellgren (1938a & b) detailed specific sites of referred pain to teeth, joints, and organs occurring from a focus of irritation within a muscle using local novocaine injections. From the 1940s (Kelly 1941) to the 1980s this approach was built upon and culminated in the first edition of the descriptive publication by Travell and Simons (1983) in applying digital pressure, 'spray and stretch', or local novocaine to deactivate MTPs. Currently MTP treatment is conducted by practitioners treating musculoskeletal problems with digital pressure, dry needling, injection therapy or neuromyotomy.

Myofascial trigger points can be located within the muscle belly or at musculotendinous junctions and are classified as active or latent, primary or associated. Active MTPs are responsible for the pain generated in myofascial pain syndromes (Lucas 2007, Simons et al 1999). Latent MTPs are asymptomatic nodules that may contribute to restricted range of movement and muscle stiffness and have the potential to become active (Hong et al 1998, Lucas 2007, Lucas et al 2004). They may, however, be painful on palpation. Primary MTPs occur within the muscle responsible for causing pain and may refer symptoms to specific regions associated with that muscle. Associated MTPs may occur in the region of the referred pain zone of a primary MTP. They could also occur due to increased functional demands of the associated musculature (Simons et al 1999). The development of MTPs is described in Chapter 24.

Myofascial trigger points in the cervical and temporomandibular regions can be caused by direct trauma or muscle imbalance (Dommerholt et al 2006, Simons et al 1999). They may also be elicited by overactivity of muscles, sustained postural stresses, emotional stresses, intervertebral disc dysfunction, and articular and neural conditions (Brukner et al 2006, Dommerholt et al 2006, Huguenin 2004, Okeson 2005, Lucas 2007, Lucas et al 2004, Simons et al 1999). Other causes of MTPs include bruxism, sleep apnea, asthma, sustained dental procedures, visual disturbance, automobile accidents, altered cervical positions required in playing the violin or flute, cervical traction treatment, or pre-existing cervical injury (Lavigne et al 2006, Okeson 2005, Simons et al 1999). Thus, MTPs can develop on their own or due to other causative factors.

The contribution of non-musculoskeletal structures or specific medical conditions to MTPs in patients with headache and TMD needs to be considered. Authors in this book have described the contribution of hormonal changes, food sensitivity, nutritional deficiencies, anxiety, depression, fibromyalgia, central sensitization, and neoplastic changes to headache and TMD. As the scientific literature provides evidence that these conditions can cause MTPs (Dommerholt et al 2006), it is important to evaluate the likelihood that MTPs may be secondary to other medical conditions.

Active inflammatory biochemicals can be present in MTPs. Shah et al (2005) conducted an *in vivo* biochemical analysis within normal muscle and on active and latent MTPs in real time at sub-nanogram level of concentration. Active MTPs demonstrated significantly increased levels of norepinephrine, serotonin, bradykinin, interleukin-1, calcitonin-gene-related-peptide (CGRP), tumor necrosis factor, and substance P in its immediate milieu. Latent MTPs showed lower concentrations of CGRP and substance P than active MTPs but higher than normal muscle tissue. In regard to the other chemical concentrations, latent MTPs and normal muscle tissue were not significantly different. This investigation confirms the clinical difference between active MTPs, latent MTPs and normal muscle tissue, and suggests that biochemicals could contribute to persistent active MTP activity, pain, tenderness and hyperalgesia (Dommerholt et al 2006).

Some clinicians argue that taut bands and myofascial trigger points are elicited due to central nervous system activity (Cohen 2005). Fernandez de las Penas et al (2007) argue that nociceptive input from peripheral tender muscles contributes to chronic tension type headache and central sensitization. They observed a higher concentration of chemical mediators in active MTPs and lower ph levels compared to control tender points. On the basis of this evidence, the investigators hypothesized that MTPs are the primary hyperalgesic region responsible for the development of central sensitization in chronic tension type headache. Further investigations with event-related functional MRI suggest that patients with myofascial pain have an abnormal brain response to pain stimulus (Niddam et al 2008). The activation patterns from the left upper trapezius in 16 fibromyalgic patients were compared to healthy controls when evoked from an 'equivalent site' with stimulus intensity matched and pain intensity matched stimuli. The imaging was conducted in all subjects during needle and digital stimulation of the trapezius. Patients revealed significantly enhanced somatosensory (SI, SII, inferior parietal, mid-insula) and limbic (anterior insula) activity and suppressed right dorsal hippocampal activity compared to asymptomatic people. At matched pain intensity, increased brain activity was observed in the same somatosensory regions but not in limbic regions. The findings indicated that patients with hyperalgesia had abnormal brain activity in areas that processed stimulus intensity and negative affect. The authors speculated that suppressed hippocampal activity may reflect secondary stress-related changes in patients with chronic pain. Future studies need to evaluate whether the abnormal brain response triggers MTPs or if MTPs trigger the brain response leading to central sensitization.

The inter-examiner reliability of identifying MTPs has traditionally been poor (Gerwin et al 2000, Hsieh et al 2000, Lew et al 1997). In contrast, one clinical study found good inter-examiner reliability, reporting that key factors in improving identification of MTPs were specific training in the examination process and increased clinical experience (Gerwin et al 1997) – criteria that should not be underestimated. In an effort to improve the identification process, more recent studies have used an algometer to measure pressure pain thresholds of latent MTPs (Lucas et al 2004, Sciotti et al 2001). Having acknowledged the difficulties with accurate MTP identification between clinicians, intra-examiner reliability is usually good and therefore useful when evaluating the de-activation of MTPs. However, clinicians are reminded that overall treatment must be evaluated by functional outcome measures such as those described for headache in Chapter 13, or for TMD by Stegenga et al (1993), or by patient-specific outcome measures (Cleland et al 2006).

The following discussion, though not exhaustive, provides guidelines to evaluate MTPs in patients with headache and/or TMD.

Assessment

A detailed history of the etiology and onset of the patient's headache/TMD, referred pain patterns, intensity, frequency and duration of symptoms, and aggravating and easing factors needs to be assessed to rule out sinister pathology and other non-musculoskeletal factors that may contribute to the headache/TMD.

Posture

Postural observation of the spine and temporomandibular regions in standing and sitting positions should be performed to ascertain whether altering the patient's posture produces a change in symptoms as described in Chapter 19. Patients should be advised to modify their ergonomic environment, and be reviewed if their symptoms alter over a two weeks.

Cervical region

Active and passive movement examination of the cervical region can then be performed (including passive physiological and accessory movements) to evaluate if the headache/TMD has a cervical component (Jull et al 2002, 2004, Maitland 1986, Niere et al 1995, Trott 1985, Zito et al 2006, 2007). The spatula test described in Chapter 19 may also assist in differentiating whether the headache/TMD has cervical or orofacial components. The craniocervical flexor test described in Chapter 14 can be performed to evaluate the endurance of the flexor muscle and whether the detected impairments could be a factor in contributing to headache. The length of cervical axio-scapular muscles can also be evaluated in the sitting or supine positions (Janda 1985). The contribution of the shortened muscle can be established by altering the length of the muscle and then reassessing the patient's symptoms.

Temporomandibular region

Active movements of the TMJ can be evaluated (Chapter 19) while observing the patient's pain response, the quality of mandibular excursion, any deviation in its motion, and whether any movement dysfunction correlates to functional incapacity. Crepitus or clicking of the TMJs, and retrodiscitis (Okeson 2005) can be assessed by placing the fifth finger in each external auditory meatus (preferably with gloved hands) or with a stethoscope over the pre-auricular region. The range of opening the mouth can be assessed by measuring interincisor opening between the central incisors with a millimeter/inch ruler in the sitting or supine positions.

Trigger point examination

The following section describes the examination of MTPs in the cervical and masticatory muscles. Intra-oral examination is performed with a gloved hand. In identifying the primary MTPs, it is important to consider the cause of

the condition, initial pain pattern, pain referral zone, associated symptoms, aggravating factors and whether these findings correlate with muscle function.

The authors observe that normal tissue resistance can be felt immediately upon palpating beyond the skin, when compared to the pathological increased resistance provided by MTPs or taut bands. In our experience, the MTP locations and pain referred from MTPs to distal regions are not restricted to regions listed in texts (Simons et al 1999). They often vary significantly and cover larger or unexpected areas, sometimes even giving rise to false neural type paresthesia.

Careful palpation of the whole muscle is required to identify MTPs. The muscle fiber direction needs to be considered while palpating over a small group of muscle fibers from their origin to insertion for taut bands or firm nodules. Following this the adjacent groups of muscle fibers are examined until the whole muscle is examined. Digital pressure directly over the MTP may produce a local twitch response (muscle fasciculation), a jump sign, or reproduce the patient's pain locally or distally in its myofascial pain referral zone (Simons et al 1999). Eliciting local twitch response/s is the most objective sign of the presence of an MTP, though the most difficult to elicit (Simons et al 2002). However, reproduction of the patient's pain requires less clinical skill and is more reliable than the jump sign (Huguenin 2004). The authors recommend that pressure on a MTP may need to be sustained for up to 10 to 30 seconds before it is eliminated as a potential source of symptoms.

The identification of an MTP and reproduction of pain does not indicate that it is the source of the pain. The pain may be arising from articular (Bogduk 2001, Govind et al 2005, Okeson 2005), cervical discogenic, and neural (peripheral/central) structures (see Ch. 9), or other pathology that may have sensitized the somatic pain pathway to provide a false positive. Deactivating the MTP needs to be accompanied by lasting change in symptoms to verify the contribution of the MTP. If the MTP is deactivated by 50% but the symptoms change only 10% the clinician needs to suspect other source/s of the symptoms. In contrast, the MTP treatment may reduce the symptoms significantly but the improvement is not maintained. The clinician then needs to consider if the muscle extensibility should be fully restored for long term improvement. They also need to consider that lasting changes may only be gained by addressing the ergonomic environment at work and/or home and lifestyle stressors which can contribute to muscle tension.

Grading of MTPs

MTPs can be graded according to the depth of the muscle during palpation of an MTP (Selvaratnam 2008). Maitland (1986) described similar grading of articular structures based on amplitude of movement. Grading of MTPs as Grades I to IV (Fig. 23.1) refers to the depth

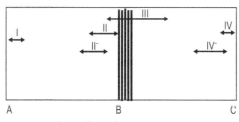

Depth of a myofascial trigger point

Figure 23.1 • Schematic diagram showing grading of MTPs based on depth. Grade I is a gentle sustained pressure on the skin to elicit a pain response at the beginning of the range before resistance from an MTP is encountered. Grade II is a deeper pressure at the point of initial resistance provided by an MTP. Grade II⁻ is a gentle pressure just prior to initial resistance. Grade III is a sustained pressure to moderate depth, about midway through the MTP. Grade IV is deep pressure at the end of the MTP. Grade IV⁻ is gentle pressure applied just before end range of the MTP (see text). **A** = external surface of skin, **B** = region where palpation of an MTP encounters initial resistance, **C** = end range of MTP resistance.

of palpation applied through the skin, subcutaneous tissue and muscles overlying the MTP.

Grade I is a gentle sustained pressure on the skin to elicit a pain response at the beginning of the range before resistance from a MTP is encountered. Grade I can be applied in patients with acute pain, hyperalgesia or allodynia. In some patients with hyperalgesia/allodynia, the palpatory pressure might reproduce their pain with very gentle pressure on the skin.

Grade II is a deeper pressure at the point of initial resistance provided by an MTP. It is important to establish if this is normal tissue resistance or pathological resistance of the MTP. Grade II pressure can be applied in patients with sub-acute pain or pain that is easily reproduced or referred from the MTP.

Grade III is a sustained pressure to moderate depth, about midway through the available range of the MTP. It can be applied in patients with chronic conditions or when referred pain is not easily reproduced.

Grade IV is a deep pressure at the end of the available range of the MTP. It can be applied in patients with chronic conditions or conditions requiring firm pressure.

Variations to these grades can also be applied. For instance, a Grade II⁻ depth can be palpated just prior to initial resistance. Similarly a Grade IV⁻ depth can be palpated just before end range.

The pain response during and following MTP palpation needs to be evaluated with a verbal analogue scale (e.g., where 0 is no pain, 1 mild pain, 5 moderate pain, and 10 their most severe imaginable pain) and constantly communicating with the patient regarding their pain (Selvaratnam et al, 1994). Apart from subjective assessment, movement signs need to be re-assessed to evaluate if objective signs have changed. The patient needs to be warned of the likelihood of post-examination pain lasting up to 72 hours.

Muscles contributing to headache or TMD

Temporalis

The temporalis arises from the floor of temporal fossa and deep surface of temporal fascia and inserts onto the tip and medial surface of coronoid process and anterior border of ramus of mandible (Moore et al 2002). It assists in closing the mouth, and its posterior fibers retrude the mandible (Moore et al 2002).

Trigger point location

Temporalis may develop MTPs (see Fig. 7.3) in the mid-section of the muscle and may refer pain to the upper incisors and premolars. A MTP in the anterior aspect of temporalis can refer pain in an arc above the orbit of the eye and inferiorly along the line of the mandible. The MTP can also refer pain posteriorly in finger-like projections over the temporal region (Simons et al 1999).

Palpatory examination

The index, middle, and ring fingers are used to outline the border of the temporal fossa while the patient clenches their teeth to contract the temporalis. The muscle is then palpated over the temporal bone to identify MTPs and any pain reproduction.

Masseter

The masseter originates from the inferior border and medial surface of zygomatic arch and inserts on the lateral surface of ramus of mandible and is coronoid process (see Fig. 20.3a). It closes the mouth, and its deep fibers retrude the mandible (Moore et al 2002).

Trigger point location

Myofascial trigger points in the superficial masseter (Fig. 23.2) can refer pain to the lower jaw, molar teeth and maxilla. The MTP in the deep portion may refer pain deep into the ear and may also cause tinnitus (Simons et al 1999).

Palpatory examination

The patient is instructed to clench their teeth to identify the masseter. The index and middle fingers are used to perform external palpation of the masseter from the zygomatic arch to the ramus of the mandible. The muscle can be palpated immediately above the angle of the mandible.

Intra-oral palpation enables direct palpation of the anterior fibers of masseter. The patient is instructed to open the mouth to approximately 20–30 mm. The thumb and index finger are

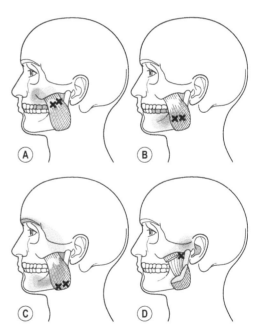

Figure 23.2 ● Trigger points and pain referral zone in masseter. The Xs locate trigger points in various parts of the masseter muscle. A = superficial layer, upper portion. B = superficial layer, mid-belly. C = superficial layer, lower portion. D = deep layer, upper part – just below the temporomandibular joint.

positioned intra-orally in a pincer grip to palpate masseter from the zygomatic arch to the ramus of the mandible. Once the MTP is identified the presence of any referred pain is confirmed. The deep portion of the masseter can be palpated with the same intra-oral pincer grip by moving posteriorly over the soft tissues anterior to the TMJ (Simons et al 1999).

Occipitofrontalis

Occipitofrontalis runs from the nuchal lines to the eyebrows. From above it draws the scalp backwards to raise the eyebrows. From below it draws the scalp forwards creating transverse wrinkles (Moore et al 2002).

Trigger point location

An MTP in the occipitofrontalis (Fig. 23.3) may occur just superior to the eyebrow and reproduce pain over the same region. Referred pain

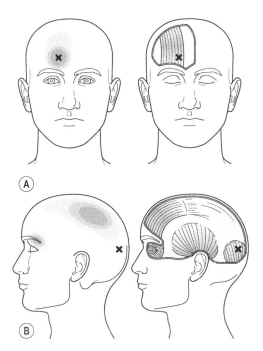

Figure 23.3 • Trigger points and pain referral zone in occiptofrontalis.

may spread upwards over the forehead towards the vertex of the head on the ipsilateral side. The MTP in occipitalis may give rise to a more classic muscular headache pattern over the posterior aspect of the head or through the head causing an intense deep pain in the orbit of the ipsilateral eye (Simons et al 1999).

Palpatory examination

Palpation of taut bands and firm nodules is particularly difficult in these broad thin muscles. Frontalis is palpated above the eyebrow to the hairline or just superiorly with the index and middle fingers in line with the eye. Small circular frictions with moderate (Grade III) pressure are applied inferiorly towards the eyebrow. The patient can be asked to raise their eyebrows to contract the muscle during this procedure.

The occipitalis is palpated with the patient in the prone or supine positions. When the frontalis is involved, the prone position may aggravate the patient's symptoms due to direct pressure of the forehead against the examination couch. In the supine position, the cervical spine is contralaterally rotated to access the muscle belly. The fingers are used to palpate the occiput ipsilaterally from behind the ears to the midline evaluating for pain or discomfort from the MTP.

Medial pterygoid

The superficial head arises from the tuberosity of the maxilla and the deep head from the medial surface of the lateral pterygoid plate and pyramidal process of palatine bone. It inserts into the medial surface of ramus of the mandible (Moore et al 2002). Acting together the medial pterygoid closes the mouth and protrudes the mandible; acting alone it protrudes the mandible to the side (Moore et al 2002). Muscle imbalance would therefore cause deviation of the mandible to the contralateral side.

Trigger point location

Trigger points are located in the mid-belly and refer to the hard palate (Fig 23.4). They can also cause a blocked feeling in the ear (Simons et al 1999).

Palpatory examination

Extra-oral palpation of the inferior fibers is performed by placing the index and middle fingers on the ramus of the mandible and sliding the fingers posteriorly and medially under the ramus to palpate for a 'sling-like taut band' of muscle. The patient is then requested to laterally deviate to the contralateral side whilst palpating for increased muscle tone and if the MTP is consistent with the patient's pain.

Intra-oral palpation of the superior fibers is performed with the patient opening their mouth (as far as comfortable) to assess for a 'webbed shaped' soft tissue at the back of the palate running in an oblique longitudinal arc. Following this, the tip of the index/little finger is placed against the mid portion of the muscle. The examination

may cause the patient to gag. The clinician can then remove their finger and when comfortable resume the examination (Simons et al 1999).

Lateral pterygoid

The inferior head arises from the lateral surface of lateral pterygoid plate and the superior head from the infratemporal surface and infratemporal crest of greater wing of sphenoid bone. The muscle inserts to the articular disc, the neck of the mandible, and the TMJ capsule. Acting together they open the mouth. Acting alone and alternatively they produce side-to-side movements of mandible (Moore et al 2002). Muscle imbalance would therefore cause deviation of the mandible to the contralateral side.

Trigger point location

Trigger points are located within the mid-belly and refer over the zygomatic arch and deep into the TMJ just anterior to the ear (Fig. 23.5). Pain may mimic sinusitis or sinus headache (Simons et al 1999).

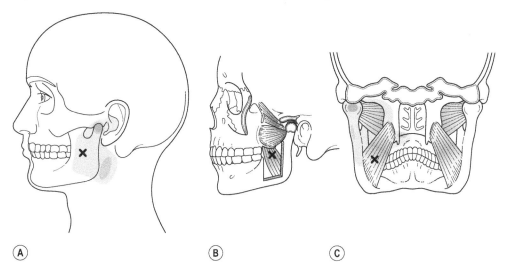

(A)   (B)   (C)

Figure 23.4 • Trigger point location and pain referral zone in medial pterygoid. Referred pain pattern (dark) and location of the responsible trigger point (X) in the left medial pterygoid muscle. **A** = external areas of pain to which the patient can point. **B** = anatomical cut-away to show the location of the trigger point area in the muscle, which lies on the inner side of the mandible. **C** = coronal section of the head through the temporomandibular joint, looking forward, showing internal areas of pain.

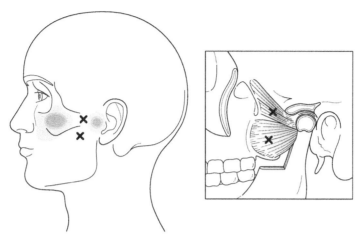

Figure 23.5 • Trigger point location and pain referral zone of lateral pterygoid. A trigger point can be located in the mid-belly of both superior and inferior divisions of the lateral pterygoid muscle. Pain is referred deep into the TMJ and to the region of the maxilla sinus. The pain is strongly associated with functional disorders of that joint. Active trigger points may mimic sinusitis or sinus headache.

Palpatory examination

Direct external palpation of the muscle is not possible due to its depth. However, it can be palpated externally through the masseter. The patient is initially requested to open their mouth while the clinician applies gentle pressure with the tip of their index or middle finger through the aperture between the mandibular notch and zygomatic process. If the patient's pain is elicited, evaluate whether it is consistent with the lateral pterygoid pain distribution or masseter distribution (Simons et al 1999). Dry needling through this aperture may enable access to the lateral pterygoid but needs to be performed with care and should be avoided in those whose condition is irritable or hypersensitive.

Intra-oral palpation of the inferior head of the lateral pterygoid may be performed while the patient opens the mouth by approximately 20–25 mm. The patient is requested to laterally deviate the mandible to the same side. The clinician's index/little finger then palpates along the contact surface of the upper teeth until the finger is positioned posterior to the last molar or wisdom tooth. From this position, the uppermost rear corner of the cheek pouch is pressed inward to palpate the muscle (Murray G, personal communication 2008, Phanachet et al 2001).

Digastric

The anterior belly arises from the digastric fossa of mandible and the posterior belly from mastoid notch of temporal bone. They attach via an intermediate tendon to the body and greater horn of the hyoid bone. It depresses the mandible and assists in opening the mouth. With the hyoid fixed it assists in swallowing (Moore et al 2002).

Trigger point location

The anterior and posterior bellies of digastric may contain an MTP. The MTP in the posterior belly may refer pain over the mastoid process and occasionally to the throat under the

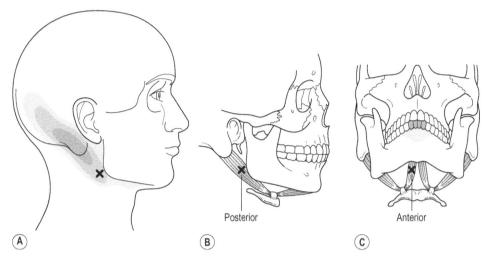

Figure 23.6 ● Trigger point location and referred pain pattern in the right digastric muscle (essential portion, solid dark; spill over portion, stippled) of trigger points (X s). **A** and **B** = posterior belly, side view. **C** = anterior belly, front view.

chin (Fig. 23.6). The anterior belly refers to the lower central incisors and to the alveolar ridge below (Simons et al 1999).

Palpatory examination

Direct external palpation of posterior digastric is difficult due to the depth of the muscle. The anterior digastric is examined by identifying the lateral margins of the hyoid, and then palpating the inferior surface of the mandible by placing the thumbs on either side of the midline. To confirm the location of the anterior digastric, the patient is requested to swallow; a prominence of the anterior belly can be palpated under the thumb tips as the hyoid is drawn superiorly. The muscle is then palpated with the thumb/fingers from the mandible (caudally and slightly laterally) to the hyoid.

The anterior digastric test has been described to evaluate if this muscle refers pain to the lower teeth. The patient is requested to strongly draw the corners of their mouth to tense the anterior neck muscles. If pain is reproduced in the lower teeth the anterior digastric is implicated. (Simons et al 1999).

Intra-oral palpation of the anterior digastric is performed with the patient opening their mouth by approximately 20–25 mm. The clinician's index finger is placed over the inner surface of the lower incisors below the alveolar ridge to palpate the soft tissue overlying the digastric. The thumb or index finger of the clinician's other hand then palpates extra-orally along the anterior belly for the MTP.

Mylohyoid

Arises from mylohyoid line of mandible and inserts onto raphe and body of hyoid (Fig 23.7). It elevates the floor of mouth, the hyoid bone and tongue during swallowing and speaking (Moore et al 2002).

Trigger point location

Myofascial trigger points in mylohyoid can refer pain to the tongue although specific pain patterns have not been clearly established (Simons et al 1999).

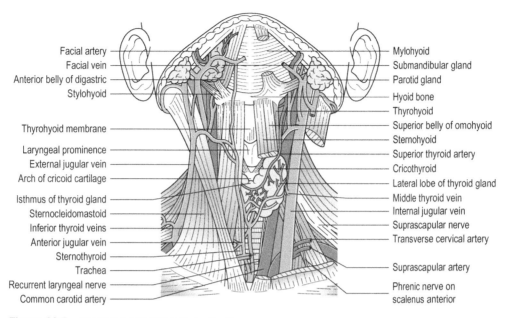

Figure 23.7 • Mylohyoid and adjacent structures.

Palpatory examination

The patient is positioned in the supine position with the cervical spine in neutral position. Extra-oral examination is initially performed with the thumb or index finger 'hooked' under the anterior digastric muscle belly. The finger then gently glides over the mylohyoid along the inner aspect of the mandible towards the angle of the mandible. To identify the location of the muscle and MTPs, the patient is requested to press their tongue into the roof of their mouth. From clinical experience, palpation of MTP in this region can produce a dry tickly or itchy sensation in the region of the soft palate and upper throat.

Additional considerations

The authors observe (that once sinister pathology has been ruled out), treatment of mylohyoid benefits patients who describe a tight choking sensation or difficulty swallowing in association with headache or TMD symptoms.

Sternocleidomastoid

The sternocleidomastoid (SCM) arises from the lateral surface of mastoid process of the temporal bone and lateral half of superior nuchal line. The sternal head attaches to the anterior surface of manubrium or sternum; the clavicular head to the superior surface of medial third of clavicle.

The SCM laterally flexes neck to the same side and rotates the neck towards the opposite side. Both SCM act together and flexes the neck. (Moore et al 2002).

Trigger point location

The muscle bellies of the sternal (medial) and clavicular (lateral) heads of the SCM may contain MTPs (see Fig. 7.2). The most inferior MTP in the sternal head can refer to the superior aspect of the sternum. The mid two MTPs can refer to the cheek, the maxilla, over the supraorbital ridge and deep within the orbit of the eye. They can also refer to the pharynx and to the posterior aspect of the tongue. MTPs in the superior aspect of SCM can refer pain to the occipital region behind the ear (Simons et al 1999).

The superior MTP in the clavicular head may refer pain deep into the ear and to the posterior auricular region with occasional referral to the ipsilateral cheek or molar teeth. The MTP in the mid-belly may refer pain across the frontal region (Simons et al 1999).

Palpatory examination

The patient lies in the supine position and is instructed to rotate the neck to the contralateral side and slightly flex forward in order to identify the border of the sternal head and return to the neutral position. The MTPs are identified with a pincer grip between the thumb and index finger. A hold-release technique is then applied along the sternal muscle belly commencing at the sternal notch while evaluating for MTP and pain reproduction. The clavicular head is more difficult to palpate. Once the hypertonicity in the sternal head is reduced, palpation of the lateral border may be achieved by progressing superiorly from the tendon insertion in the clavicle to the mastoid process by applying oscillating pressure with the fingers. MTP activation may reproduce the patient's symptoms.

Additional considerations

Receptors in the clavicular head provide spatial feedback. It is possible that dysfunction of this muscle may contribute to dizziness (Simons et al 1999).

The authors observe that dysfunction of the scalenes and levator scapulae muscles may affect the ability of the SCM to function optimally. Thus in the presence of MTPs in the SCM it is important to assess the function of the scalenes and levator scapulae.

Upper trapezius

The trapezius arises from the medial third of superior nuchal line, external occipital protuberance, nuchal ligament, spinous processes of C7–T12 vertebrae and lumbar and sacral spinous processes. It inserts onto the lateral third of clavicle, acromion, and spine of scapula. The upper trapezius elevates the scapula (Moore et al 2002).

Trigger point location

Upper trapezius may have MTPs located in the mid-section of the muscle belly approximately mid-way between the angle of the neck and the acromion (Fig. 23.8). Pain can emanate from this MTP unilaterally in a question mark shaped distribution radiating from the upper trapezius to the posterolateral aspect of the neck, the mastoid process, and when intense to the temple and the back of the orbit. Occasionally pain

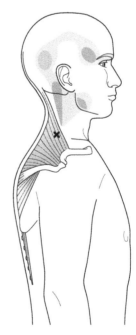

Figure 23.8 ● Trigger point and pain referral zone in upper trapezius.

may radiate to the occiput and to the angle of the mandible (Simons et al 1999). This MTP may be present in patients with tension type headache (Fernandez de las Penas et al 2006b). A second MTP may be located more posteriorly and laterally to this MTP. It refers predominantly to the posterolateral cervical region behind the ear (Simons et al 1999).

Palpatory examination

The upper trapezius can be palpated in the prone or supine positions. A mild to moderate pincer grip can be applied with the thumb and index or middle fingers while palpating from the lateral attachment of upper trapezius towards the angle of the neck. The clinician may identify taut bands or a local twitch response upon direct pressure of the MTP (Simons et al 1999).

Levator scapulae

Arises from transverse process of C1–C2, posterior tubercles of transverse processes of C3–C4 vertebrae and attaches to the superior part of medial border of the scapula. It elevates and rotates the scapula (Moore et al 2002).

Trigger point location

Levator scapulae may have MTPs at its midbelly or located just superior to its attachment at the superior angle of the scapula (Fig. 23.9). Both can refer pain ipsilaterally over the posterolateral angle of the neck. The lower MTP may occasionally refer pain inferiorly along the medial border of the scapula or along the distal border of the spine of the scapula to the posterior aspect of the shoulder (Simons et al 1999).

Palpatory examination

Direct palpation of levator scapulae is difficult due to the overlying upper trapezius. The levator scapulae may be palpated in the prone or

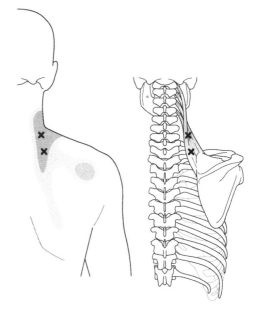

Fig. 23.9 • Trigger point location and referral zone in levator scapulae.

side-lying position with the affected side uppermost. In order to relax upper trapezius, the clinician supports the patient's ipsilateral elbow with one hand (while the patient's elbow is flexed to 90°), and then passively elevates the shoulder girdle. Following this, the index or middle finger of the other hand palpates anteriorly under the border of the upper trapezius just above the superior angle of the scapula to identify the distal aspect of the levator scapulae. The muscle is then followed superiorly until it disappears under the overlying muscles.

Additional considerations

In the authors' experience myofascial pain from levator scapulae can often reproduce pain in the subacromial region and limit shoulder elevation. Similarly it can limit cervical rotation. If left untreated, MTPs in levator scapulae can become precursors for associated MTPs in the SCM and may lead to poor scapula control

(Simons et al 1999). The shoulder girdle stabilizers also need to be assessed and treated to reduce the presence of chronic MTPs in levator scapulae.

Splenius capitis

Arises from inferior half of nuchal ligament and spinous processes of C7–T3 vertebrae and supraspinous ligament and inserts into the lateral aspect of mastoid process and lateral third of superior nuchal line. It laterally flexes and rotates head and neck to same side; acting bilaterally, they extend head and neck (Moore et al 2002).

Trigger point location

A MTP may be located just superior to the mid-belly of splenius capitis (Fig. 23.10) which could refer pain to the vertex of the head on the ipsilateral side (Simons et al 1999). Hypertonicity of splenius capitis may occur with a wry neck, lifting heavy loads, a forward head posture, shortening of the anterior cervical muscles, whiplash associated disorders, and cervical articular or neural dysfunction (Simons et al 1999).

Palpatory examination

The patient is positioned in the prone position with the arms resting under the hips and their palms facing upwards. The upper trapezius can be relaxed in this position. The clinician then places the index and middle fingers over the posterior aspect of the mastoid process. Following this, the fingers palpate inferiorly toward the mid to lower cervical spine. The splenius capitis can be palpated superiorly; inferiorly the muscle disappears under the overlying musculature. It is important to identify the splenius capitis fiber direction and potential regions of hypertonicity. To define the border of this muscle, the patient is requested to initiate extension of the head and neck with rotation to the same side. Correlation with referred pain patterns should be evaluated.

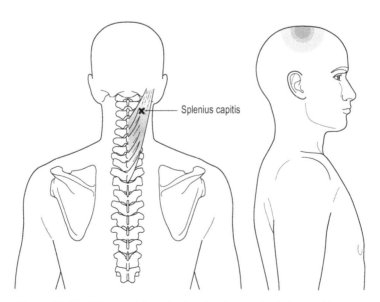

Splenius capitis

Figure 23.10 ● Trigger points and pain referral zone of splenius capitis.

Additional considerations

Active MTPs in splenius capitis and levator scapulae on the ipsilateral side can limit cervical rotation in patients with a wry neck. Active MTPs in splenius capitis and upper trapezius can present with symptoms similar to occipital neuralgia (Simons et al 1999).

The sub-occipital group

The sub-occipital group comprises rectus capitis posterior (RCP) major, rectus capitis posterior minor, inferior oblique and superior oblique (Fig. 23.11)

The rectus capitis posterior major arises from the spinous process of the C2 vertebra and attaches to the lateral aspect of the inferior nuchal line of the occipital bone. The RCP minor arises from the posterior tubercle on the posterior arch of C1 vertebra and inserts onto the medial third of the inferior nuchal line. The inferior oblique arises from the spinous process of C2 vertebra and inserts onto the transverse process of C1 vertebra. The superior oblique arises from the transverse process of C1 vertebra and attaches to the

occipital bone between superior and inferior nuchal lines. Action of sub-occipital group is to extend the head on C1 and rotate the head on C1 and C2 (Moore et al 2002).

Trigger point location

Myofascial trigger points may occur in the mid belly of both RCP major and minor and inferior oblique. The MTPs in the sub-occipital muscles may refer pain to the occiput and temporal region and cause bilateral headache (Simons et al 1999). Clinical investigations demonstrate that MTPs in the sub-occipital muscles may be associated with episodic tension-type headache (ETTH) (Fernandez de las Penas et al 2006c). In one study, 10 patients with ETTH were compared with 10 asymptomatic controls for the presence of sub-occipital MTPs. Of the ETTH patients, 60% had active MTPs which reproduced their symptoms while the rest had latent MTPs. Latent MTPs were found in 2 controls. A subsequent study was conducted in 11 subjects to evaluate the cross-sectional area of the RCP major and minor with MRI and its relationship with active MTPs in chronic tension-type headache (CTTH) patients (Fernandez de las

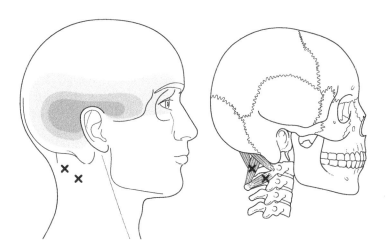

Figure 23.11 • Trigger points and pain referral zone of the sub-occipital group-rectus capitis posterior major (RCP), rectus capitis posterior (RCP) minor, inferior oblique and superior oblique.

Penas et al 2008). Active MTPs were found in 55% of patients and the rest had latent MTPs. The cross-sectional area of RCP minor was significantly smaller in those with active MTPs compared to those with latent MTPs. It was hypothesized that muscle atrophy of the RCP minor was associated with active MTPs and CTTH. These investigations support previous inference that active MTPs in sub-occipital muscles might contribute to headache. The presence of muscle atrophy in RCP minor suggests that such atrophy could occur in other active MTPs. However, further MRI needs to be conducted in other muscle groups before reaching firm conclusions.

Palpatory examination

Direct palpation of these muscles is not possible. Reproduction of the patient's pain, confirmation of the location of the most tender point, and awareness of structures underlying and overlying the palpated area is the most effective way to perform examination of this region.

The patient is positioned in the supine position with the cervical region and shoulders relaxed and requested to perform deep expiration to relax muscles. The clinician places the palm of their hand under the patient's head just above the occiput to position the head and neck in upper cervical flexion and about 10° of contralateral lateral flexion. To palpate over RCP major, the thumb or finger tip is placed just adjacent to the C2 spinous process at a 45° angle to the spine. The fingers are then moved superiorly and laterally towards the occiput. The same starting position is used to palpate over inferior oblique just adjacent to the C2 spinous process. The thumb or fingers are moved obliquely into a region of soft tissue towards the transverse process of C1.

Treatment of trigger points

Digital pressure can be applied to deactivate MTPs (Simons et al 1999) and is described in Table 23.1. Similarly dry needling can also be applied to deactivate MTPs and is described in Chapter 24.

Treatment of MTPs needs to be evaluated with outcome measures described in Chapter 13 and by Stegenga et al (1993) However, MTP therapy may be only part of the treatment program. Management strategies may include postural and ergonomic considerations, articular and neural interventions (Bogduk 2001, Govind et al 2005, Jull & Niere 2004, Niere & Selvaratnam 1995), appropriate medication, psychological support and relaxation skills with cognitive behavioral therapy (Raphael et al 2008). Self-management programs may include cervical and lumbar stabilization programs (Jull et al 2002, Richardson et al 1999), exercises for masticatory muscles (de Wijer 2005) (see also Chapters 19, 20 and 25), and appropriate aerobic exercise programs.

Conclusion

Examination of patients presenting with headache or TMD should include muscular, articular, and neurological evaluation to determine the patient's functional level. Particular attention should be paid to identification of MTPs, craniocervical flexors, and the length of the muscles examined. It is important to evaluate whether treatment of MTPs alters the patient's physical and functional outcomes. When the response to treatment is slow, or non-musculoskeletal pathology is suspected, patients need to be referred to their medical practitioner.

Table 23.1 Treatment of myofascial trigger points.

Muscle	Treatment
Temporalis	Treatment can be performed by applying small circular frictions on MTPs for 10–20 sec with the index or middle finger (Grade II technique). The patient is instructed to slowly open their mouth during the intervention. Treatment can be progressed by moving transversally over temporalis. A firm resistance will be initially felt over MTPs. Confirm with the patient the presence of any referred pain. As the resistance decreases the digital pressure can be increased (Grade III to Grade IV). A reduction in MTP resistance should correspond with a reduction in pain.
Masseters	Treatment can be performed by applying direct pressure extra/intra-orally on a masseter MTP for 10–20 seconds and then releasing the pressure (Grade II technique).
Occipitofrontalis	The MTP can be treated by the moving fingers in a cross-fiber direction applying small circular frictions (Grade II). The pressure can be gradually increased (Grade III) until the patient's pain is reduced or the MTP is deactivated.
Medial pterygoid	Extra-oral treatment can be performed under the postero-medial aspect of the ramus by applying small circular frictions with the thumb or fingers to the inferior aspect of the muscle. The intra-oral procedure can be performed on the superior fibers by placing the index finger on the MTP and applying 1 sec hold-release pressure on the muscle belly from the ramus of the mandible towards the medial pterygoid plate for 10–20 sec. This intervention may cause the patient to gag. The clinician then needs to remove their finger and resume treatment when the patient is comfortable.
Lateral pterygoid	The intra-oral procedure described in the text is performed by palpating the muscle. A 1-sec hold-release pressure is applied on the muscle for 10–20 sec. The patient's pain response and opening of the mouth are re-assessed. Dry needling can be performed extra-orally through the mandibular notch and left in-situ for 5 minutes.
Digastric	The clinician's finger tips are placed intra-orally and extra-orally immediately above the MTP. The MTP is oscillated extra-orally by applying small circular frictions for 10–20 sec to deactivate the MTP (Grade II depth). A firm resistance may be felt initially against the finger tips. Confirm with the patient if this reproduces their pain. If the patient is able to tolerate it, increase the digital pressure (Grade IV⁻) as the resistance within the MTP abates. The reduction in MTP resistance should correspond with reduction of pain.
Mylohyoid	The patient is requested to open their mouth to mid-range. The clinician then slides their index or middle finger along the inner surface of the lower incisors below the alveolar ridge to the soft tissue where the mylohyoid is located. The thumb and index finger of the other hand is placed extra-orally just lateral to the midline and adjacent to the anterior digastric (this position sandwiches the mylohyoid intra and extra-orally between the fingers). The thumb and index finger (extra-orally) then glide together over the mylohyoid towards the angle of the mandible. On identification of any MTPs, gently apply small circular frictions for 10–20 sec. A reduction in MTP resistance should correspond with a reduction in pain. Repeat the technique as required.
Sternocleidomastoid	The MTP in the sternal head can be deactivated from the sternal notch to the mastoid process by maintaining a pincer-grip (Grade II) on the muscle with the cervical spine in the neutral position. From clinical experience the sternocleidomastoid MTPs can be very hyperalgesic, especially when attempting to reproduce frontal headache in patients. The clinician will need to reduce the pressure applied or treat with gentle oscillating hold-release technique (Grade II⁻) for 10–20 sec.

Continued

Table 23.1 Treatment of myofascial trigger points—Cont'd

Muscle	Treatment
	Clinicians need to take care in the vicinity of the internal carotid artery. The technique can be progressed while applying the pincer grip and the patient actively rotating their neck to the contralateral side and then returning to the neutral position.
Upper trapezius	A moderate pincer grip is used to deactivate the MTPs in the supine or side-lying positions. The patient is requested to actively elevate the scapula and then depress it while deactivating the upper trapezius. Alternatively, in the supine position the patient is requested to slowly rotate their neck to the opposite side as the pincer grip is maintained. The MTP can also be deactivated in the prone position with the patient's hands positioned under their hips with the elbows flexed and the shoulders relaxed. The clinician then performs small circular frictions with their thumb or fingers using a pincer grip. Initially a firm resistance may be palpated against the finger tips. Direct pressure can be increased as resistance in the MTP and muscle tautness abates. This procedure should correspond with the patient reporting a reduction in their pain. The presence of any referred pain should be assessed. Assessment of scapula position and shoulder girdle stabilization programs will be beneficial in those with chronic MTPs. In the author's experience deactivation of MTPs in infraspinatus and teres minor may reduce MTP activity in upper trapezius.
Levator scapulae	The inferior MTP is deactivated in the prone or side-lying positions with gentle pressure (Grade II⁻) applied over the MTP while the patient actively elevates and then depresses the shoulder girdle. The procedure is repeated until the pain reduces significantly or the MTP becomes less sensitive. The clinician can also slide their thumb or index and middle fingers transversely across the taut levator scapulae fibers as they passively elevate and depress the patient's shoulder girdle while supporting their elbow. The presence of an MTP near the attachment at the superior angle is most probably an attachment MTP and may be relieved by deactivating the MTP at the muscle belly.
Splenius capitis	The index, middle and ring fingers are initially aligned over the mastoid process. Following this the splenius capitis is palpated transversely over taut bands. Once the MTP is identified, firm pressure is applied over it for apporximately 20 sec. The pressure is then released, and reapplied until pain dissipates or the MTP is deactivated.
Sub-occipital group	
Rectus capitis posterior major and minor	The recti can be treated in the supine position by gently rocking the chin further into upper cervical flexion as digital pressure is applied with the thumb or fingers. When the head returns to its neutral position a firm resistance may be experienced initially against the finger tips. As the resistance in the tissues abates the procedure is progressed by increasing direct pressure. A reduction in MTP resistance should correspond with a reduction in pain.
Inferior oblique	The same technique as the recti can be applied to treat inferior oblique. The head can be gently rocked into further lateral flexion as an oscillating pressure is applied with the fingers.

MTP = myofascial trigger point.

References

Benoliel R, Sharav Y 2008 Masticatory myofascial pain, and tension-type and chronic daily headache. In: Sharav Y, Benoliel R (eds) Orofacial pain and headache. Elsevier, Edinburgh, p 109-148.

Bogduk N 2001 Cervicogenic headache: anatomic basis and pathophysiologic mechanisms. Curr Pain Headache Rep 5:382-386.

Brukner P, Khan K 2006 Clinical Sports Medicine (3rd edn). McGraw-Hill Professional, Sydney.

Cleland JA, Fritz JM, Whitman JM et al 2006 The reliability and construct validity of the Neck Disability Index and patient specific functional scale in patients with cervical radiculopathy. Spine 31 598-602.

Cohen M 2005 (Abstract) Masticatory muscle function and Pain. In The 4th international conference of orofacial pain and temporomandibular disorders. The scientific basis of clinical decision making. Kleinberg I (ed). August 26-28, 2005. Sydney, Australia, p.21.

de Wijer A 2005 (Abstract) Clinical issues in the TMD-the evidence base. In: the 4th international conference of orofacial pain and temporomandibular disorders. The scientific basis of clinical decision making. Ed: Kleinberg I. August 26-28, 2005. Sydney, Australia, 14-15.

Dommerholt J, Bron C, Franssen J 2006 Myofascial trigger points: an evidence-informed review. J Manual Manip Therapy 14(4):203-221.

Fernandez de las Penas C, Cuadrado ML et al 2006a Myofascial disorders in the trochlear region in unilateral migraine: a possible initiating or perpetuating factor. Clin J Pain 22:548-553.

Fernandez de las Penas C, Alonso-Blanco C, Cuadrado et al 2006b Myofascial trigger points and their relationship to headache clinical parameters in chronic tension-type headache. Headache 46(8): 1264-1272.

Fernandez de las Penas C, Alonso-Blanco C, Cuadrado ML et al 2006c Myofascial trigger points in the suboccipital muscles in episodic tension-type headache. Man Ther 11(3):225-230.

Fernandez de las Penas C, Cuadrado ML, Arendt-Nielsen L et al 2007 Myofascial trigger points and sensitization: an updated pain model for tension-type headache. Cephalgia 27(5):383-393.

Fernandez de las Penas C, Cuadrado ML, Arendt-Nielsen L et al 2008 Association of cross-sectional area of the rectus capitis posterior minor muscle with active trigger points in chronic tension-type headache: a pilot study. Am J Phys Med Rehabil 87(3):197-203.

Gerwin R, Shannon S 2000 Interexaminer reliability and myofascial trigger points. Arch Phys Med Rehabil 81(9):1257-1258.

Gerwin RD, Shannon S, Hong CZ et al 1997 Inter-rater reliability in myofascial trigger point examination. Pain 69(1-2):65-73.

Govind J, King W, Giles P et al 2005 Headache and the Cervical Zygapophyseal Joints (Cervicogenic Headache). (Orthopaedic Proceedings). J Bone Joint Surg, 87B:399-340.

Hong CZ, Simons DG 1998 Pathophysiologic and electrophysiologic mechanisms of myofascial trigger points. Arch Phys Med Rehabil 79(7):863-872.

Huguenin LK 2004 Myofascial trigger points: the current evidence. Physical Therapy in Sport 5:2-12.

Hsieh CY, Hong CZ, Adams AH et al 2000 Interexaminer reliability of the palpation of trigger points in the trunk and lower limb muscles. Arch Phys Med Rehabil 81(3): 258-264.

Janda V 1985 Muscle weakness and inhibition (pseudoparesis) in back pain syndromes. In: Grieve G (ed) Modern manual therapy of the vertebral column. Churchill Livingstone, Edinburgh, p 197-201.

Jerjes WG, Madland et al 2007 A psychological comparison of temporomandibular disorder and chronic daily headache: are there targets for therapeutic interventions? Oral Surg Oral Med Oral Pathol Oral Radiol Endod 103(3):367-373.

Jull GA, Trott P, Potter H et al 2002 A randomized controlled trial of exercise and manipulative therapy for cervicogenic headache Spine 27:1835-1843.

Jull GA, Niere K 2004 The cervical spine and headache. In: Boyling G, Jull G (eds) Grieve's modern manual therapy – the vertebral column, 3rd edn. Churchill Livingstone, Edinburgh, p 291-309.

Kellgren JH 1938a Observations on referred pain arising from muscle. Clin Sci 3:175-190.

Kellgren JH 1938b A preliminary account of referred pains arising from muscle. Br Med J 1:325-327.

Kelly M 1941 The treatment of fibrositis and allied disorders by local Anaesthesia. Med J Aust 1:294-298.

Lavigne G, Morisson, F, Khoury S et al 2006 Sleep-related pain complaints: morning headaches and tooth grinding Insom, 7:4-11.

Lew PC, Lewis J et al 1997 Inter-therapist reliability in locating latent myofascial trigger points using palpation. Man Ther 2(2):87-90.

Lewis T 1938 Suggestions relating to the study of somatic pain. BMJ 1:321-325.

Lucas KR, Polus BI, Rich PA 2004 Latent myofascial trigger points: their effects on muscle activation and movement efficiency. JBMT 8(3): 160-166.

Lucas 2007 The effects of latent myofascial trigger points on muscle activation patterns during scapular plane elevation. PhD thesis. Australasian Digital Thesis Network.

Maitland G 1986 Vertebral manipulation. Butterworths, London.

Moore KL, Agur AMR 2002 Essential Clinical Anatomy, 2nd edn. Lippincott Williams and Wilkins, Philadelphia.

Niddam DM, Chan RC, Lee SH et al 2008 Central representation of hyperalgesia from myofascial trigger point. Neuroimage 39(3):1299-1306.

Niere K, Selvaratnam PJ 1995 The cervical region. In: Zuluaga M et al (eds) Sports physiotherapy-applied science and practice. Churchill Livingstone, Edinburgh, p 325-341.

Okeson J 2005 The clinical management of orofacial pain. Bell's orofacial pain. Quintessence Publishing Company Inc., Chicago.

Phanachet I, Whittle T, Wanigaratne K, Murray GM 2001 Functional properties of single motor units in inferior head of human lateral pterygoid muscle: task relations and threshold. Neurophysiology 86:2204-2218.

Raphael KG, Ciccone DS 2008 Psychological aspects of chronic orofacial pain. In: Sharav Y, Benoliel R (eds) Orofacial pain and headache. Elsevier, Edinburgh, p 57-74.

Richardson C, Jull G, Hodges P, Hides J 1999 Therapeutic exercise for spinal segmental stabilization in low back pain. Scientific basis and clinical approach. Churchill Livingstone, Edinburgh.

Sackett D, Richardson W 1997 Evidence-based medicine. How to practice & Teach EBM. Churchill Livingstone, New York.

Sciotti VM, Mittak VL, DiMarco L et al 2001 Clinical precision of myofascial trigger point location in the trapezius muscle. Pain 93:259-266.

Selvaratnam PJ, Matyas TA, Glasgow EF 1994 Noninvasive discrimination of brachial plexus involvement in upper limb pain. Spine 19:26-33.

Selvaratnam PJ 2008 Dry needling for Physiotherapists. Handbook of the clinical doctorate program in dry needling. The University of Melbourne, School of Physiotherapy, Department of Medicine, Dentistry and Health Sciences, Parkville, Victoria, Australia.

Shah JP, Phillips TM, Danoff JV et al 2005 An in-vivo microanalytical technique for measuring the local biochemical milieu of human skeletal muscle. J App Physiol 99:1980-1987.

Simons DG, Hong CZ et al 2002 Endplate potentials are common to midfiber myofascial trigger points. Am J Phys Med Rehabil 81(3): 212-222.

Simons D, Travell J, Simons LS 1999 Myofascial pain and dysfunction: the trigger point manual. Upper half of the body. Lippincott Williams and Wilkins, Philadelphia.

Stegenga B, de Bont LGM, de Leeuw R, Boering G 1993 Assessment of mandibular function impairment associated with temporomandibular joint osteoarthrosis and internal derangement. Journal of Orofacial Pain 7:183-195.

Travell JG, Simons DG, 1983 Myofascial pain and dysfunction: The trigger point manual, vol 1. Williams & Wilkins, Philadelphia.

Trott P 1985 Examination of the temporomandibular joint. In: Grieve G (ed) Modern manual therapy of the vertebral column. Churchill Livingstone, Edinburgh, p 521-529.

Zito G 2007 Diagnostic criteria used by physiotherapists to differentiate cervicogenic headache from temporomandibular headache. Clinical doctorate thesis. Brownless Medical library. The University of Melbourne, Parkville, Melbourne, Australia.

Zito G, Jull G, Story I 2006 Clinical tests of musculoskeletal dysfunction in the diagnosis of cervicogenic headache. Man Ther 11:118-129.

Zito G, Morris M, Selvaratnam PJ 2008 Characteristics of TMD headache – systematic review. Physical Therapy Reviews 13(5):324-332.

24

Dry needling, acupuncture and laser

Peter Selvaratnam and Philip Gabel

Dry needling and laser can benefit patients with headache and TMD. In this chapter the authors, a musculoskeletal physiotherapist-anatomist and a sports physiotherapist, present medical theories and research on these modalities and provide case studies to guide practitioners in the treatment of patients.

The treatment modalities of dry needling (DN), acupuncture, and low level laser therapy (LLLT), have been shown to be beneficial in the management of various musculoskeletal conditions including headache and myofascial pain (Bjordal et al 2001, Brukner & Khan 2006, Ilbuldu et al 2004). This chapter explores the treatment of myofascial trigger points (MTPs) as a source of cervical pain and headache using dry needling, through direct application of acupuncture needles and LLLT. Both techniques use as their core approach the application of a second stimulus; for DN it is noxious or counter-stimulatory (Huguenin 2004) and for laser it is bioregulatory (Chow et al 2006). The concept of treating peripheral nerve pathways in the management of pain is also discussed.

It must be emphasized that, though similar in technique, dry needling differs from acupuncture and the treatment effects will not always be the same (Davies & Davies 2006). Acupuncture has been inferred to embrace a holistic approach. Needling of acupuncture points (acupoints) has a systemic effect that is not physiologically or directly related to the area under treatment as in DN. Practitioners of Traditional Chinese Medicine (TCM) infer the presence of sensation pathways that correspond to meridians (MacDonald 1982). This concept is contrary to that of western medicine practitioners who have a modern biological and physiological approach and dispute the complexity of the philosophies of TCM and the spiritual paradigm of energy pathways and meridians (Baldry 2005, Dommerholt et al 2006, Tong 2003).

In contrast to acupuncture, dry needling can also be applied to muscle origins and insertions, tendons, ligaments, periosteum, and tender skin (Baldry 2005). These musculoskeletal structures provide the practitioner greater scope to palpate and evaluate the presence of MTPs in conjunction with active movements of the spine and limbs, and neurological examination, rather than relying solely on the site of MTPs. Some authors infer that the use of systemic points (that affect the whole body) and distal points in the TCM model invokes both a central and segmental neurological effect (Fang et al 2004, Lui et al 2004). Dry needling may also involve treatment of proximal and distal points following the segmental neurological model (Gunn 1977a & b). The arrival of event-related functional MRI (fMRI) also confirmed that needling MTPs in the upper trapezius resulted in altered brain activity and response level (Niddam al 2008). Dry needling and acupuncture therefore have significantly different philosophies of assessment and treatment.

Myofascial trigger points

The classical definition of the myofascial trigger point is provided by Simons et al (1999) as 'a hyperirritable spot in skeletal muscle that is associated with a hypersensitive palpable nodule in a taut band. The spot is painful on compression and can give rise to characteristic referred pain, referred tenderness, motor dysfunction, and autonomic phenomena'. The MTP may elicit a local twitch response (muscle fasciculation) or jump sign (whole body movement) with digital pressure or dry needling (Huguenin 2004). The twitch response is considered an objective sign of the presence of a MTP (Simons et al 2002); however, reproduction of the patient's pain is more reliable. Myofascial trigger points are classified as active or latent, primary or associated. Active MTPs reproduce local or referred pain including headache or neurological signs. Latent MTPs are tender only on compression and are considered to be caused by muscle shortening from poor posture or cumulative trauma. Primary and associated MTPs are described in Chapter 23. It is believed that application of DN to the affected muscle belly can deactivate these MTPs and reduce both local and referred symptoms such as those found with headache (Baldry 2005, Simons et al 1999).

Some authors suggest that acupoints correlate with myofascial trigger points. Melzack et al (1977) reported that 71% of 'channel' and 'extra' acupoints correlated with MTPs. Dorsher (2006) compared the 255 MTPs described by Travell and Simons (1983) and the 386 acupoints described by the Shanghai College of Traditional Medicine and other acupuncture texts. Dorsher stated that there was a strong relationship between MTPs and acupoints. The MTPs reported by Travell and Simons (1983) and subsequently by Simons et al (1999) suggest that they have distinct anatomical locations and numbered them in the order of their appearance (Dommerholt et al 2006). In practice, MTPs vary in each patient and do not always correlate with the distinct anatomical locations described in texts. Similarly, both correlation studies infer that acupoints have point specificity (Dommerholt et al 2006). However, there has not been any scientific validation of the anatomical location of MTPs and acupoints (Dommerholt et al 2006) or any inter-examiner reliability studies to correlate MTPs and acupoints. Thus clinicians need to interpret these findings on MTPs and acupoints with care.

Birch (2003) refuted the findings of Melzack and colleagues (1977) and reported that their methodology was based on 'questionable assumptions'. Melzack et al (1977) assumed that acupoints must exhibit pressure pain and such pain reproduction was sufficient to correlate with MTPs (Birch 2003, Dommerholt et al 2006). Birch found that only 18–19% of channel and extra acupoints examined by Melzack et al (1977) correlated with MTPs but they did not examine tender 'Ah Shi' acupoints. Hong (2000) and Audette et al (2003) surmise that acupuncturists may be treating MTPs when they needle 'Ah Shi' points. Dommerholt et al (2006) also emphasized that acupoints do not display the 'twitch' response of active MTPs and so cannot be categorized as the same. Active MTPs therefore have a clinical distinction from channel or extra acupoints.

Development of myofascial trigger points

Several mechanisms have been postulated to explain the presence of myofascial trigger points (Simons & Travell 1981). A myofascial trigger point is activated when damage or over activity causes spasm of the sarcoplasmic reticulum (the calcium repository surrounding the myofibril), which results in calcium ion release. These free ionized calcium molecules activate the actin-myosin contractile mechanism in the sarcomeres with the assistance of locally generated adenosine triphosphate (ATP). This action is self-perpetuating as the spasm or sustained contraction ultimately results in compromise of the local muscle fiber circulation that in turn leads to a vasoconstrictor reflex response. The phenomenon is due partially to a local accumulation of metabolites coupled with the inability of the calcium ions to diffuse immediately.

This subsequent circulatory compromise leads to ATP depletion that in turn prevents calcium ions returning to the sarcoplasmic reticulum repository. Consequently, the tissue calcium concentration continues despite the lack of ATP. This causes the sarcomere shortening to persist as the myosin heads do not release from the actin filaments. In addition there is a generated reflexive release of acetylcholine at the motor endplate along with the release of calcium from the stretched sarcoplasmic reticulum neighboring the MTP.

However, some authors argue that central sensitization or peripheral nervous system sensitization trigger MTPs and maintain their activity (Baldry 2005, Cohen 2005, Gunn 1977a). Although there are no definitive studies to support this claim, imaging studies with needling may lend support to this hypothesis (Fang et al 2004, Lui et al 2004, Niddam et al 2008).

Research evidence

Myofascial trigger points in the upper cervical region can cause headache or refer pain to the head (Kellgren 1938a, Lewis 1938). The injection of novocaine locally into a focus of irritation within a muscle of the upper cervical region has been shown to cause pain in the teeth, and in the occipital, vertex, and frontal regions (Kellgren 1938a). Based on this work, western medicine advocates of MTPs recommend treatment using local novocaine injections (Kellgren 1938b). Gunn (1977a) initially introduced the term 'dry needling' based on the radiculopathy model. He hypothesized that painful muscular conditions were due to nerve root dysfunction. He recommended DN proximally the paraspinal muscles innervated by the posterior primary rami, and distally the peripheral muscles supplied by the anterior primary rami in their segmental or myotomal distribution. Later, Baldry (1989) advocated both dry needling and local injection to MTPs and 'acupoints' as '... an effective treatment method for myofascial or other pain that is either local or referred from a hypersensitive focus'.

Evidence for the efficacy of dry needling and acupuncture varies from supportive (Berman et al 2004, Huguenin et al 2005, Langevin et al 2006, Lucas 2007, Lucas et al 2004, Melchart et al 2001, Shah et al 2005), to inconclusive (Griggs & Jensen 2006, White et al 2004), or ineffective (Vas et al 2005). The quality of the research and type of investigations vary considerably. Meta-analysis from the Cochrane Foundation suggests that acupuncture and dry needling may be useful adjuncts to other therapies for chronic low back pain (Furlan et al., 2005, Young and Jewell, 2002) and the treatment of 'idiopathic headaches' (Melchart et al 2001). However, the Foundation and its review process have been criticized for methodological and inherent bias against complementary and alternative medicine (Bjordal et al 2006, Sood et al 2005). Most findings by the Cochrane Foundation state that the evidence on needling is inconclusive and that further research and systematic reviews are needed due to the unique problems of an inadequate placebo and blinding.

The benefits of acupuncture and dry needling to both patient and society have been demonstrated through several randomized controlled trials on headache and cervical pain. Vickers et al (2004) conducted a randomized controlled clinical study of 401 patients with headache. One group received standard general practitioner care; the second group received 12 acupuncture treatments from physiotherapists trained in acupuncture in addition to standard care. Those who received acupuncture reported a 15% reduction in medication use and days off work as well as 25% fewer medical visits compared to controls. This investigation lends some support to the management of headache with needling intervention.

The effect of superficial and deep acupuncture needling in patients with cervical disorder has been investigated. Irnich (2002) and co-workers conducted a prospective, sham, controlled cross-over trial comparing superficial acupuncture needling and deep needling in 36 patients with chronic neck pain and limited cervical mobility. The changes in pain rating and neck mobility were evaluated following a single needling treatment or sham treatment. Superficial acupuncture needling and sham laser treatment was performed on distal acupoints in the upper and lower limbs. Deep acupuncture needling was performed on cervical muscles. The results indicated that superficial needling produced immediate analgesia and improved mobility. These therapeutic effects were not observed in those receiving localized deep needling or sham laser treatment. They postulated that deep acupuncture needling caused post treatment pain from repeated stimulation of the affected region compared to superficial distal needling of distal points. While these findings indicate that superficial needling produces analgesia, the study design has shortcomings since patients with chronic pain require evaluation over a 12 to 24 month period.

In contrast, other randomly controlled studies demonstrate that deep dry needling of lumbar MTPs produced significantly better analgesia than superficial dry needling (Ceccherelli et al 2002) and might be more effective in the management of low back pain (Gunn et al 1980, Itoh et al 2004). These findings suggest that superficial and deep DN may be both effective depending on the severity, irritability, and nature of the patient's condition (Selvaratnam & Knight 1995).

Dry needling has been found to produce physiological changes. DN skin and muscle A-δ and C afferent fibers of anesthetized rats has been observed to increase cerebral blood flow (Uchida et al 2000). Superficial needling of patients with chronic low back pain has also been observed to increase cortical blood flow (Alavi et al 1997). Langevin et al (2006) observed that superficial needle rotation of subcutaneous tissue with an acupuncture needle altered the shape of fibroblasts from a rounded appearance to a more spindle-like shape. They hypothesized that this altered shape following needling could lead to cellular and extra-cellular events including mechanoreceptor and nociceptive stimulation, variation in gene expression and extracellular matrix and eventually to neuromodulation. These physiological findings lend support to the clinical utility of dry needling.

Dry needling also has therapeutic benefits to patients. Case studies have demonstrated that dry needling MTPs produces analgesia (Lewit 1979), and reduces shoulder pain (Ingber 1989) and post-herpetic neuralgia (Weiner et al 2006). Needling can also be applied at sites distant to the region of pain. Such analgesia may be explained by the neurophysiological phenomenon of diffuse noxious inhibitory controls (Le Bars et al 1983, NHMRC 1989, Selvaratnam & Knight 1995). In this phenomenon needling is considered to block the transmission of nociception by the application of a second new noxious stimulus at a site distal from the site of injury. Investigations conducted on rats support the concept of diffuse noxious inhibitory controls (Bing et al 1990, Boucher et al 1998). It was observed that stimulation of their hindlimb with acupuncture needles at acupoints, non-acupoints and with a noxious thermal stimulus evoked inhibition of the trigeminal nucleus caudalis. This inhibition was significantly reduced by systemic nalaxone, an opiate antagonist, suggesting that needle stimulation produces an analgesic effect.

The effect of DN on 59 male Australian Rules footballers with hamstring pain was investigated by Huguenin et al (2005). In one group the gluteal muscles were dry needled with 30 mm needles and in another group placebo superficial needling was performed. Patients and controls demonstrated similar improvement on straight leg raise test, internal rotation and a running task. Though there was no significant difference, the investigation supports the notion that DN to approximately 30 mm depth and superficial needling have a therapeutic effect and need to be considered in treating other regions. Future studies are needed to evaluate the effect of DN deep gluteal and piriformis muscles with longer needles.

The effect of dry needling latent myofascial trigger points in shoulder girdle muscles and their activation pattern were investigated by Lucas et al (2004). Electromyography was used to assess the time of onset of the upper and lower trapezius, serratus anterior, infraspinatus and middle deltoid muscle activity during shoulder elevation in 154 asymptomatic subjects. The presence of latent MTPs was evaluated in subjects who exhibited abnormal muscle activation. These patients were randomly assigned to two groups. The treatment group received deep DN of latent MTPs and passive stretching. The placebo group received

sham ultrasound. The muscle activation of those who received deep DN returned to normal. The placebo group did not demonstrate any change. This investigation demonstrated that DN latent MTPs improved the activation pattern of upper trapezius and shoulder girdle muscles. This study lends support to the assessment and management of latent MTPs in patients presenting with headache.

Currently there is no gold standard for clinical diagnosis of MTPs or acupoints as imaging is inconclusive and invasive techniques are not practical (Brukner et al 2006, Huguenin 2004). Previous investigations have not demonstrated any histological changes in MTPs (Huguenin 2004). However, subsequent investigations demonstrate the presence of an inflammatory biochemical milieu in MTPs. Shah et al (2005) investigated the upper trapezius for the presence of pain-influencing chemical mediators within MTPs and normal muscle tissue. An in vivo investigation of 9 subjects was conducted in near real time at sub-nanogram level of concentration. The study included 3 subjects who had neck pain and active MTPs, 3 asymptomatic subjects with latent MTPs and 3 asymptomatic subjects who did not exhibit MTPs. They observed that active MTPs had significantly higher concentrations of norepinephrine, serotonin, bradykinin, interleukin-1, calcitonin-gene-related-peptide (CGRP), tumor necrosis factor, and substance P in its immediate milieu compared to normal muscle tissue. In contrast, latent MTPs showed lower concentrations of CGRP and substance P than active MTPs but higher than normal muscle tissue. A needle was then applied to elicit a twitch response at the active and latent MTPs. The researchers observed that the concentration of the biochemical milieu in the immediate vicinity of the active MTPs reduced to normal levels. In a subsequent study Shah et al (2008) conducted a similar study in

9 subjects comparing the upper trapezius with gastrocnemius. They reported the presence of the biochemical milieu in those with active and latent MTPs in the upper trapezius. The concentration of the selected inflammatory mediators in those with active MTPs differed quantitatively from a remote uninvolved region in the gastrocnemius. These studies demonstrate the clinical difference between active and latent MTPs (Shah et al 2005, 2008) and that eliciting a local twitch response can normalize the selected inflammatory mediators in active MTPs (Shah et al 2005).

The effect on the CNS of needling acupoints and myofascial trigger points has been investigated. Hsieh et al (2001) evaluated the effect of needling the acupuncture point in the first dorsal interosseous muscle (referred to in TCM as Large Intestine 4, or LI4) and a nearby non-classical/non analgesic point in 16 healthy subjects. Positron emission tomography was performed assessing regional blood flow as an index of brain activity. Acupuncture stimulation of LI4 activated the hypothalamus with an extension to midbrain, the insula, the anterior cingulate cortex, and the cerebellum. They hypothesized that the classical analgesic point mediated the analgesic effects of acupuncture stimulation. Functional MRI (fMRI) has also been employed to evaluate the effect of needling on pain modulating centers (Fang et al 2004, Lui et al 2004). These studies compared 'real' acupoints to sham acupoints. The investigation by Fang et al (2004) indicated that stimulation of real acupoints increased activation of the thalamus, cerebellum and somatosensory cortex but not of the sham acupoints. A subsequent fMRI study by Lui et al (2004) demonstrated that 'real' acupuncture point stimulation increased activation of the same somatosensory cortical areas and the periaqueductal grey but not of the sham acupoints. These studies suggest that acupuncture increases activity of pain modulating centers

which produce pain relieving hormones such as beta endorphin, enkephalin, serotonin, and oxytocin. However, needle stimulation of the upper trapezius in healthy controls can also evoke brain activity (Niddam et al 2008). Thus, future studies need to compare the effect of needle stimulation of acupoints with another noxious stimulation on pain modulatory centers in the central nervous system (CNS).

Dry needling has also been shown to have an effect on the CNS. Niddam et al (2008) investigated brain activity in 16 patients with MTPs in the left upper trapezius and 16 healthy controls with event-related fMRI. Electrical stimulation was applied to upper trapezius MTPs in patients and to the same muscle in controls. The patients demonstrated significantly enhanced somatosensory and limbic activity and suppressed right dorsal hippocampal activity compared to controls. The increased brain activity was observed in the same somatosensory regions but not in limbic regions at matched pain intensity. The authors hypothesized that the suppressed hippocampal activity may have been due to secondary stress-related changes in patients with chronic pain. This study confirms that dry needling MTPs activates pain modulatory regions in the CNS. Future studies on MTPs need also to compare dry needling with another noxious stimulus and evaluate the effect on pain modulating centers in the CNS.

Guidelines for dry needling

Dry needling can be applied to deactivate active myofascial trigger points in the cervical or craniomandibular muscles when a patient's headache is reproduced by digital pressure or needling. Dry needling can also be applied to latent MTPs which are tender on palpation. These muscles may include the suboccipital muscles, trapezii, sternocleidomastoid, splenius capitis, masseters, temporalis and occipitofrontalis and are described in Chapter 23. Similarly, if digital pressure or needling of MTPs eases the headaches, DN may be considered as a treatment option. However, MTPs do not occur in isolation and may exist in response to changes in joint mechanics, neurodynamics, localized muscle dysfunction, neurological problems or sinister pathology. Thus, it is important to assess the cause of the MTP and rule out any sinister pathology prior to considering DN.

Dry needling can be applied in patients with an acute or irritable condition when other manual therapy procedures may easily exacerbate the patient's headaches (Selvaratnam & Knight 1995). Needling has been reported to promote analgesia at points distal to the site of stimulation. For instance, if a patient experiences headaches in the temporal region, and they are sensitive to palpation of the temporalis, dry needling can be applied to MTPs in the upper cervical region due to the neural connections of the trigeminocervical nucleus (TCN) (Zhao et al 2005).

Dry needling can be performed in patients with tension headache or cervicogenic headache who have cervical or masseter muscle hypertonicity. Needling is considered to have a local segmental effect by depolarizing large diameter afferents in lamina V of the dorsal horn and thereby inhibiting nociceptive information (Le Bars et al 1983, NHMRC 1989). The segmental effect is postulated to contribute to local analgesia and reduction of muscle hypertonicity. Some experimental evidence supports the analgesic effect of needling anatomical structures which are innervated by the TCN (Zhao et al 2005). Although the exact mechanism is unclear, it is suggested that analgesia could be due to inhibitory effects on the TCN and spinal dorsal horn neuron, central modulation of the spinal dorsal horn neuron, peripheral modulation, or descending inhibitory effects on pain processing

(Zhao et al 2005). Thus, DN can be used in headache sufferers, with muscle guarding or MTPs in the cervical or craniomandibular muscles.

Dry needling may be beneficial in patients with long term headaches when other therapeutic modalities or medication have had limited effects. Needling has neurophysiological effects in the acute and chronic stages of a condition (Selvaratnam & Knight 1995). Acupuncture needling releases opiate peptides such as beta-endorphins, enkephalins and dynorphins. These neurotransmitters block the transmission of pain information (He 1987, Ulett et al 1998). Enkephalins and dynorphins are considered to block nociceptive transmission between primary afferents and the spinal cord neurons and thereby inhibit the experience of pain being activated in the CNS. The descending modulatory pathways may be regulated by beta-endorphins released from the pituitary gland that in turn might prevent impulses reaching the gland and affect the inhibitory impulses from the brain centers. Nalaxone, reduces the effect of acupuncture analgesia suggesting that needling procedures increase endorphin levels (Ulett et al 1998).

Cross perfusion/infusion experiments also indicate that needling has analgesic effects which could benefit headache sufferers. This effect following acupuncture was demonstrated when cerebrospinal fluid (CSF) was transferred from a donor rabbit to a recipient rabbit (Ulett et al 1998). It has also been observed that electroacupuncture induces stronger analgesic effects than needling alone. Release of endorphins in the CSF has been measured after electroacupuncture. High frequency (100 Hz) and low frequency (2 Hz) electroacupuncture are reported to selectively activate the release of enkephalins and dynorphins in animal and human experimental studies (Sluka et al 1998, Ulett et al 1998). Nalaxone prevented electroacupuncture-induced analgesia, inferring that endorphins are involved. These studies further support the concept that needling could provide analgesia to headache sufferers.

Needling and peripheral neural pathways

In the treatment of pain, clinicians can also follow the distribution of the peripheral nerve in the treatment of pain and headache. Stimulation of cutaneous nerve receptors either directly or through palpated tender points or MTPs along the nerve pathway will influence the peripheral nervous system, the spinal cord and thereby the CNS.

For example, in a patient with pain in the distribution of the sciatic nerve, DN can be performed on tender points or MTPs along the buttock or posterior leg (Selvaratnam 2008). Similarly in patients with occipital headache or mandibular pain, DN can be performed in the distribution of the greater occipital nerve or the mandibular branch of the trigeminal nerve (Fig. 24.1) at the palpated tender points or MTPs. It may be argued that the course of the nerves may vary in each patient. However, palpating for tender points along nerve pathways based on evidence-informed neuroanatomy enables clinicians to have an anatomical approach to DN as opposed to adopting TCM principles, which follow energy pathways along meridians which continue to remain elusive and have not been anatomically proven.

The effect of applying dry needling along neural pathways may also be explained by the neurophysiological phenomenon of diffuse noxious inhibitory controls. In this principle, transmission of nociceptive information or headache can be blocked by the application of a second new noxious stimulus along the peripheral

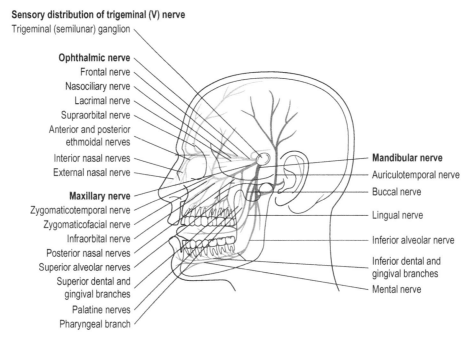

Sensory distribution of trigeminal (V) nerve
Trigeminal (semilunar) ganglion

Ophthalmic nerve
Frontal nerve
Nasociliary nerve
Lacrimal nerve
Supraorbital nerve
Anterior and posterior ethmoidal nerves
Interior nasal nerves
External nasal nerve

Maxillary nerve
Zygomaticotemporal nerve
Zygomaticofacial nerve
Infraorbital nerve
Posterior nasal nerves
Superior alveolar nerves
Superior dental and gingival branches
Palatine nerves
Pharyngeal branch

Mandibular nerve
Auriculotemporal nerve
Buccal nerve
Lingual nerve
Inferior alveolar nerve
Inferior dental and gingival branches
Mental nerve

Figure 24.1 • Distribution of the branches of the trigeminal nerve.

neural pathway which in turn activates brain stem centers and descending modulatory pathways (Le Bars et al 1983, NHMRC 1989, Selvaratnam & Knight 1995). Needling peripheral nerve pathways is also supported by Gunn's (1977a & b) neuropathic model where DN is performed in the dermatomal segment supplied by the peripheral nerve. Similarly, peripheral nerves can be dry needled in the myotomal distribution of the nerve. Following Gunn's model (1977a & b), needling can be performed proximally in tender regions/MTPs supplied by the posterior primary rami and distal regions of the nerve supplied by the anterior primary rami (Gunn 1977a & b).

Contraindications and precautions

Contraindications and precautions must be considered before application of dry needling. Dry needling has no curative effect in headache sufferers with cancer or other malignant disorders but may assist in easing the headache (Jayasuriya 1981). Patients need to be made aware of the non-curative effect of DN to avoid misunderstanding. Secondary effects such as pain and lack of sleep may be safely managed by superficial DN but needling directly into cancerous or malignant tissue must be avoided. Dry needling is also contraindicated when acute medical care is required, such as with a fractured mandible, dislocated temporomandibular joint (TMJ), meningitis, or raised intra-cranial pressure (Jayasuriya 1981).

Practitioners need to take great care needling myofascial trigger points in the upper and middle trapezius muscles (Simons et al 1999). A pneumothorax can occur if the apex of the lung is punctured. It is therefore recommended that, in this region, needles be inserted

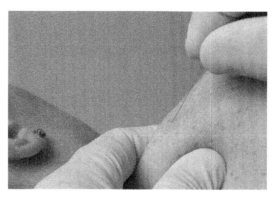

Figure 24.2 • Dry needling the upper trapezius in a posteroanterior and partially cephalad direction.

in a posteroanterior and partially cephalad direction (Fig. 24.2). Needling the thoracic region should be performed superficially in an oblique caudad direction over bony prominences where possible and perpendicular needling avoided. Needling in the vicinity of the carotid and vertebral arteries and the suboccipital region should be performed with consideration to the anatomy of the region and only after considerable experience. It is a generally accepted recommendation to avoid DN to patients who are intoxicated, drug affected, emotional, or overly anxious.

Consideration should be given to patients with hemorrhagic diseases, and those taking anticoagulants, medication for diabetes (there is a possibility of hypoglycemia following acupuncture needling), and hypertension (a sudden fall in blood pressure may be experienced when needling at Liver 3, a point between the 1st and 2nd metatarsal bases) (Jayasuriya 1981).

Patients with a history of rheumatic fever and insufficiency of heart valves should be needled carefully to avoid bleeding and thereby infection. Needling lymphedematous limbs such as after breast surgery may carry added risk of infection, and is therefore contraindicated. Clinicians should consider the use of DN during the first and last trimester of

> **Box 24.1**
>
> **Potential complications of acupuncture and dry needling.**
>
> 1. Vasovagal attacks
> 2. Infection
> 3. Damage to viscera
> 4. Capillary hemorrhage/bruising.
> 5. Post-treatment drowsiness or fatigue
> 6. Allergic reactions including angioedema and hives
> 7. Convulsions
> 8. Sympathetic nervous system activation
> 9. Pneumothorax
>
> (Adapted from: Macpherson et al (2004) and Baldry (2005).)

pregnancy carefully since needling may induce premature delivery. Box 24.1 illustrates some potential complications of acupuncture and DN (Baldry 2005, MacPherson et al 2004).

Management with dry needling

It is essential to take a detailed patient history that includes a subjective and objective examination (Maitland et al 2001). Any pathology requiring urgent medical attention or management must be ruled out. Clinical and neurological examination is important to assess the cause of headaches since MTPs could be secondary to central sensitization, peripheral nervous system involvement, or cervical pathology. Patients with cervical pain, headache, or temporomandibular joint (TMJ) pain need to have a detailed examination of active and passive movements of the cervical spine, the TMJ region (Ch. 19), and associated MTPs. Patients need to be sub-grouped as described in Chapter 19 based on the clinical assessment to provide the best treatment and management

strategy in which the use of needling techniques may form a part.

Patient consent must be obtained prior to needling. The authors recommend that if it is the patient's first needling experience, or in acute conditions, that superficial cutaneous needling be applied to the cervical region without needle stimulation. The needles can be left *in situ* for 5 to 30 minutes depending on the nature of the condition. The procedure can be progressed later to cutaneous stimulation of myofascial trigger points in muscles, tendons, or ligaments for 2 to 5 seconds (Baldry 2005). Cutaneous stimulation can be performed by rotating the needle in a clockwise and/or anti-clockwise direction. The needles can then be left *in situ* for 5 to 30 minutes.

When the patient's condition is slow to respond, deeper stimulation of MTPs can be performed. The depth, duration, and frequency of DN should be considered prior to treatment. The needle can be inserted as a single insertion to deactivate the MTP and then removed. It is important for the clinician to 'feel' the needle penetrating the skin, the subcutaneous tissue, the entrance of the MTP, and the MTP itself.

Deep needling can also be performed to activate a 'twitch' response in the MTP (Brukner & Khan 2006, Huguenin 2004, Simons et al 1999) by inserting the needle and partially releasing it or rotating the needle in a clockwise and/or anti-clockwise direction. Once a twitch response is activated the needle may be left in the patient for 5 to 20 minutes. When dry needling does not produce a twitch response, the trigger point can be deactivated by deep stimulation for 2 to 5 minutes and the needle left *in situ* for 5 to 20 minutes. The patient should be provided with a bell to call for attention if the practitioner is leaving the room, and a timer should be used for the duration of the treatment. At the completion of treatment, the patient should be warned of post-treatment drowsiness and requested to walk for 5 minutes before driving.

Progression of treatment

Treatment progression could include different MTPs in the cervical, cranial (e.g., temporalis, frontalis), or facial region (masseters). Alternatively, treatment can be progressed following the neural pathway of the greater occipital nerve or the maxillary or mandibular branches of the trigeminal nerve. Treatment can also be performed in the dermatomal (Fig. 24.3) and myotomal segmental distribution of the peripheral nerve (Gunn 1977a & b). In some patients electrostimulation of the needles can be performed (Niddam et al 2008).

Thus, the procedure of dry needling patients may need to be sub-grouped according to whether they require needling of MTPs, musculotendinous junctions, ligaments, skin or periosteum. Patients can also be sub-grouped if the condition requires needling along the pathway of the peripheral nerves, the dermatomal or myotomal segments of the nerve. Once this decision has been made, the clinician needs to assess whether DN is to be performed superficially with or without manual stimulation or deep stimulation at the entrance of the MTP or within the MTP. Treatment can be further sub-grouped as to whether electrical stimulation is performed with superficial or deep needling and the frequency that is best for the patient's condition.

The following case study illustrates how dry needling can be applied in the management of headache.

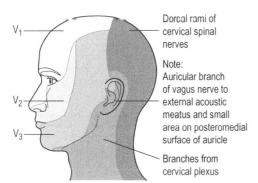

Figure 24.3 • Dermatomal supply of the head, face and upper neck. V1-ophthalmic, V2-maxillary and V3-mandibular branches of the trigeminal nerve.

V1

Dorsal rami of cervical spinal nerves

Note:
Auricular branch of vagus nerve to external acoustic meatus and small area on posteromedial surface of auricle

V2

V3

Branches from cervical plexus

Case study 1

Tilly, a 25-year-old administrator, presented with a 5-year history of frontal, vertex, and occipital headache, described as a 'pressure cooker' sensation. The headache commenced insidiously a month after her father died. The headaches were exacerbated on awakening, while reading with cervical flexion, and by work pressures.

The CT scan of the brain was normal. A neurologist had ruled out sinister pathology and diagnosed 'tension headache'. A dentist had provided an occlusal splint for suspected bruxism but with no effect. Spinal mobilization had been provided by a variety of health professionals. Over-the-counter medication of antidepressants did not benefit her, neither did psychological cognitive counseling. Yoga meditation provided only temporary relief. Tilly reported that she had coped well following her father's death five years previously.

Cervical flexion in the sitting position reproduced her headache, as did palpation of the MTP in the posterior aspect of the temporalis (see Fig. 7.3). In the supine position, palpation of the suboccipital region (bilaterally), and unilateral palpation over the right C2 articular pillar reproduced her headache. The MTP in the right upper trapezius was tender. Manual distraction of the upper cervical region diminished the headache intensity. There were signs of bruxing facets in the lower incisors and interincisor excursion was limited to 33 mm (normal range in women: 35–45 mm).

Clinical reasoning. The clinical impression was that the tension headaches had an affective component due to difficulties in dealing with psychological stressors leading to secondary cervical disorder and temporomandibular disorder (TMD).

Treatment

Treatment 1 (Day 1). Cognitive strategies and progressive muscle relaxation strategies were implemented (Jacobsen 1929). Manual cervical distraction in supine was instituted (7 sec Hold, 3 sec Rest) (Kaltenborn 1970) for 2 minutes. The headache intensity was only minimally reduced.

Treatment 2 (2 weeks later). Tilly reported that headaches continued to be triggered by cervical flexion and work pressures. Postural management was instituted to reduce cervical flexion. Treatment was progressed to sustained pressure to the suboccipital region (bilaterally) in the supine position, followed by the right C2 articular pillar in the prone position for 30 seconds in addition to the intervention of Day 1.

Tilly's headaches were unaltered. Superficial DN (without stimulation) was therefore applied in left side-lying to MTPs that reproduced the headache; the suboccipital region (lateral needle placement, bilaterally) (see Fig. 23.11), over the right C2 articular pillar (superolaterally), and the right temporalis (posteroanteriorly). DN was also applied to the right trapezius (posteroanteriorly and cephalad) (Fig 24.2). Needles were left inserted for 30 minutes.

Treatment 3 (2 weeks later). Tilly reported that the headaches were relieved for 2 days. Manual therapy as per Treatment 2 was continued. Superficial cutaneous stimulation was applied to all the points as per Treatment 2 for 10 seconds. Superficial DN (without stimulation) was also applied to a tender point in the region of the vertex of the head.

Treatment 4 (4 weeks later). Tilly reported that she was headache free for 4 weeks until she had to deal with a work conflict. Psychotherapy was recommended but she was not keen to pursue further psychological management. Intervention as per Treatment 3 was continued and she presented headache-free 4 weeks later. Tilly was examined 6 weeks later and reported that she had not experienced headaches in this period. Intervention as per Treatment 4 was continued.

In summary, Tilly's headache had an affective component with physical manifestation. She had sought medical treatment, psychological counseling, and hands-on treatment from a variety of practitioners. It was hypothesized that DN had an effect on the peripheral and central nervous system to reduce the intensity and frequency of her long-term headaches.

Laser phototherapy

A number of approaches to the management of active MTPs and myofascial pain have been taught in Australian medical and allied health tertiary courses; these include massage, ischemic or acupressure techniques, ice, stretching and low level laser therapy (LLLT) or phototherapy (Laakso et al 2002). Laser is an electrotherapy modality that results in biostimulation of living tissue (Karu 1989). Laser emits photons that are polarized, monochromatic, and colluminated, usually within the range of 623.8 to 904 nm at a power range less than 1W (Gabel 1995).

Indications for laser as an alternative to dry needling and acupuncture

In many countries, including China, Japan, Hungary, and Russia, it is an accepted non-invasive alternative technique to DN – particularly for patients with risk factors such as blood-based conditions including HIV and hepatitis, anxiety, or needle phobia, and with children (Baxter 1994). In several Western countries, including Australia, its use in treating MTPs and acupoints is recognized and documented (Laakso et al 1997) but remains controversial (NHMRC 1994a & b).

Research evidence

The means of action of low level laser therapy and its effectiveness as a legitimate treatment modality is disputed by some western medicine practitioners. Most often this is in response to methodologically flawed studies where subtherapeutic doses have been utilized (Aigner et al 2006, Gur et al 2004). In addition the criteria in some investigations have not excluded patients with concurrent medication, such as cardiac drugs with beta blocker effects or anti-inflammatory medications, that counters the biomodulatory effect of LLLT (Altan et al 2005, Bjordal et al 2001).

It is generally accepted that the effects of LLLT occur through several mechanisms (Bjordal et al 2003) with the primary and essential mechanism being the stimulation of the mitochondrial respiratory chain within cells. This action in turn leads to an increase in cellular ATP and consequently improvement or normalization of cellular activity (Karu 1989, Smith 1990). Further biostimulatory mechanisms are through alteration of the cellular membrane lipid bipolar layer affecting the ion channel activity and viability (Djordjevic 1990, Fenyo 1990), or simply alteration of the cell membrane surface which contributes to strengthening cell to cell contacts (Kubasova et al 1988). Reported systemic effects are hypothesized to occur as a result of endogenous opioid production (Laakso et al 1994), messenger neurotransmitter circulation within the neural axoplasmic flow (Gabel 1997), alterations to neural peripheral and central pathways (Chow et al 2006), and through the changes and modulation of cells and plasma within circulating blood (Samoiliva 2002).

The known action of LLLT stimulating ATP and affecting the cellular membrane would, if one subscribes to the Simons and Travell myofascial trigger point model (Simons et al 1999), explain why LLLT therapy has been found effective as an alternative form of stimulation or deactivation of MTPs (Bjordal et al 2003, Hakguder et al 2003). The effect is a direct bioactivation through the stimulation of local cellular ATP production and changes to the cell membrane that affects the passage of calcium ions. Consequently, LLLT does not require an immediate direct action on the neural tissue to produce its effect. This theory counters reports that LLLT is ineffective at deactivating MTPs as it is athermal with no immediate pain response (Lundeberg et al 1987), and it has no

influence on either A-δ or C-nerve fibers (Jarvis et al 1990). Subsequent research has shown the contrary with neural inhibition and analgesic actions being demonstrated (Chow et al 2006). The theoretical model outlined above supports the role of LLLT in trigger point deactivation and as an effective alternative to DN though the mechanism is quite different.

What type of laser is best?

The initial consideration in using low level laser therapy for MTP deactivation is to ensure that the light source is truly laser and not a Light Emitting Diode (LED) which has limited penetration to only the first few millimeters of the epidermis (Tuner & Hode 2000). Light for the treatment of MTPs must penetrate up to several centimeters if it is to be effective in providing biostimulation of target tissue. The optimal wave length is between 670 and 904 nm, with 830 nm the preferred option due to its reduced absorption by melanin, hemoglobin, and water (Kert & Rose 1989). In addition, the power of the unit in milliwatts must be considered, since higher power means less time required to produce a therapeutic dose and possibly an increased penetration depth. However, excessive power can provide a suboptimal effect and a balance is therefore required (Tuner & Hode 2000). A further consideration is the type of probe; a single probe will provide treatment precision and lower cost compared to most multiple-diode array (cluster) units that treat larger areas using multiple wavelengths and power levels.

Contraindications

Low level laser therapy is contraindicated and should not be applied to malignant tumors, skin infections, severe arterial or venous pathology, or in the area of the pregnant uterus (De Dominico et al 1990, Tuner & Hode 2000). Care must also be taken with eye exposure. The eyes must be protected with appropriate laser-resistant glasses due to the risk of retinal damage.

An excessive dose at the initial treatment may cause a 'treatment effect' which may include provocation of the symptoms, localized throbbing, and discomfort; physical changes to the skin or tissue are extremely rare (Kert and Rose 1989, Tuner & Hode 2000). A 'rule of thumb' for this can be considered as: total dose of 1 joule (J) per kg for a pale skinned patient; and up to 2 J/kg for a dark skinned patient (Baxter 1994, Gabel 1995).

Treatment guidelines

The aim of laser therapy in the treatment of MTPs is to deliver a therapeutic dose to the target tissue. There is general agreement that the desired dose is 4 joules (J) where 1 J = 1 Watt per second (Baxter 1994, Tuner & Hode 2000). Most units have probes that are calibrated in milliWatts (mW), such as a 200 mW or 500 mW probe which would require 5 and 2 seconds respectively to produce 1J.

To deliver the therapeutic dose at the skin, 'incident irradiation' must allow for penetration depth of the light based on wavelength, absorption by surrounding tissue, and the type of tissue it must pass through; tissue with higher vascularity will absorb more light and reduce penetration. A further 'rule of thumb' is that approximately 25% of the initial dose will be present at 5 mm of less vascularized tissue, e.g. skin, ligament, and capsule, with this reducing to around 15–20% with muscle (Gabel 1995, Tuner & Hode 2000). Hence,

to achieve the required dose the 'incident' or skin dose must be increased four-fold for each 0.5 cm or 16-fold for each cm that lies between the probe and the target tissue accounting for probe pressure and depth. For example, superficial areas such as MTPs in occipitalis or temporalis (see Ch. 23) may require 16 J (which would take 80 seconds for a 200 mW probe and 32 seconds for a 500 mW probe) to the skin in a lean, pale-skinned patient, and 32 J in a darker skinned patient.

Deeper structures, such as the TMJ may require 128 J, and the cochlear apparatus of the ear, considered for the treatment of tinnitus, may need up to a 256 J incident dose to provide a 4 J therapeutic dose at the target tissue. Thus, as higher dosage treatments are needed, the treatment time increases significantly and a higher powered (e.g. 500 mW) probe becomes more practical in the clinical setting.

Progression of treatment

Treatment progression should always err on the side of caution with a maximum of approximately 1 J per kg of body weight to a total dose limit of 100 J when commencing therapy. Dose can be increased incrementally by 25–50% based upon body mass and size. For example, a smaller elderly individual with no consequence or negative effects from an initial treatment dose may receive increased doses by 25% from a total of 60 J to 75 J; whereas a rugged, younger, muscular individual could progress by an increase of 50% from 90 J to 135 J (Baxter 1994, Kert & Rose 1989, Tuner & Hode 2000).

The following case study illustrates how LLLT can be applied in the management of headache.

Case study 2

Libby, a 42-year-old mother and supermarket worker, is a light-framed fair-skinned female who was concurrently referred to a physiotherapist and dentist by a medical practitioner with reported bruxism, headache, TMJ pain, abrasion to the molar enamel, and bilateral restriction of cervical rotation. Tenderness was associated with a 'twitch' response and headache reproduction on palpation at the MTPs of the occipitalis, sternocleidomastoid (SCM), and middle trapezius, each being recognized referral sources of cervicogenic headache (Simons et al 1999). The patient was needle phobic with a previous history of Hepatitis C. Some temporary relief was gained from analgesics and prescription anti-inflammatories.

There were no additional confounding factors though specific life stressors relating to family and the construction of a new house were felt to be contributors and responsible for some affective contribution. X-ray and CT scan were both normal with minimal vertebral sclerotic changes noted. Cervical movements were normal apart from bilateral painful restriction of rotation to 30°.

Clinical reasoning The clinical impression was that the headache was of a combined myofascial and joint source which was likely to be perpetuated by the presence of the affective component. The restricted painful rotation range was leading to the three principle overactive muscle groups and subsequent headaches. A treatment plan was developed by the physiotherapist with sequential laser to the MTPs followed by manual therapy to the cervical region and TMJ combined with the initiation of an occlusal splint.

Treatment

Treatment 1 (Day 1). Two primary myofascial trigger points at the occipitalis (see Fig. 23.3) and SCM (see Fig. 7.2) were initially treated using an 810 nm 500 mW single probe gallium aluminium arsenide (GaALAr) diode laser. The less sensitive and deeper occipital MTP was irradiated for 90 seconds (as 1 joule is 1 Watt/second, a 500 mW laser will provide 1 joule in 2 seconds, so the total dose provided was 45 J) and the highly sensitive and superficial sternocleidomastoid MTP was

irradiated for 30 seconds (15 J). The total dose delivered to the patient at the first treatment was 60 J. A review appointment was made for further treatment after two days. A night splint was ordered by the patient's dentist who assessed the patient on the following day.

Treatment 2 (2 days later). The patient reported no adverse effects such as throbbing or aching in the region. Following treatment the headache had temporarily diminished that evening but resumed 36 hours after initial treatment. Cervical range of motion remained restricted, TMJ soreness continued, but the MTPs were reduced in tenderness with no twitch response apart from the mid-trapezius. The night splint was on order.

The doses to the two MTPs were repeated and the mid-trapezius and the TMJ were irradiated at 15 J each; total dose increased by 50% to 90 J. In addition manual therapy was initiated with posterior-anterior mobilization of the upper cervical spine and mobilization of the TMJ. LLLT was continued to the MTPs. Cervical range for rotation, posture, and active upper cervical retraction along with craniocervical flexor exercises (see Ch. 15) were demonstrated as a home program to be performed twice daily, six times per week until symptoms ceased. The exercises were then continued for an additional fortnight on a daily basis.

Treatment 3 (5 days later). The headache, cervical range, and MTP tenderness was improved but the TMJ remained tender. Treatment was continued to the MTP with the same LLLT dosage but the LLLT dosage to the TMJ was increased to 30 J. This treatment was initiated in conjunction with ongoing manual therapy.

Treatments 4 and 5 (8 and 11 days later). Two further treatments were provided over the subsequent week with the same combination of LLLT and manual therapy, with the patient reporting of full cervical range of motion and only mild TMJ and MTP tenderness. The night splint was supplied at the end of the first week and was adjusted by the dentist at the end of the second week with a provisional review in a month. At the final treatment the symptoms were minimal and cervical movements were full range. The patient demonstrated that she was performing the exercise program correctly and her postural control was satisfactory.

This case study illustrates the application of laser for cervical and craniomandibular dysfunction and the benefits of combining LLLT with occlusal therapy and manual therapy to achieve the best outcome for the patient.

Conclusion

Dry needling and low level laser therapy can complement manual therapy, dental, and medical management of patients with headache and TMD. The use of DN and LLLT does not preclude the use of normal clinical protocols such as education and exercises. Regardless of the treatment chosen, it is imperative to remember that MTPs are rarely an isolated phenomenon, and the key to successful long-term outcomes from any treatment regime is a thorough history and clinical examination to confirm the patient's diagnosis and identify precipitating and predisposing factors for each patient.

References

Aigner N, Fialka C, Radda C, Vecsei V 2006 Adjuvant laser acupuncture in the treatment of whiplash injuries: a prospective, randomized placebo-controlled trial. Wien Klin Wochenschr 118:95-99.

Alavi A, Lariccia PJ, Sadek AH et al 1997 Neuroimaging of acupuncture in patients with chronic pain. J Altern Complement Med 3(suppl 1): S47-S53.

Altan L, Bingol U, Aykac M, Yurtkuran M 2005 Investigation of the effect of gaas laser therapy on cervical myofascial pain syndrome. Rheumatol Int 25:23-27.

Audette JF, Binder RA 2003 Acupuncture The management of myofascial pain and headache. Curr Pain Headache Rep 7(5 suppl):395-401.

Baldry PE 1989 Acupuncture, trigger points and musculoskeletal pain. Elsevier, Edinburgh.

Baldry PE 2005 Acupuncture, trigger points and musculoskeletal pain, 2nd edn. Elsevier Churchill Livingstone, Edinburgh.

Baxter GD 1994 Therapeutic lasers. Theory and practice. Churchill Livingstone, Edinburgh.

Berman BM, Lao L, Langenberg P et al 2004 Effectiveness of acupuncture as adjunctive therapy in osteoarthritis of the knee: a randomized, controlled trial. Ann Intern Med 141:901-910.

Bing Z, Villanueva L, Le Bars D 1990 Acupuncture and diffuse noxious inhibitory controls: naloxone-reversible depression of activities of trigeminal convergent neurons. Neuroscience 37(3):809-818.

Birch S 2003 Trigger point: acupuncture point correlations revisited. J Altern Complement Med 9:91-103.

Bjordal JM, Couppe C, Ljunggren AE 2001 Low level laser therapy for tendinopathy. Evidence of a dose response pattern. Physical Therapy Reviews 6:91–99.

Bjordal JM, Couppé C, Chow RT et al 2003 A systematic review of low level laser therapy with location-specific doses for pain from joint disorders. Australian Journal Of Physiotherapy 49:107-116.

Bjordal JM, Lopes-Martins RA, Iversen VV 2006 A randomised, placebo controlled trial of low level laser therapy for activated achilles tendonitis with microdialysis measurement of peritendinous prostaglandin E2 concentrations. Br J Sports Med 40:76-80.

Boucher T, Jennings E, Fitzgerald M 1998 The onset of diffuse noxious inhibitory controls in postnatal rat pups: A C-Fos Study. Neuroscience Lett 257(1):9-12.

Brukner P, Khan K 2006 Clinical sports medicine (3rd edn). Mcgraw-Hill, Sydney.

Ceccherelli F, Rigoni MT, Gagliardi G, Ruzzante L 2002 Comparison between superficial and deep acupuncture in the treatment of lumbar myofascial pain: a double-blind randomized controlled study. Clin J Pain 18:149-153.

Cohen M 2005 (Abstract) Masticatory muscle function and pain. In: Kleinberg I (ed) The 4th International Conference of Orofacial Pain and Temporomandibular Disorders. The Scientific Basis of Clinical Decision Making. August 26-28, 2005. Sydney, Australia. p 21.

Chow R, Heller GZ, Barnsley L 2006 The effect of 300 Mw, 830 nm laser on chronic neck pain: a double-blind, randomized, placebo-controlled study. Pain 124:201-210.

Davies C, Davies A 2006 The trigger point therapy workbook. Your self-treatment guide for pain relief. New Harbinger Publications, Oakland.

De Dominico G, Foord I, Hadley J et al 1990 Clinical standards for the use of electrophysical agents. Australian Journal of Physiotherapy 36:39-49.

Djordjevic Z 1990 Summary of clinical tests done with the bioptron lamp. Bioptron Ag, Monchaltorf, Switzerland.

Dommerholt J, Del Moral OM, Gröbli C 2006 Trigger point dry needling. J Manual Manip Therapy 14 (4):70-87.

Dorsher P 2006 Trigger points and acupoints: anatomic and clinical correlations. Med Acupunct 17 (3):21-25.

Fang JL, Krings T, Weidemann J et al 2004 Functional MRI in healthy subjects during acupuncture: different effects of needle rotation in real and false acupoints. Neuroradiology 46:359-362.

Fenyo M 1990 Theoretical and experimental basis of biostimulation by Bioptron. Bioptron Ag, Monchaltorf, Switzerland.

Furlan AD, Van Tulder MW, Cherkin DC et al 2005 Acupuncture and dry-needling for low back pain. John Wiley, Chichester.

Gabel CP 1995 The effect of LLLT on slow healing wounds and ulcers. Health Sciences, Darwin, Northern Territory.

Gabel CP 1997 LLLT – a proposed mechanism for systemic and latent effects. Laser Therapy 9:53-54.

Griggs GC, Jensen J 2006 Effectiveness of acupuncture for migraine: critical literature review. J Adv Nurs 54:491-501.

Gunn CC 1997a The Gunn approach to the treatment of chronic pain, 2nd edn, Churchill Livingstone, New York.

Gunn CC 1997b Radiculopathic pain: diagnosis, treatment of segmental irritation or sensitization. J Musculoskeletal Pain 5(4):119-134.

Gunn CC, Milbrandt WE, Little AS, Mason KE 1980 Dry needling of muscle motor points for chronic low-back pain: a randomized clinical trail with long-term follow-up. Spine 5:279-291.

Gur A, Sarac AJ, Cevik R et al 2004 Efficacy of 904 nm gallium arsenide low level laser therapy in the management of chronic myofascial pain in the neck: a double-blind and randomized-controlled trial. Lasers Surg Med 35:229-235.

Hakguder A, Birtane M, Gurcan S et al 2003 Efficacy of low level laser therapy in myofascial pain syndrome: an algometric and thermographic evaluation. Lasers Surg Med 33:339-343.

He L 1987 Involvement of endogenous opioid peptides in acupuncture analgesia. Pain 31:99-121.

Hong CZ 2000 Myofascial trigger points: pathophysiology and correlation with acupoints. Acupunct Med 18(1):41-47.

Hsieh J, Tu C, Chen F et al 2001 Activation of the hypothalamus characterizes the acupuncture stimulation at the analgesic point in human: a positron emission tomography study. Neuroscience Letters 307:105-108.

Huguenin LK 2004 Myofascial trigger points: the current evidence. Physical Therapy in Sport 5(1):2-12.

Huguenin L, Brukner PD, Mccrory P et al 2005 Effect of dry needling of gluteal muscles on straight leg raise: a randomised, placebo-controlled, double-blind trial. Br J Sports Med 39:84-90.

Ilbuldu E, Cakmak A, Disci R, Aydin R 2004 Comparison of laser, dry needling, and placebo laser treatments in myofascial pain syndrome. Photomed Laser Surg: 22:306-311.

Ingber RS 1989 Iliopsoas myofascial dysfunction: a treatable cause of 'failed' low back syndrome. Arch Phys Med Rehabil 70:382-386.

Irnich D, Behrens N, Gleditsch J et al 2002 Immediate effects of dry needling and acupuncture at distal points in chronic neck pain: results of a randomised, double blind, sham-controlled crossover trial. Pain 99:83-89.

Itoh K, Katsumi Y, Kitakoji H 2004 Trigger point acupuncture treatment of chronic low back pain in elderly patients: a blinded RCT. Acupunct Med 2(4):170-177.

Jacobsen E 1929 Progressive Relaxation. University of Chicago Press, Chicago.

Jarvis D, Maciver MB, Tanelian DL 1990 Electrophysiologic recording and thermodynamic modeling demonstrate that helium-neon laser irradiation does not affect peripheral a delta-or c-fiber nociceptors. Pain 43:235-242.

Jayasuriya A 1981 Clinical Acupuncture Colombo, The Acupuncture Foundation of Sri Lanka.

Kaltenborn F 1970 Mobilisation of the spinal column. New Zealand University Press, Wellington.

Karu TI 1989 Photobiology of low power laser effects. Health Physics 56:691-704.

Kellgren JH 1938a Observations on referred pain arising from muscle. Clin Sci 3:175-190.

Kellgren JH 1938b A preliminary account of referred pains arising from muscle. Br Med J 1:325-327.

Kert J, Rose L 1989 Clinical laser therapy: low level laser therapy.

Scandinavian Medical Laser Technology, Copenhagen.

Kubasova T, Fenyo M, Somosy Z et al 1988 Investigations on biological effects of polarised light. Photochemistry and Photobiology 48:505-509.

Laakso EL, Cramond T, Richardson C, Galligan JP 1994 Endogenous opioids induced by laser and their effects on pain. Laser Therapy 6:133-142.

Laakso L, Richardson C, Crammond T 1997 Pain scores and side effects in response to low level laser therapy (LLLT) for myofascial myofascial trigger points. Laser Therapy 9:67-72.

Laakso EL, Robertson VJ, Chipchase LS 2002 The place of electrophysical agents in Australian and New Zealand entry-level curricula: is there evidence for their inclusion?. Australian Journal of Physiotherapy 48:251-254.

Langevin HM, Bouffard NA, Badger GJ et al 2006 Subcutaneous tissue fibroblast cytoskeletal remodeling induced by acupuncture: evidence for a mechanotransduction-based mechanism. J Cell Physiol 207:767-774.

Le Bars D, Dickenson AH, Besson JM 1983 Opiate analgesia and descending control systems. In: Bonica JJ, Lindblom V, Iggo A (eds) Advances in pain research therapy. Raven Press, New York.

Lewis T 1938 Suggestions relating to the study of somatic pain. BMJ 1:321-325.

Lewit K 1979 The needle effect in the relief of myofascial pain. Pain 6:83-90.

Lucas KR, Polus BI, Rich PA 2004 Latent myofascial trigger points: their effects on muscle activation and movement efficiency. JBMT 8 (3):160-166.

Lucas 2007 The effects of latent myofascial trigger points on muscle activation patterns during scapular plane elevation. PhD Thesis. Australasian Digital Thesis Network.

Lui WC, Feldman SC, Cook DB et al 2004 Functional MRI study of acupuncture-induced periaqueductal grey activity in humans. Neuroreport 15:1937-1940.

Lundeberg T, Hode L, Zhou J 1987 A comparative study of the pain relieving effect of laser therapy and acupuncture. Acta Physiologica Scandinavia 131:161-162.

MacDonald 1982 Acupuncture from ancient art to modern medicine. Allen and Unwin, London.

Macpherson H, Scullion A, Thomas KJ, Walters S 2004 Patient reports of adverse events associated with acupuncture treatment: a prospective national survey. Quality And Safety In Health Care 13:349-355.

Maitland G, Hengeveld E, Banks K, English K 2001 Maitland's vertebral manipulation. Butterworth-Heinemann, Oxford.

Melchart D, Linde K, Berman B et al 2001 Acupuncture for idiopathic headache. The Cochrane Database of Systematic Reviews. CD001218.

Melzack R, Stillwell DM, Fox EJ 1977 Myofascial trigger points and acupuncture points for pain: correlation and implications. Pain 3:3-23.

NHMRC 1994a A report by The Australian Health Technology Advisory Committee (AHTAC) June 1994. Australian Journal of Science and Medicine In Sport 3:73-76.

NHMRC 1994b Low-power lasers in medicine. A report by The Australian Health Technology Advisory Committee (AHTAC) June 1994. Australian Journal of Science and Medicine in Sport. 3:73-76.

NHMRC 1989 Acupuncture. Canberra, Australia, Australian Government Printing Service.

Niddam DM, Chan RC, Lee SH et al 2008 Central representation of hyperalgesia from myofascial trigger point. Neuroimage 39(3):1299-1306.

Norton N, Carter K, Craig JA, Netter F et al 2006 Netter's head and neck anatomy for dentistry. W B Saunders, Philadelphia.

Samoiliva K 2002 Systemic mechanisms of anti-inflammatory, immunomodulating, and wound healing effects of visible and infrared light. In: Kazuo H (ed) World association of laser therapy (WALT). WALT, Tsukuba, Tokyo Japan.

Selvaratnam PJ, Knight K 1995 Acupuncture. In: Zuluaga et al (eds) Sports physiotherapy applied science and practice. Churchill Livingstone, Edinburgh.

Selvaratnam PJ 2008 Dry needling for physiotherapists. Handbook of the clinical doctorate program in dry needling. University Of Melbourne, School Of Physiotherapy, Department Of Medicine, Dentistry And Health Sciences, Parkville, Victoria, Australia.

Shah JP, Phillips TM, Danoff JV et al 2005 An in-vivo microanalytical technique for measuring the local biochemical milieu of human skeletal muscle. J Appl Physiol 99:1980-1987.

Shah JP, Danoff JV, Desai MJ et al 2008 Biochemicals associated with pain and inflammation are elevated in sites near to and remote from active myofascial trigger points. Arch Phys Med Rehabil 89(1):16-23.

Simons DG, Travell JG 1981 Myofascial trigger points, a possible explanation. Pain 10:106-109.

Simons DG, Travell JG, Simons LS 1999 Myofascial pain and dysfunction: the trigger point manual vol 1, Williams And Wilkins, Baltimore.

Simons DG, Hong CZ, Simons LS 2002 Endplate potentials are common to midfiber myofascial trigger points. Am J Phys Med Rehabil 81(3): 212-222.

Sluka KA, Bailey K, Bogush J et al 1998 Treatment with either high or low frequency TENS reduces the secondary hyperalgesia observed after injection of kaolin and carrageenan into the knee joint. Pain 77:97-102.

Smith KC 1990 Light and life: the photobiological basis of the therapeutic use of radiation from lasers. International Laser Therapy Association Conference, Osaka.

Sood A, Sood R, Bauer BA et al 2005 Cochrane Systematic Reviews In Acupuncture: methodological diversity in database searching.

J Altern Complement Med 11:719-722.

Tong D 2003 Chinese traditions and beliefs. Armour Publishing, Singapore.

Travell JG, Simons DG 1983 Myofascial pain and dysfunction: the trigger point manual. Williams & Wilkins, Baltimore.

Tuner VJ, Hode L 2000 Laser therapy – clinical practice and scientific background. Prima Books, Grangesburg, Sweden.

Uchida S, Kagitani F, Suzuki A et al 2000 Effect of acupuncture-like stimulation on cortical cerebral blood flow in anesthetized rats. Jpn J Physiol 50:495-507.

Ulett GA, Han S, Han J 1998 Electroacupuncture: mechanisms and clinical application. Biol Psychiatry 44:129-138.

Vas J, Perea-Milla E, Mendez C 2005 Acupuncture and rehabilitation of the painful shoulder: study protocol of an ongoing multicentre randomised controlled clinical trial. BMC Complement Altern Med Oct 14, 19.

Vickers AJ, Ellis N, Fisher P et al 2004 Acupuncture for chronic headache in primary care: large, pragmatic, randomised trial. British Medical Journal 328:744-747.

Weiner DK, Schmader KE 2006 Post-herpetic pain: more than sensory neuralgia? Pain Med 7:243-249.

White P, Lewith G, Prescott P, Conway J 2004 Acupuncture versus placebo for the treatment of chronic mechanical neck pain: a randomized, controlled trial. Ann Intern Med 141:911-919.

Young C, Jewell D 2002 Interventions for preventing and treating pelvic and back pain in pregnancy. In (1): Cd001139., C. D. S. R. (Ed.).

Zhao CH, Stillman MJ, Rozen TD 2005 Traditional and evidence-based acupuncture in headache management: theory, mechanism and practice. Headache 45:716-730.

The Feldenkrais Method

Karol Connors, Lisa Campbell and Diana Svendsen

The Feldenkrais Method aims to improve human function using an exploratory motor learning approach. The Method has been found to be effective in the management of conditions such as chronic pain, multiple sclerosis, and non-specific musculoskeletal disorders. In this chapter, the authors, three Feldenkrais practioners who are also physiotherapists, discuss the Feldenkrais Method with reference to headaches and jaw dysfunction.

Moshe Feldenkrais (1904–1984), an Israeli scientist, developed the Feldenkrais Method. He combined his knowledge of mechanics, physics, electrical engineering, neurophysiology and learning theory with his personal experience in martial arts and interest in the human body to develop a unique system of movement education. The Feldenkrais Method is now taught and practiced in many countries, and is overseen by the International Feldenkrais Federation (www.feldenkrais-method.org).

The Feldenkrais Method is considered an education system rather than a therapy aimed at 'curing disease'. It is designed to allow people to learn how to improve the organization and efficiency of their movement and their ability to act out their lives (Feldenkrais 1972). The Method uses an exploratory learning model. People are not asked to imitate movements, but rather are presented with movement 'problems'

and are guided to find 'solutions' which open up new possibilities for movement.

The Feldenkrais Method has been found to be useful in a range of conditions, from a person with multiple sclerosis trying to improve balance (Stephens 2001), to factory workers with neck-shoulder complaints (Lundblad et al 1999). Another study demonstrated its effectiveness in management of chronic pain where participants reported reduced pain for at least a year following completion of a Feldenkrais program (Bearman & Shafarman 1999). Bearman and Shaferman also found that the Medicaid costs for these patients over that year dropped by 40% (1999). Another study found the Feldenkrais Method was at least as effective as conventional physiotherapy for a group of patients with non-specific musculoskeletal disorders (Malmgren Illsson and Branholm 2002). In this chapter the application of the Feldenkrais Method for people with headaches and jaw dysfunction is discussed.

The Feldenkrais Method in practice

The movement exploration sessions may either be one to one with a practitioner involving touch and guided movements (Functional Integration), or as part of a group, where the class is guided verbally through movement sequences (Awareness through Movement). Feldenkrais devised hundreds of these lessons that address all parts of the body in various movement patterns and relate to a wide spectrum of everyday activities.

'Awareness through Movement' lessons

Clients perform movement sequences (lessons) guided by verbal instructions. Lessons can vary in structure, speed, levels of physical exertion and cognitive attention, and in positions used. Some lessons involve small, subtle movements, others larger, more demanding movements and activities such as rolling, or moving between sitting and lying. To maximize learning, it is important for the person to be as comfortable as possible throughout, to have frequent rests, to do the movements slowly, within an easy range, and to pay close attention to how the movement is being performed.

'Functional Integration' lessons

The aim of functional integration is to clarify how the person moves within their comfortable range of movement. Once this is achieved, the practitioner uses subtle techniques to enlarge this range. By staying within the parameters of comfort, the practitioner aims to engage the person's deep attention without triggering protective or pain responses.

This is a 'hands on' process that guides movement through precise touch. The type of touch used in the Feldenkrais Method is distinctive and is used to inform both the practitioner and the client. Through the Feldenkrais practitioner's hands, a silent 'conversation' can take place: 'Can you feel this part of you? Is it easy to move in this direction? What about this direction? What happens if this other part joins in? Let's vary that combination. Now how is that movement? Is it easier than before?'

The Feldenkrais Method and headache

The Feldenkrais practitioner sees headache and bruxism as part of a total psychophysiological behavioral pattern. All people have habitual patterns of using their bodies, and each of which is distinctive and developed over a lifetime. The Feldenkrais Method offers the practitioner a way of perceiving and understanding individuals and their difficulties, limitations, and potential. It provides a framework of movement exploration to allow individuals to become aware of their own patterns, and develop greater choice and possibilities in the way they function.

There are no specific protocols for dealing with headache or any other condition. However, recurring themes that are usually addressed when someone presents with headache include:

- overuse of musculature around neck, jaw and face, shoulder girdle and chest
- increased muscle tone
- lack of support/stability from feet, legs, pelvis and spine
- disturbed breathing patterns including use of accessory inspiratory muscles for stabilization of the head and neck
- restricted head and neck movements and poor coordination between these movements with movements of the thorax and rest of the body
- postural problems, with the head held in uneasy alignment with the rest of the spine, inefficient organization of spinal curves
- undifferentiated movement of the eyes and head.

The case studies below provide examples of applications of the Feldenkrais Method.

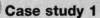
Case study 1

Julie sustained a workplace injury involving soft tissue damage to the neck and shoulder girdle. Her neck/shoulder/jaw pain and headaches persisted despite various treatment interventions. After 18 months, she presented to a Feldenkrais practitioner with severely restricted movement in neck, jaw and shoulder, asymmetric posture, limited function, sleep disruption and increased sympathetic nervous system arousal. There was a strong guarding/anxiety component to her limitations of movement and function and she was unable to work.

The Feldenkrais approach began with helping Julie to recognise the behavioral and movement patterns she had developed, particularly the relationship between movement, pain, thoughts, and emotional responses. Using specific breathing awareness techniques and fully supporting her body in the most comfortable position, gentle movement was begun away from the painful area, to avoid triggering pain and spasms.

Over several sessions, as she learned to move comfortably and safely, her fear of moving her right shoulder, neck, and jaw gradually diminished as muscular co-contraction in this area was reduced. Small, subtle movement patterns were introduced to

this area, avoiding movements that would cause discomfort or anxiety.

Gradually the range and complexity of the Feldenkrais movements was expanded and discrete movements were integrated into 'patterns of movement' that mimicked everyday activities. Activities involving pain-free shoulder elevation, reaching, and turning were incorporated into domestic, personal care and work activities. These integrated movements helped to reduce the bio-mechanical stresses and overload on her injured neck and shoulder girdle. Her headaches and pain gradually reduced in frequency, duration and intensity.

Towards the end of her Feldenkrais treatment program weight-bearing activities were included to provide resistance and graduated strengthening.

Julie attended for 9 months. She regained full independence and eventually resumed full-time work.

Electromyographic (EMG) recordings have been used in clinical and research settings to demonstrate muscle activation patterns. EMG is not a standard part of the Feldenkrais method, but has been used to illustrate the effect of the Feldenkrais Method on Julie's muscle activation (Fig. 25.1a and b).

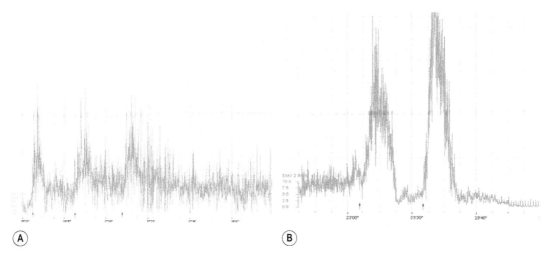

(A) (B)

Figure 25.1 • Surface EMG recordings from right upper trapezius during shoulder shrugging. (X axis: time in minutes and seconds, Y axis: electrical activity in microvolts). Arrows indicate the start of each shrug. (A) Note elevated 'resting' baseline activity, which further increases with each shoulder shrug. (B) Same patient, several sessions later. Activity rises sharply with each shrug, and then falls again to baseline. Patient is now able to reduce muscle activity after each contraction. Note lower baseline of muscle activity after the shoulder shrugs.

Case study 2

Kate was referred by her dentist who noticed her difficulty in holding her mouth open for dental procedures. She had also been suffering headaches and pain around the jaw and face. An occlusal splint had not been successful in reducing teeth grinding at night.

The Feldenkrais practitioner began by exploring in detail the patterns of available movement in the jaw, neck, and tongue and helped Kate to become aware of these. By introducing unusual, non-habitual movements to this area (as demonstrated in Fig. 25.2),

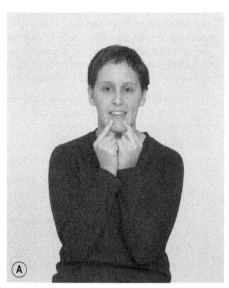
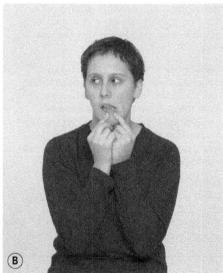
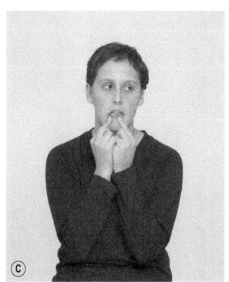

Figure 25.2 • Jaw lesson in sitting. Moving the skull on the mandible (a novel, non-habitual movement). The client stabilizes the jaw between the thumb and fingers (A), and gently moves the head from right (B) to left (C). By reversing the usual relationship between the jaw and the skull, a new neuromuscular organization is introduced.

Kate's habitual neuromuscular patterns were bypassed to create new opportunities for freer, more comfortable mouth opening and neck movement.

Attention was then expanded to include her sitting and standing posture. Anterior and posterior pelvic tilt movements were used to change the position of the chest and head to allow the mandible to hang more comfortably in the fossae. She was also able to feel her pelvis supporting her body weight, and the internal support of her skeletal structure, which enabled her head to feel more balanced and supported.

After two sessions her pain had resolved, but she was keen to continue for several more sessions, to understand her movement and postural patterns, aiming to prevent recurrence. Over this time she also came to understand the link between her compulsive 'overthinking' (worrying, catastrophizing, procrastinating) and her compulsive excessive muscle activity in the musculature around her neck and mouth; she learnt to modify both her thinking and movement behaviors.

How does the Feldenkrais Method work?

The Feldenkrais Method is not simply a series of techniques, but a multi dimensional approach to working with clients (Box 25.1). This section introduces some of the principles of the Method and discusses the theory underlying these principles.

Altering habitual movement patterns

All people adopt movement habits that become entrenched over time. Each person's movement is as individual as their fingerprint or, as expressed through movement, in their handwriting or gait pattern. Some habits serve us well, but others do not. The Feldenkrais Method assists the individual to develop new movement patterns that over-ride engrained motor habits that are no longer beneficial.

Dynamic systems thinking is useful for understanding concepts concerned with changing how we move, as all movement is described as 'emergent' – not set in fixed patterns, but the product of an organism's response at any moment in time (Thelen & Smith 1996). Movement emerges from an interaction between the individual, the task and the environment (Shumway-Cook & Woollacott 2001). The Feldenkrais Method manipulates these three factors to produce new movements – novel movements that bypass a person's habitual patterns and defenses. From these novel movements, the person may find an easier way to perform an action or function that has previously been difficult. Butler, who has studied clients with chronic pain, describes, 'Movements that are feared, avoided and context dependent will have to be presented to the brain in different ways...' (Butler 2000 p. 37). This can be illustrated by an example of a lesson that helped Kate, who experienced pain and tension in her jaw, improve movement of this area (Fig. 25.2).

Box 25.1

Features of the Feldenkrais Method

- Is an education system, not a therapy
- Develops awareness of how we move
- Uses an exploratory learning approach
- Engages the whole skeleton in movement
- Spreads effort throughout the whole body
- Shifts the focus away from pain
- Uses neurodevelopmental movement sequences
- Understands that emotions are embodied in movement
- Changes muscle activation patterns
- Alters habitual movement patterns

Changing muscle activation patterns (neural plasticity)

The Feldenkrais Method aims to allow a person to move more easily by improving the ability of the agonists and antagonists to work together. Tight muscles are seen as a consequence of the ongoing functioning of the nervous system rather than the cause of the problem (Goldfarb 1994). The problem is not at the level of the muscles in the neck or the jaw, but in the brain – in the body schemata there that we operate from. It is our self image in the brain's motor control system which holds the key to easier movement. Recent neuroscience is confirming that the brain does change in response to experience and training. Learning and experience can alter cortical sensory and motor maps (Bayona et al 2005). It is at this level that the Feldenkrais Method attempts to influence.

The movement lessons enable the self image, as represented in the brain, to be modified by expanding the person's body awareness away from the painful areas. These ideas of neural plasticity are similar to those proposed by Butler in his explanations of central sensitization as the cause for chronic pain (Butler 2000).

Developing body awareness

It is essential that the individual improve self-awareness so that they may be able to understand their habitual movement patterns and muscle over-activity. This muscle over-activity may contribute to ischemic nociceptive pain, which can be a major contributor to a person's pain experience (Butler 2000). They must learn to feel/sense what it is that they are doing when they are attempting certain movements or performing activities. For example a person with symptoms around the jaw frequently is not be able to discriminate fine movements of the temperomandibular joints and they may be unaware that they are

clenching their teeth. Lessons directed to the region of the jaw are often aimed at giving the person an experience of 'softer' jaw musculature that they can then incorporate into everyday function.

Engaging the whole skeleton

Another key feature of the Feldenkrais Method is the relationship of each part of the body to the whole. From his martial arts background, Feldenkrais understood that power and efficiency in movement demand that the whole body is engaged in every activity. Lessons are designed to assist the individual to engage the whole skeleton in each movement, resulting in greater efficiency of movement and reduced stress on individual body parts.

A common problem experienced by people with headaches is over-activity of the cervical region and under-activity in the thoracic region (slump posture) (Fig. 25.3a). This places excessive strain on the neck and can contribute to headache. Through Feldenkrais lessons, the individual learns to engage more of their trunk in movement, to spread the load across more of the body and reduce stress on the neck and shoulder girdle (Fig. 25.3b).

Understanding emotions and movement

There is a growing understanding that the whole brain acts as an integrated system (Butler 2000, Carter 2002, Damasio 2003). Feldenkrais proposed that thinking/feeling/sensing and moving were completely integrated, simultaneous events (Feldenkrais 1972). Recent neuroscience research has shown that an individual's emotional state will influence their movement (Berthoz 2000), and that thoughts can alter perception (Damasio 2003).

The emotional context is considered as the Feldenkrais practitioner assists the individual

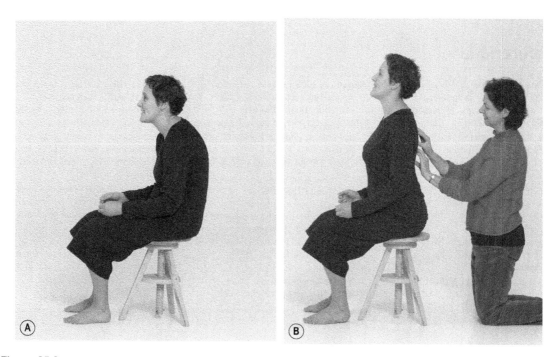

Figure 25.3 • Normalizing cervical and thoracic activity. (A) The slump position places excessive strain on the neck. (B) The Feldenkrais practitioner makes contact with the client's thoracic spine, as she looks up. The physical contact brings her attention to this area, which is habitually held in flexion, and facilitates movement in this part of her spine.

to explore movement. It is not the Feldenkrais practitioner's role to provide counseling, but often the individual may be led to make discoveries about these matters as they allow themselves to explore their movement, and indeed themselves, in a sensitive way in a supportive, non judgmental environment.

These discoveries can result in shifts in understanding about how a habitual emotional response is related to a habitual movement response (e.g. grinding teeth in certain stressful situations). Sometimes the movement response is easier to detect than the emotional feeling, so the person can learn to start to read their emotions by tracking their movements. Once the person can identify these habitual responses, and they have learnt other options for responding, their sense of control can improve.

Conclusion

In cases of headache and jaw problems, the Feldenkrais Method offers an approach that can be useful on its own or as part of a multidisciplinary team approach to treatment. It is particularly valuable in cases where: there are associated postural disturbances; movement dysfunctions are present; strong guarding/protective muscle activity is present; or there appears to be an emotional component to the physical presentation. Practitioners of the Feldenkrais Method seek to be aware of the person as a whole and to recognize that people presenting with pain or discomfort present with behavioral patterns that have developed in response to lifetime experiences. Some of these patterns will probably be contributing to the person's difficulties. Intervention is directed towards changing these patterns through a process of deep experiential learning.

References

Bayona N, Bitensky J, Teasell R et al 2005 Plasticity and reorganisation of the uninjured brain. Topics in Stroke Rehabilitation 12(3):1-10.

Bearman D, Shafarman S 1999 The Feldenkrais Method in the treatment of chronic pain: a study of efficacy and cost effectiveness. American Journal of Pain Management 9:22-27.

Berthoz A 2000 The brain's sense of movement. Harvard University Press, USA.

Butler D 2000 The sensitive nervous system. Noigroup Publications, Australia.

Carter R 2002 Mapping the mind, 2nd edn Orion Books Ltd, London.

Damasio A 2003 Looking for Spinoza: joy, sorrow and the feeling brain. Hartcourt Books, Florida.

Feldenkrais M 1972 Awareness through movement. Penguin Books, Great Britain.

Goldfarb L 1994 Why robots fall down. Feldenkrais Journal 19:5-14, p 11.

Lundblad et al 1999 RCT of physiotherapy and Feldenkrais interventions in female workers with neck-shoulder complaints Journal of Occupational Rehabilitation 19(3):179-94.

Malmgren-Illssen E, Branholm I 2002 A comparison between three physiotherapy approaches with regard to health-related factors in patients with non-specific musculoskeletal disorders. Disability and Rehab 24(6);308-317.

Shumway-Cook A, Woollacott M 2001 Motor control: theory and practical applications, 2nd edn. Lippincott Williams & Wilkins, USA.

Stephens J (ed) 2001 Research studies compilation (revised). Feldenkrais Educational Foundation of North America, USA.

Thelen E, Smith L 1996 Dynamic systems theory and the development of cognition and action. MIT Press, USA.

26

Botox injections

Robert Delcanho

Botox injections have been controversial in the management of headache and temporomandibular disorders. In this chapter the author, a dental practitioner, discusses the indications for and effects of Botox injections and those patient groups likely to benefit.

The anaerobic bacterium *Clostridium botulinum* was once best known as a cause of severe food poisoning associated with rapid onset paralysis and respiratory arrest. In the 1920s, the exotoxins produced by the bacteria were isolated and demonstrated to cause muscle paralysis by blocking the release of acetylcholine from motor nerve endings. With the passage of time, seven separate serotypes of botulinum neurotoxins (A–G) have been identified with all serotypes blocking acetylcholine release but varying in their potency and other biological properties. Some serotypes have been purified and developed for therapeutic injections into hyperactive muscles. Botulinum neurotoxin-A (BoNT-A) is the most widely used in clinical practice and is considered the most potent. Since the 1980s, the highly specific cholinergic neuromuscular blocking action of BoNT has been utilized to treat an increasing number of conditions involving involuntary or unwanted muscle contractions. In 1989, a commercial BoNT-A preparation, Botox was approved by the US FDA for use in strabismus and blepharospasm. Further clinical applications including spasmodic torticollis and cervical dystonia were approved in 2000. Neurologists have also effectively used BoNT to treat spasticity, focal dystonias and tremor where, in addition to the muscle relaxant action, some analgesic effects were noted. In cosmetic medicine, BoNT has gained wide acceptance for treatment of facial wrinkles such as crow's feet and forehead lines. It was from such a group of patients that in 2000 Binder et al (2000a) published an open label study of the quite serendipitous finding of the beneficial effects of BoNT injections in the brow upon migraine headaches. Since that time, there has been a growing evidence base on the analgesic effects of BoNT in other primary headache disorders such as chronic tension-type headache and chronic daily headache. Additionally, BoNT-A has been studied in the treatment of other painful conditions including myofascial pain, fibromyalgia, low back pain, and post herpetic neuralgia. In the orofacial region, BoNT has also been used to help treat primary and secondary masticatory and facial muscle spasm, chronic myogenous facial pain, temporomandibular disorders (TMD), severe bruxism, facial tics, orofacial dyskinesias/dystonias, and idiopathic hypertrophy of the masticatory muscles (Clark 2003).

This chapter reviews the clinical use of BoNT including mode of action and clinical protocol(s). The current literature relating to the use of BoNT in treating primary headache conditions and other facial pain disorders is also reviewed.

Mechanism of action

Clostridium botulinum type A neurotoxin protein comprises a 100 kD heavy chain disulphide linked to a 50 kD light chain peptide. The heavy chain binds with high affinity and specificity to the presynaptic membrane of the neuromuscular junction. The light chain becomes internalised and cleaves an intracellular protein SNAP-25, which is involved in the exocytosis of the neurotransmitter acetylcholine. This inhibits acetylcholine release from vesicles at the neuromuscular junction which in turn prevents muscle contraction of the muscle fibers associated with that motor unit. Restoration of muscle action occurs due to sprouting of additional motor end plates and recovery of the neurotoxin affected nerve terminal. It appears to take about six months for full recovery of muscle function to occur (Brin 1997). More recently it has been established that autonomic nerves are also affected by BoNT causing an inhibition of acetylcholine release in glands and smooth muscle (Bhidayasiri & Truong 2005).

An analgesic effect of BoNT-A was noted early in patients treated for dystonia and spasticity. Although reduction of muscle hyperactivity through inhibition of activity at the neuromuscular junction may alleviate some of the pain associated with these conditions, it does not fully explain the analgesic actions of BoNT-A,

particularly in headaches. An increasing body of scientific data suggests that the analgesic effects of BoNT-A may be mediated by neural mechanisms rather than muscle paralysis. For example, as BoNT-A does not cross the blood–brainbarrier and is inactivated during its retrograde axonal transport, any analgesic effect is likely mediated by first order sensory neurons rather than by central mechanisms (Dressler et al 2005). Other research data suggest that BoNT-A may inhibit the release and block antidromic flow of glutamate, substance P and calcitonin gene related peptide (CGRP) from trigeminal nociceptive primary afferent neurons (Aoki 2003, Durham et al 2004). Theoretically, this could result in a decrease in peripheral sensitization of nociceptive fibers, thereby indirectly reducing central sensitization. A beneficial effect of BoNT-A may be through blocking stimulated CGRP release from sensory ganglionic neurons (Fielder & Durham 2003).

The antinociceptive effect of BoNT-A was examined using a rat model of carrageenan (1%) and capsaicin (0.1%) induced paw pain (Bach-Rojecky & Lackovic 2005). The study reported the mechanical and thermal responses to BoNT-A (5 U/kg) applied either 6 days or 1 day before irritant carrageenan or capsaicin injections into rat paws. The injection given 6 days prior significantly reduced or abolished the enhanced sensitivity to mechanical and thermal stimuli caused by injection of the irritants. BoNT-A has also been demonstrated to reduce wide dynamic range neuronal firing within the dorsal horn of the spinal cord and reduce activity of central nociceptive neurons as measured by decreased c-fos expression after stimulation of nociceptors (Cui et al 2004). Oshinsky et al (2004) found peripheral application of BoNT-A prevented both central sensitization and increased cutaneous receptive fields of second order neurons in rat trigeminal nucleus caudalis whilst Cui and co-workers

(2004) demonstrated that BoNT-A resulted in reduced firing of wide dynamic range neurons in spinal nerves. BoNT was also found to block sensitization and expansion of receptive fields of wide dynamic range neurons.

Clinical procedures

Training in the use of BoNT-A usually occurs at short courses or workshops offered under the direction of an experienced practitioner, under the auspices of the manufacturer. It is strongly recommended that prospective users undergo appropriate training that includes local anatomy, injection techniques, handling of the materials, appropriate dosing, side effects, complications, and follow-up procedures. As for any procedure involving injection of medications, it is strongly recommended that, before proceeding, a qualified healthcare professional thoroughly reviews the procedure with the patient, including a discussion of the indications, expectations, post injection instructions, known side effects and expected duration of the treatment. It is also recommended that a signed informed consent be obtained from the patient.

Available preparations

BoNT-A is manufactured in the US as Botox purified neurotoxin complex. This agent is supplied within glass vials in sterile, vacuum dried white powder form for reconstitution. Each vial contains 100 units (U) of Clostridium botulinum toxin type A with an expiration date of 24 months when stored at −5° to −20°C. Another BoNT-A formulation, Dysport, is marketed outside of the US. It should be noted that the various BoNT-A preparations, Botox, and Dysport differ in formulation, potency and side effect profile, hence, their dosage

units cannot be used interchangeably. Another serotype, BoNT-B, marketed as Myobloc also has different dosage units.

Technique

The vial of 100U powdered BoNT-A is kept refrigerated until use and normal saline (preservative-free 0.9% sterile saline solution) is used to reconstitute the neurotoxin for injection. The dilution method should follow the manufacturer's guidelines for Botox and MyoBloc. The author dilutes 100 units Botox by injecting 4ml of saline into the vial which results in 2.5 units Botox per 0.1 ml solution. The solution is then drawn up into a calibrated 1.0 ml tuberculin syringe to which a 26–30 gauge needle is attached. Once prepared, the solution should be used within 4 hours although recent data suggest that refrigerated, reconstituted BoNT-A can be used as long as six weeks later without loss of efficacy (Hexsel et al 2003). Skin preparation involves alcohol wipes and dry sterile gauze sponges. Once the skin has been prepared, the planned injection site should not be touched. Aspiration before injection is mandatory.

In the orofacial area, the frontalis, procerus, corrugators, temporalis and masseter muscles are most frequently injected. These muscles should be injected bilaterally to minimize the risk of asymmetrical cosmetically undesirable side effects. The dose at each site into these smaller muscles is usually between 5 and 10 units. Other muscles which are frequently injected for headaches include the suboccipital, sternomastoid, splenius capitis and trapczius. The reader is referred to standard anatomy textbooks and reference anatomical material made available by the BoNT manufacturers.

Appropriate selection and accurate targeting of muscles is a crucial factor in achieving efficacy and reducing untoward effects from

BoNT-A injections. A 26 to 30 gauge needle is usually placed subdermally or into the target muscle. In the orofacial region, the target muscles are quite superficial and can usually be identified by asking the patient to frown, grimace, or clench the teeth. In the larger jaw, neck, and shoulder girdle muscles, the patient is asked to contract the muscle by the appropriate action as the muscle is palpated manually. Where it is wished to inject certain deeper muscles that are difficult or impossible to palpate, for example lateral pterygoid muscle, correct needle position before injection can be confirmed by use of a monopolar injection needle that also has the ability to record the electromyographic (EMG) signal from the muscle. By following meticulous injection technique and asking patients not to massage the area for 4 hours, the risk of BoNT-A dispersion through tissue into adjacent sites can be minimized. This will also allow the toxin to penetrate the target nerves. It is also recommended that the patient restrict physical activity to minimum for 24–48 hours.

Injection paradigms

For the treatment of headache with BoNT-A, two separate injection paradigms have been suggested (Blumenfeld 2003). The first is the so-called 'Fixed Site' approach whereby the injection sites are predetermined. The second is the 'Follow-the-Pain' approach whereby injections are made into the regions where the patient reports pain and tenderness. To date, most of the published studies looking at the use of BoNT-A in headache have utilized a fixed site approach, however the studies have varied widely in terms of parameters such as injection sites, number of units per site of injection, dilution of neurotoxin and total administered neurotoxin dose. Neither paradigm has been proven scientifically to be superior to the other.

A recent study found fixed-site injections into the glabellar muscles alone was no less effective in reducing migraine headaches than the higher dose, multi-site follow-the-pain approach (Bechmand et al 2003). Theoretically, however, to facilitate wider delivery of BoNT-A to peripheral trigeminal nerve terminals, it may be more appropriate to inject a greater number of sites with smaller doses. Intuitively, however, one would suspect that increasing the number of injection sites would not only be more painful for the patient but would also increase the risk of undesirable cosmetic side effects such as drooping of the brow or ptosis. Further studies are required to identify which groups of headache patients are most likely to respond to the various injection paradigms as well as to identify optimal dosing and injection sites. Additionally, some data suggest that chronic headache patients who receive a repeat BoNT-A administration report better improvement than patients who only received a single appointment of injections (Ondo et al 2002).

Effect duration

The US FDA recommends that injections be no more frequent than once every 3 months, and to use the lowest effective dose. A small group of patients who receive multiple injections may over time develop antibodies to BoNT-A that may reduce its effect by inactivating the biological activity of the toxin. In 2000, the US FDA approved Myobloc (BoNT-B) for the treatment of cervical dystonia for patients who developed BoNT-A resistance. A recently reformulated Botox preparation has a lower protein content that may decrease the risk of antibody formation and the development of resistance. It appears that the risk for antibody formation can be reduced by using the lowest effective dose of BoNT-A at less frequent intervals. Following injection, the therapeutic effects first appear in 1–3 days, peak in 1–4 weeks, and decline after 3–4 months. Pharmacokinetic studies in rats suggest rapid systemic metabolism and total excretion of the neurotoxin itself within 2–3 days.

Adverse events and side effects

Most published trials have reported minimal and transient adverse events which have included blepharoptosis, diplopia, and injection site weakness. The most common side effects include local injection site discomfort and bruising. Transient facial muscle weakness causing brow ptosis, particularly if asymmetrical, can cause cosmetic concerns. No long term systemic safety problems have been reported with BoNT-A treatment. Botox is classified as a Category C drug by the US FDA due to lack of experience with pregnant and lactating women and should probably be avoided in that group. Approximately 1% of patients receiving BoNT-A injections may experience severe, debilitating headaches which may last for 2–4 weeks before gradually fading.

Cautions and contraindications

BoNT-A treatment is contraindicated in the presence of infection at the injection site(s) and in individuals with myasthenia gravis, Eton Lambert Syndrome, or known hypersensitivity to any ingredient in the formulation. Individuals with peripheral motor neuropathic diseases or neuromuscular junctional disorders should receive BoNT-A treatment with caution. Drugs that interfere with neuromuscular transmission, such as aminoglycoside antibiotics, polymyxins, tetracyclines and tubocurarine-type muscle relaxants, can potentiate the effect of BoNT-A. Patients who have injections in the cervical region, tongue, or posterior region of the mouth with BoNT-A can experience dysphagia. Cardiac

arrhythmia and myocardial infarction have rarely been reported. Some of these patients had pre-existing cardiovascular disease. As mentioned above, administration is not recommended during pregnancy or lactation. Caution is advised if injecting patients with excessive atrophy or weakness in target muscle, ptosis, deep dermal scarring, thick sebaceous skin, marked facial asymmetry, and inflammatory skin disorders at the planned injection site.

Botulinum neurotoxin use in primary headache

Migraine

Migraine is a chronic neurovascular disorder characterized by recurrent episodes of headache, nausea, aura, and sensory disturbances. Migraine affects approximately 10% of the population (6% females and 4% males) with attacks causing significant impact upon the individual's function and quality of life. There is a concomitant heavy personal and societal burden including loss of earnings and productivity (Lipton & Bigal 2005).

The pathophysiology of migraine has been recently reviewed (Goadsby 2005) and appears to involve the trigeminovascular system and central nervous system modulation of the nociceptive signals emanating from the pain-producing intracranial structures. The relative degree to which pain is caused directly by activation of nociceptors within pain sensitive intracranial structures, or the more indirect centrally mediated facilitation (or lack of inhibition) of the afferent signals, is not clear at this time.

Unfortunately, to date the acute and prophylactic medications used to reduce migraine attacks are not totally effective and in general are poorly tolerated. Moderate to severe side effects are common with the available prophylactic medications, and clinicians treating headaches require improved and novel prophylactic agents in particular. The first double blinded placebo controlled study of Botox in episodic migraine was by Silberstein et al (Silberstein et al 2000). In this study 123 patients with a mean 4–5 moderate to severe migraine attacks per month were assigned to receive placebo, Botox 25 units, or Botox 75 units in a fixed dose, fixed site approach. Four injections were made into frontalis muscle: two into the corrugators, and one each into the procerus and temporalis muscles. There was a statistically significant reduction in the primary end point of moderate to severe attack frequency per month in months 2 and 3 in the Botox 25 unit group but, surprisingly, not in the Botox 75 unit group. The Botox 25 units group also demonstrated reduced maximum severity of migraines, a reduced number of days using acute migraine medications, and reduced incidence of migraine-associated vomiting. The Botox was very well tolerated although the 75 unit group had significantly more adverse events than the placebo group.

Several studies have since concluded that BoNT-A is an effective and safe prophylactic treatment for migraine headache across a range of patient types (Barrientos et al 2003, Binder et al 2000, Blumenfeld et al 2004). Barrientos studied 30 patients with episodic migraine (Barrientos et al 2002). A fixed dose, fixed site total 50 units of Botox was injected into temporalis (2 sites), frontalis (4), glabellar (4), procerus (1), trapezius (2) and splenius capitis (2). Statistically significant reductions were seen in the number of migraine attacks per month at 30, 60, and 90 days and the overall 90 day migraine attack frequency was reduced in the Botox group when compared to the placebo group. Similarly, migraine duration was significantly reduced. The amount of acute

medication use and subject/investigator global assessments were significantly superior in the Botox versus the placebo groups. The Botox was well tolerated with only one of the 30 patients developing frontalis asymmetry that lasted about 30 days.

By contrast, Evers et al (2004), in a randomized double blinded placebo controlled study, did not find any statistically significant effect on migraine frequency or severity following injection of two different doses of Botox. Sixty patients were separated into 4 groups receiving a total of 100 units into various frontal and neck muscles, 16 units into the frontal muscles alone, or placebo saline into either all the muscles or just neck muscles. For analysis, the primary treatment outcome parameter was 50% reduction in frequency of migraine attacks at 3 months compared to the month preceding the injections. Other parameters included migraine frequency, number of days with moderate to severe pain, reduction of associated symptoms and reduction of acute medication use. Both groups that received the Botox injections achieved a 30% reduction of migraine frequency; however, the placebo group achieved a 25% reduction. No significant differences were found between the groups with respect to number of days with migraine, number of days with moderate to severe migraine or amount of acute drugs taken to treat the migraine attacks. No serious adverse events were noted and any that occurred were considered mild and transient.

Similarly, two recently published studies looking at the use of BoNT-A for episodic migraine (Aurora et al 2005, Relja et al 2005) failed to find significant differences between Botox injected and placebo saline injected groups in either frequency of migraine attacks per 30 day period, or percentage of patients with 50% or greater decrease in migraine headaches.

Two recent reviews of the literature have summarized the data on BoNT-A for migraine prophylaxis (Evers et al 2006, Gobel 2004). Almost all double blind, placebo-controlled trials had statistically insignificant findings as far as primary outcome for episodic migraine is concerned. However, it remains uncertain whether BoNT-A has a role in severely affected patients with frequent chronic migraine headaches. It appears that BoNT-A is effective in certain individuals to reduce the frequency, severity, and disability associated with migraine headaches. In the author's opinion, BoNT-A should therefore be considered another tool to be utilized in migraine patients unresponsive to other treatments, where the other treatments are contraindicated or where concomitant jaw or neck muscle spasm is identified.

Tension-type headache

Although one would suspect that BoNT-A injections would most likely benefit those headaches where pericranial muscle contractions or increased muscular tension were traditionally felt to be a primary contributory factor, studies looking at the effects of BoNT-A injections in tension-type headache (TTH) patients have been equivocal finding less effect than that found for migraine headaches. Padberg et al (2004) studied 40 patients with TTH and over a 12 week period no significant differences were found between a control group (n = 21) who received saline and a group of 19 patients who received a total of up to 100 U Botox (1 unit per kg) in various pericranial and neck muscles (10 20 units per muscle) that exhibited clinically increased muscle tone or tenderness. Some patients responded well, raising the possibility that there is a subgroup of chronic TTH sufferers who do indeed respond to BoNT-A injections. The authors concluded that further studies

are required to attempt to elucidate that subgroup.

An earlier study (Rollnick et al 2000) failed to find any significant differences between a treatment and control group of 21 episodic (majority) and chronic TTH patients. On the basis of the results the authors hypothesized that increased muscle tenderness may not play a major role in the pathophysiology of TTH. More recent randomized double blinded placebo controlled studies (Boudreau 2005, Relja & Telarovic 2004, Schulte-Mattler & Krack 2004) have been published comparing BoNT-A to placebo injections in TTH sufferers, with no significant differences being found for most outcome variables. The authors concluded that there is no clinically significant effect of BoNT-A on chronic tension-type headache.

It has been postulated that TTH sufferers may have a lesser degree of central sensitization than that which occurs in migraine sufferers. As a result, the development of scalp cutaneous allodynia found in migraine attacks (Burstein et al 2004) is absent or not as evident in TTH. If central sensitization is mediated by CGRP and glutamate, the central release of which has been demonstrated to be affected by BoNT-A, then this may explain the relative lack of response to BoNT-A in TTH.

Chronic daily headache

The term chronic daily headache (CDH) now refers to headaches experienced 15 or more days per month. Primary CDH is not related to structural or systemic illness whilst secondary CDH has an identifiable underlying cause, including medication overuse, intracranial disorders, idiopathic intracranial hypertension, cervical spinal disorders, and temporomandibular disorders. Primary CDH is by far the more common, with prevalence studies consistently finding about 4%

of the adult population are affected, it being twice as common in women as men (Scher et al 2005). CDH, in particular with a pre-existing history of migraine and associated with over use of medication, accounts for the majority of headaches seen in headache sub-specialty practices (Silberstein et al 1994). Open trials and placebo controlled trials have suggested that CDH may improve following injections of BoNT-A. Whether this is due to muscle paralysis or possible effects on peripheral and central nerve function is uncertain. Mauskop (1999) used 50–100 units to treat 12 refractory CDH patients who overused medication almost daily. Only one patient obtained good relief and had repeated injections. It was felt that the overuse of medications on a daily basis could explain the lack of effect and suggests that successful outcome of treatment in this group of patients is dependent on reducing their reliance on daily abortive type medications.

Eross and Dodick (2002) evaluated the effects of Botox injections (25–100 U) on reducing disability in 47 patients with either episodic or chronic migraine. Using a well-validated migraine-related disability tool (MIDAS), 58% of all patients reported reduced migraine associated disability; 75% of the episodic migraine patients (n = 12) reported reduced migraine frequency as compared to 53% of the chronic migraine group. Ondo and Derman (2002) conducted a randomized double blind placebo-controlled parallel clinical trial that examined the effect of BoNT-A treatment (200U or placebo) on patients with CDH, including chronic TTH and transformed migraine. The 'follow the pain' protocol was used and at 12 weeks a second open label injection of BoNT-A was provided. Following the first injection, patients treated with BoNT-A had significantly fewer headaches between weeks 8 and 12 compared to those injected with placebo.

Subjectively, 10% of patients in the BoNT-A group reported dramatic improvement and 24% reported marked improvement compared with 3% and 7% respectively in the placebo group.

Mathew and colleagues (2002) conducted a randomized double blind placebo controlled, parallel group clinical trial involving 355 patients suffering CDH. Although the primary outcome measure (change from baseline in number of headache-free days) did not reach statistical significance, the study demonstrated that BoNT-A, as compared to placebo, significantly reduced the frequency of headache episodes in migraine/CDH patients with a 50% plus decrease in headache days per month. A further subgroup analysis of patients not receiving other prophylactic medications to treat their chronic daily headaches, found even greater differences in key measures of efficacy in favour of treatment with BoNT-A compared to placebo (Dodick et al 2005). Indeed it is becoming apparent that BoNT-A may be most efficacious in the population of quite disabled and complicated headache sufferers. Phase III studies are now under way, as significant insights were gained from the earlier studies.

Temporomandibular disorders

There is currently a lack of any large scale controlled studies on the effects of BoNT-A injections on signs and symptoms of the various temporomandibular disorders (TMD). BoNT-A has been suggested as having use in the treatment of masseter and/or temporalis muscle hypertrophy, bruxism, recurrent dislocation of the temporomandibular joint, as an adjunct to oral surgical procedures involving the temporomandibular joint and to improve trismus associated with brain injury. A preliminary study (Freund et al 1999) of 15 patients with TMD failed to demonstrate any significant clinical benefit from BoNT-A injections. A more recent uncontrolled open label study (Freund & Schwartz 2002) found that following injection of 50U BoNT-A into each masseter and 25U into each temporalis muscle of 60 patients suffering myogenous TMD, resulted in improved chronic TTH symptoms.

Conclusion

On the basis of clinical research, BoNT-A appears to be a promising therapy for migraine and chronic daily headache, particularly where the headaches have proved resistant to other forms of treatment. However, for chronic tension-type headache, the use of BoNT-A is not strongly supported by the literature, nor does BoNT-A appear any more successful than local anesthetic injections for treatment of myofascial pain trigger points (although it offers a treatment option in recalcitrant cases). There is insufficient data to comment on the use of BoNT-A for the less common primary headaches and orofacial conditions. Further studies are needed to establish the best patient profiles that may predict successful use of BoNT treatment.

References

Aoki KR 2003 Evidence for antinociceptive activity of botulinum toxin type A in pain management. Headache 43(suppl 1):S9-S15.

Aurora SK, Gawel M, Brandes J et al 2005 Botulinum toxin Type A: prophylactic treatment for episodic migraine using a modified follow-the-pain treatment paradigm: a randomized double blind, placebo controlled, phase ii study. Headache 45(6):825-826. S116.

Bach-Rojecky L, Lackovic Z 2005 Antinociceptive effect of botulinum toxin type a in rat model of carrageenan and capsaicin induced pain. Croat Med J 46(2):201.

Barrientos N, Chana P 2002 Efficacy and safety of botulinum toxin type A (BOTOX) in the prophylactic treatment of migraine [abstract]. Headache 42:5:ABS S137.

Barrientos N, Chana P, De la Cerda A, Munoz G 2003 Efficacy and safety of botulinum toxin in migraine: 1-year follow-up. J Neurol Sci 214(1-2):91.

Bechmand RA, Tucker T, Guyuron B 2003 Single-site botulinum toxin type A injection for elimination of migraine trigger points. Headache 43:1085-108.

Bhidayasiri R, Truong DD 2005 Expanding use of botulinum toxin. J Neurol Sci 15:235(1-2):1-9.

Binder WJ, Brin MF, Blitzer A et al 2000 Botulinum toxin type A (BOTOX) for treatment of migraine headaches: An open-label study. Otolaryngol Head Neck Surg 123(6):669-676.

Blumenfeld A 2003 Botulinum Toxin Type A as an effective prophylactic treatment in primary headache disorders. Headache 43(8):853-885.

Blumenfeld AM, Dodick DW, Silberstein SD 2004 Botulinum neurotoxin for the treatment of migraine and other primary headache disorders. Dermatol Clin 22(2):167-175.

Boudreau G 2005 Treatment of chronic tension-type headache with botulinum toxin: a double-blind, placebo-controlled clinical trial. Cephalalgia 25(11):110.

Brin MF 1997 Botulinum toxin: chemistry, pharmacology, toxicity, and immunology. Muscle Nerve. 20(suppl 6):S146-S152.

Burstein R, Jakubowski M, Collins B 2004 Defeating migraine pain with triptans: a race against the development of cutaneous allodynia. Ann Neurol 55:19-26.

Clark GT 2003 The management of oromandibular motor disorders and facial spasms with injections of botulinum toxin. Phys Med Rehabil Clin N Am 14(4):727-748.

Cui M, Khanijou S, Rubino J, Aoki KR 2004 Subcutaneous administration of botulinum toxin A reduces formalin-induced pain. Pain 107:125-133.

Dodick DW, Mauskop A, Elkind AH et al 2005 Botulinum toxin type A (BOTOX) for the prophylactic treatment of chronic daily headache: Subgroup analysis of patients not receiving other prophylactic medications: a randomised, double-blind, placebo controlled study. Headache 45(4):315-324.

Dressler D, Adib Saberi F 2005 Botulinum toxin: mechanisms of action. Eur Neurol 53(1):3-9. Epub 2005 Jan 12.

Durham PL, Cady R, Cady R 2004 Regulation of calcitonin gene-related peptide secretion from trigeminal nerve cells by botulinum toxin type A: Implications for migraine therapy. Headache 44(1):35-41.

Eross EJ, Dodick DW 2002 The effects of botulinum toxin type A on disability in episodic and chronic migraine. Neurology 58(suppl 3):A497.

Evers S, Oleson J 2006 Botulinum Toxin in headache treatment: the end of the road? Cephalalgia 26:769-771.

Evers S, Vollmer-Haase J, Schwaag S et al 2004 Botulinum toxin A in the prophylactic treatment of migraine – a randomised, double blind, placebo controlled study. Cephalalgia 24:838-843.

Fielder T, Durham PL 2003 Stimulation of CGRP secretion from trigeminal ganglia neurons by nitric oxide and repression by botulinum toxin type A. Soc Neurosci Abstr Viewer Itiner ABS588.6.

Freund BJ, Schwartz M 2002 Relief of tension-type headache symptoms in subjects with temporomandibular disorders treated with botulinum toxin-A. Headache 42:1033-1037.

Freund B, Schwartz M, Symington J 1999 The use of botulinum toxin for the treatment of temporomandibular disorders: preliminary findings. J Oral Maxillofac Surg 8:916-921.

Goadsby PJ 2005 Migraine pathophysiology. Headache 45 (suppl 1):S14-S24.

Gobel H 2004 Botulinum toxin in migraine prophylaxis. J Neurol 251(suppl):1:I8-11.

Hexsel DM, De Almeida AT, Rutowitsch M et al 2003 Multicenter, double blind study of the efficacy of injections with botulinum toxin type A reconstituted up to six consecutive weeks before application. Dermatol Surg 29:523–529.

Lipton RB, Bigal ME 2005 Migraine: epidemiological, impact, and risk factors for progression. Headache 45(suppl 1):S3-S13.

Mathew NT, Frishberg BM Gawel M et al 2005 BOTOX CDH Study Group. Botulinum toxin Type A (BOTOX) for the prophylactic treatment of chronic daily headache; a randomized, double blind, placebo-controlled trial. Headache 45(4): 293-307.

Mauskop A 1999 Botulinum Toxin in the treatment of chronic daily headaches. Cephalalgia 19:453.

Ondo WG, Derman HS 2002 Botulinum toxin A for chronic daily headache: a 60 patient, randomised, placebo controlled, parallel design study. Headache 42:431.

Ondo WG, Vuong KD, Derman HS 2002 Botulinum toxin A (BOTOX) for chronic daily headache: a randomised placebo controlled, parallel design study. American Headache Society 44th Annual Scientific Meeting June 21-23 2002, Seattle, Wash. Abstract S131.

Oshinsky ML, Pozo-Rosich J, Luo J et al 2004 Botulinum Toxin type A blocks sensitisation of neurons in the trigeminal nucleus caudalis. Cephalalgia 24(9):781 ABS-PA.21.

Padberg M, de Bruijn SFTM, de Haan RJ et al 2004 Treatment of chronic tension type headache with botulinum toxin: a double blind, placebo controlled clinical trial. Cephalalgia 24:675-680.

Relja M, Telarovic S 2004 Botulinum toxin in tension-type headache. J Neurol 251(suppl 1):I12-I14.

Relja M, Poole AC, Schoenen J et al 2005 A multicenter, double blind, randomised, placebo controlled, parallel group study of multiple treatments of botulinum toxin type A (BoNTA) for the prophylaxis of migraine headaches. J Neurol 252(suppl 2):62 (P222).

Rollnick JD, Tanneberger O, Schubert M et al 2000 Treatment of tension type headache with botulinum toxin type A: a double blind, placebo controlled study. Headache 40: 300-305.

Scher AI, Stewart WF, Lipton RB 2005 Epidemiology of chronic headaches. In: Goadsby PJ, Silberstein SD, Dodick DW (eds) Chronic daily headache for clinicians. BC Decker Inc, Hamilton, p 3-10.

Schulte-Mattler WJ, Krack P; BoNTTH Study Group 2004 Treatment of chronic tension-type headache with botulinum toxin A: a randomized, double-blind, placebo-controlled multicenter study. Pain 109(1-2): 110-114.

Silberstein SD, Lipton RB, Solomon S et al 1994 Classification of daily and near daily headache: proposed revisions to the IHS Classification. Headache 34:1-7.

Silberstein S, Mathew N, Saper J, Jenkins S 2000 Botulinum toxin type A as a migraine preventive treatment. For the BOTOX Migraine Clinical Research Group. Headache 40(6):445-450.

27

Neurosurgery

Richard Bittar

A broad spectrum of conditions may result in pain involving the head or face. In some cases this pain becomes intractable, refractory to conventional medical and physical therapies. In this chapter the author, a neurosurgeon, provides the reader with an overview of the role of contemporary neurosurgical intervention in the management of headache and facial pain.

Neurosurgical interventions for intractable headache and facial pain may be broadly divided into three categories: decompressive, ablative, and neuromodulatory.

Decompressive surgery involves the relief of physical pressure on neural structures which may be causing the pain syndrome in question. For example, trigeminal neuralgia is frequently treated with microvascular decompression. This procedure involves interposing a small piece of Teflon between a small artery and the trigeminal nerve. By reducing the focal pressure (and particularly the arterial pulsations) on the nerve, over 90% of patients are relieved of their pain (Ashkan & Marsh 2004). Decompressive surgery is also used to relieve elevated intracranial pressure due to intracranial space-occupying lesions, such as tumors. Hydrocephalus, which often causes headaches, is treated either by ventriculoperitoneal shunting or endoscopic third ventriculostomy. Both of these techniques reduce the build-up of cerebrospinal fluid (CSF) intracranially, decreasing intracranial pressure and yielding symptomatic improvement. Benign intracranial hypertension may be treated with bilateral subtemporal decompressions or CSF diversionary procedures (Lifshutz & Johnson 2001). Chiari malformations, or herniation of the cerebellar tonsils into the spinal canal, are treated surgically by decompression of the foramen magnum (Fischer 1995).

Ablative procedures involve the destruction of pain-generating or transmitting structures, and may be accomplished using a variety of methods. These include the injection of chemicals such as glycerol or alcohol, temporary compression of neural structures using an inflatable balloon, or the physical disruption of neural structures by heating or cutting. Conditions frequently treated using one or more of these ablative techniques include trigeminal neuralgia and occipital neuralgia. Some advantages of these approaches are their relatively low morbidity, and their ability to be performed using percutaneous or minimally invasive techniques. Unfortunately the failure and recurrence rate can be significant, and the development of deafferentation pain, whilst uncommon, can be disastrous (Lopez et al 2004).

The most recent techniques used by neurosurgeons to treat intractable head and facial pain are classified as neuromodulatory or neuroaugmentative. These modalities utilize electrical stimulation of neural structures to ameliorate pain. They include peripheral nerve stimulation, spinal cord stimulation, motor cortex stimulation, and deep brain stimulation.

Peripheral nerve stimulation involves the placement of an electrode over the nerve supplying the painful region of the head. It may be effective for the treatment of cervicogenic headaches and occipital neuralgia, providing significant long-term pain and medication reduction in over 70% of patients (Weiner 2006).

Spinal cord stimulation entails the positioning of one or two electrodes extradurally over the posterior aspect of the spinal cord. These electrodes may be inserted either percutaneously or via an open surgical technique (laminotomy or laminectomy). They may be inserted under general anesthetic or under light sedation, permitting intraoperative assessment of stimulation effects. Certain types of head and facial pain may be treated with high cervical spinal cord stimulation (Osenbach 2004).

Deep brain stimulation refers to the insertion of electrodes into the sensory thalamus and/or periventricular grey matter, whereas motor cortex stimulation is performed by placing one or two paddle-type electrodes over the motor cortex, usually extradurally.

Deep brain stimulation requires the use of a stereotactic head frame to ensure a high degree of spatial accuracy. The author's practice is to perform intraoperative stimulation to confirm the presence of beneficial effects in the desired region, as well as the absence of side effects. The risks of deep brain stimulation include stroke, seizures, and death.

Motor cortex stimulation may carry lower risks than deep brain stimulation. It is particularly useful for the treatment of neuropathic facial pain, due to the large cortical representation of the face (Henderson & Lad, 2006). It does not require a stereotactic head frame; however, frameless stereotaxy, preoperative functional magnetic resonance imaging, and intraoperative cortical stimulation may improve the accuracy of electrode placement. With most neuromodulatory approaches, a trial period (usually several days) of stimulation is performed before the second stage of the surgery (implantation of the battery or pulse generator) is undertaken. If adequate pain relief is not achieved, the electrodes can be removed without adverse long term sequelae in the majority.

Conditions treated with neurosurgery

Trigeminal neuralgia

Paroxysmal, lancinating facial pain in the distribution of one or more divisions of the trigeminal nerve is known as trigeminal neuralgia. This is a common cause of facial pain, which may be extremely severe and unremitting. The usual mechanism is compression of the dorsal root entry zone of the trigeminal nerve by a small artery or, less commonly, a vein. Such vessels may be visualized preoperatively with magnetic resonance angiography. In some cases no vascular impingement on the nerve is seen, even at surgery. Trigeminal neuralgia may also occur in the setting of multiple sclerosis, as a result of demyelination, and is particularly difficult to treat.

Trigeminal neuralgia is treated pharmacologically initially, with membrane-stabilizing agents such as carbamazepine, and typically responds favorably to this medication. In those cases which are resistant to pharmacotherapy, more invasive treatment approaches may be considered. Percutaneous targeting of the trigeminal ganglion and microvascular decompression are the most frequently employed surgical approaches (Bennetto et al 2007).

Percutaneous techniques involve the insertion of a needle into Meckel's cave (which houses the trigeminal ganglion) through the cheek. This is done, often under local anesthesia, under X-ray control or with the aid of frameless stereotaxy. Once the needle is in place, one of three strategies may then be employed. Glycerol may be injected into the subarachnoid space around the ganglion (glycerol rhizolysis). Alternatively, a small balloon may be inflated to transiently compress (and damage) the ganglion. The third option involves controlled heating of the ganglion using a radiofrequency electrode (radiofrequency rhizolysis). The efficacy of most percutaneous procedures relies upon the production of a degree of facial numbness. This 'trade-off' against pain relief must be understood and accepted by the patient beforehand. Percutaneous procedures have a 70–90% success rate, but the incidence of recurrence after five years is significant (Kondziolka & Lunsford 2005). The procedure may need to be repeated at that time.

In the author's opinion, the benefits of percutaneous strategies include a relatively low morbidity, but the small risk ($< 1\%$) of stroke and anesthesia dolorosa must be considered. This is the treatment of choice for multiple sclerosis-related trigeminal neuralgia, patients unfit for craniotomy, and for patients who do not wish to undergo an open procedure.

Microvascular decompression is performed via a posterior fossa craniotomy. A window of bone behind the ear is removed, and the trigeminal nerve is approached by gently retracting the cerebellum. A small piece of teflon is interposed between a compressing artery and the nerve. If the offending vessel is a vein, this is coagulated and divided. The long-term (5–10 year) success rate of microvascular

decompression is over 90%. The risk of stroke or mortality is higher than for the percutaneous techniques ($< 2\%$), but the incidence of facial numbness is lower (Chen & Lee 2003).

In some centers, stereotactic radiosurgery is used to treat trigeminal neuralgia. This may be performed using a gamma knife or linear accelerator. The long-term results appear satisfactory, and it is reasonable to consider this option in patients who are not suitable for the above surgical techniques, or in those for whom these conventional approaches have failed (Drzymala et al 2005). The main disadvantage of this technique is the delayed onset of beneficial effect in reducing facial pain.

Glossopharyngeal neuralgia is a much less common similar condition caused by compression of the glossopharyngeal nerve. It causes pain in the tongue and throat. The treatment of choice for medically-intractable glossopharyngeal neuralgia is microvascular decompression (Pearce 2006).

Cervicogenic headache

Headache arising from the cervical spine is relatively common and under-recognized. These may occur as a consequence of degenerative cervical spine disease or following a whiplash-type injury to the neck. Cervicogenic headaches are typically occipital; however, they may radiate to the vertex of the skull and may also be associated with retro-orbital pain (Haldeman & Dagenais 2001). There is often, but not always, associated neck pain or discomfort. The headache may resemble true occipital neuralgia. It is important to attempt to determine the anatomical substrate of these headaches. In the author's opinion, cervicogenic headache arising from the facet joints may respond to percutaneous radiofrequency denervation, whilst those secondary to cervical disc prolapse often (but not reliably) improve with microsurgical discectomy and fusion. C2 radio-frequency pulse ganglionotomy is another percutaneous technique which may benefit some patients, particularly if C2 nerve root compression is thought to be involved in the pathogenesis of the headache. More recently, peripheral nerve stimulation of the greater and lesser occipital nerves has emerged as a potentially efficacious technique in patients with cervicogenic headache resistant to all conventional therapies (Weiner 2006).

Occipital neuralgia

Sharp, shooting pain arising in the occipital region and radiating either to the vertex of the skull, or to the temporal region, is typical of occipital neuralgia. This is frequently associated with a dull or throbbing retro-orbital pain. The pain is often reproduced by percussion over the greater or lesser occipital nerve. Occipital neuralgia may follow trauma, surgery, atlantoaxial subluxation (for example in rheumatoid arthritis), neuromas, or C2 root entrapment by a hypertrophied ligamentous structure between C1 and C2. Traditional neurosurgical strategies to manage this difficult condition have included sectioning or avulsion of the occipital nerves. In the author's experience, this procedure frequently fails, may cause significant scalp numbness, and may occasionally lead to deafferentation pain. It is not recommended by the author as an initial surgical approach. Radiofrequency ablation of the offending nerve may yield substantial symptomatic benefit, but the recurrence rate is high. If C2 root is thought to be compressed between the C1 arch and C2 lamina, surgical decompression may be beneficial. Symptomatic atlantoaxial subluxation may warrant a C1–C2 fusion. Peripheral nerve stimulation of occipital nerves has emerged as an efficacious technique in patients with intractable occipital neuralgia (Weiner 2006).

Chiari malformation

Herniation of the cerebellar tonsils through the foramen magnum is a well-described cause of headache. These are typically impulse headaches, precipitated by coughing or straining. They are usually occipital in location. There may be associated ataxia, and motor and sensory deficits. Some Chiari malformations may be associated with hydrocephalus, which may also cause headache. The treatment of symptomatic Chiari malformation requires surgical decompression (Fischer 1995). The posterior rim of the foramen magnum and arch of the C1 vertebra are removed. Most surgeons open the dura and insert a patulous fascial graft to ensure adequate decompression of the brainstem. In the majority of patients, surgery results in symptomatic improvement, however the primary goal of surgery is to arrest further deterioration.

Hydrocephalus

Hydrocephalus (dilation of the ventricular system) may result from blockage of the cerebrospinal fluid (CSF) pathways or impaired reabsorption of CSF. Hydrocephalus may cause headache due to elevated intracranial pressure. Raised intracranial pressure headaches are typically global or bifrontal, are worse in the early hours of the morning, and are exacerbated by recumbency or straining. They are frequently associated with nausea or vomiting. Hydrocephalus may be treated by ventriculoperitoneal shunting. This involves the placement of a catheter into one of the lateral ventricles, and threading a connected longer catheter subcutaneously to the abdomen, where it is inserted into the peritoneal cavity. Cerebrospinal fluid is thereby diverted from the cranium to the abdomen, where it is reabsorbed. In some cases of obstructive hydrocephalus, such as where the flow of CSF is impeded by stenosis of the cerebral aqueduct, tumors (usually non-aggressive) of the tectal plate, and posterior fossa tumors, an endoscopic third ventriculostomy may be performed. This procedure is done through a burr hole in the skull, using an endoscope. A small hole is created in the floor of the third ventricle, thereby allowing CSF to bypass the area of obstruction and flow directly into the basal cisterns. Endoscopic third ventriculostomy is highly effective and generally safe, however there is a small risk of serious complications including basilar artery rupture and post-operative memory impairment (Greenberg 2001).

Benign intracranial hypertension

Benign intracranial hypertension (pseudotumor cerebri) usually afflicts female children and young adults, many of whom are obese. The headache in benign intracranial hypertension is due to raised intracranial pressure. Papilledema (swelling of the optic discs) is seen, and blindness may occur if this condition is untreated. The treatment of medically refractory benign intracranial hypertension includes serial lumbar punctures (to reduce intracranial pressure), and lumboperitoneal or ventriculopertioneal shunting. The latter procedures involve the diversion of cerebrospinal fluid from either the lumbar subarachnoid space or the lateral ventricles to the abdomen. Ventricular catheterization may be very difficult due to the presence of small lateral ventricles, but the placement of a ventriculoperitoneal shunt in these patients is aided by the employment of stereotactic techniques. In patients with progressive visual loss, blindness may be averted by optic nerve sheath fenestration (Greenberg 2001).

Cluster headache

Cluster headaches typically comprise episodic unilateral frontal and retro-orbital pain, lacrimation, nasal congestion, and vasomotor changes resulting in scleral injection and periorbital swelling. They most frequently affect males in early- to mid-adulthood. Cluster headaches may be treated with a variety of medical therapies, including antimigraine agents, lithium, and oxygen. Most cases are able to be controlled with such measures. Where cluster headache becomes refractory to conventional therapies, and is so severe as to cause a significant degradation in the patient's quality of life, surgical intervention may be considered. Previous surgical approaches to the treatment of this frequently devastating condition have involved percutaneous interference with the trigeminal or sphenopalatine ganglion. Overall, the success rate of such strategies has been low, although some practitioners report reasonable efficacy. More recently, following the observation of discrete metabolic changes within the ipsilateral posterior hypothalamus during cluster headache, deep brain stimulation has emerged as a promising way to treat these individuals. Deep brain stimulation for cluster headache involves the placement of an electrode in the ipsilateral posterior hypothalamus, and the delivery of a high frequency current to inactivate this area. In small series, with greater than 12 months follow-up, approximately two-thirds of patients have been rendered pain-free, and around half have been able to cease pharmacological treatment (Franzini et al 2003). These results are extremely encouraging, however confirmation that these benefits persist for several years will be required before deep brain stimulation for cluster headaches becomes a standard therapy.

Neuropathic facial pain

Neuropathic facial pain, in contrast to trigeminal neuralgia, is typically a constant, burning-type pain. It is frequently associated with numbness, hypersensitivity, and allodynia. It may be severe and debilitating, as is the case with anesthesia dolorosa. Neuropathic facial pain may follow a number of conditions and interventions, including surgical attempts to treat trigeminal neuralgia, dental procedures, trauma to the supraorbital and supratrochlear nerves at the supraorbital rim and over the frontal sinus, herpes zoster, and stroke. Patients who have not responded to medical and cognitive behavioral therapies may be considered for neuromodulatory intervention. Motor cortex stimulation may be particularly useful for intractable facial pain, due to the large representation of the face on the cerebral cortex. Deep brain stimulation, targeting the sensory thalamus or periventricular grey region, may also produce a dramatic benefit in many, but has a higher risk of stroke and mortality than motor cortex stimulation. The author offers motor cortex stimulation as a treatment option before recommending deep brain stimulation. Peripheral nerve stimulation may be effective in some patients with neuropathic facial pain, and carries very low surgical risks. Neuropathic pain in the distribution of the first division of the trigeminal nerve may respond to peripheral nerve stimulation targeting the supraorbital and supratrochlear nerves. Neuropathic facial pain may also respond to high cervical spinal cord stimulation, due to capture of the descending loop of trigeminothalamic fibers which may extend as caudally as C2 or C3 (Follett 2004).

Space-occupying lesions

Space-occupying lesions, or intracranial masses, frequently present with headache. Such headaches are usually the result of raised intracranial pressure. Common causes include tumors, trauma, vascular abnormalities, and infection.

Intracranial tumors may be malignant or benign. Cerebral metastases (most frequently emanating from primary tumors in the breasts, lungs, bowel, kidneys, or cutaneous melanoma) and gliomas (primary brain tumors) are the most common intracranial malignancies. Benign tumors include meningioma, acoustic neuroma (vestibular schwannoma), and pituitary adenoma. Brain tumors may cause raised intracranial pressure due to their volume or mass effect, by inciting vasogenic edema (increased water content in surrounding brain tissue), or obstruction of CSF flow (i.e., hydrocephalus). Treatment of tumor-related headache includes steroids (dexamethasone) to decrease vasogenic edema, and surgical resection (Greenberg 2001).

Cranial trauma may result in headache as a result of raised intracranial pressure. Such trauma is frequently trivial, particularly in the elderly, alcoholics, and in people taking anticoagulants or antiplatelet agents. Subdural hematoma and intracerebral hematoma may evolve over days to weeks. Symptomatic subdural hematomas are treated with surgical drainage. Post-traumatic intracerebral hematomas are usually managed conservatively (Greenberg 2001).

Sudden-onset headache is the hallmark of an intracranial vascular event, and should be investigated and treated with urgency. Ruptured cerebral aneurysm typically causes subarachnoid hemorrhage, with resulting meningism (headache, neck stiffness, photophobia, nausea, and vomiting). Spontaneous intracerebral bleeding may be a consequence of an arteriovenous malformation, hypertension, tumor, coagulopathy, or amyloid angiopathy. Treatment depends upon the underlying cause (Greenberg 2001).

Infective causes of headaches which may require neurosurgical intervention include brain abscess and subdural empyema. Postoperative intracranial infections are a rare but important complication of cranial neurosurgery. Treatment usually comprises surgical drainage as well as antibiotic therapy (Greenberg 2001).

Conclusion

Head and facial pain may result from a variety of underlying conditions. A proportion of sufferers will fail to experience satisfactory long-term pain relief with conventional medical and interventional strategies, and may be considered for more invasive treatment. A number of surgical approaches may be employed by the neurosurgeon with expertise in the treatment of intractable chronic pain. The approach should be tailored to the individual's condition, and should only be offered in the context of a multidisciplinary pain management setting. The evolution of neuromodulatory techniques offers new hope to many sufferers who have not or would not benefit from more traditional approaches to pain management.

References

Ashkan K, Marsh H 2004 Microvascular decompression for trigeminal neuralgia in the elderly: a review of the safety and efficacy. Neurosurgery. 55:840-848.

Bennetto L, Patel NK, Fuller G 2007 Trigeminal neuralgia and its management. BMJ 334: 201-205.

Chen JF, Lee ST 2003 Comparison of percutaneous trigeminal ganglion compression and microvascular decompression for the management of trigeminal neuralgia. Clinical Neurology and Neurosurgery 105: 203-208.

Drzymala RE, Malyapa RS, Dowling JL et al 2005 Gamma knife radiosurgery for trigeminal neuralgia: the Washington University initial experience. Stereotactic and Functional Neurosurgery 83: 148-152.

Fischer EG 1995 Posterior fossa decompression for Chiari I deformity, including resection of the cerebellar tonsils. Childs Nerv Syst. 11:625-629.

Follett KA 2004 Neurosurgical pain management. 2004 Elsevier Saunders, Philadelphia.

Franzini A, Ferroli P, Leone M et al 2003 Stimulation of the posterior hypothalamus for treatment of chronic intractable cluster headaches: first reported series. Neurosurgery 52:1095-1099.

Greenberg MS 2001 Handbook of neurosurgery, 5th edn. Thieme, Florida.

Haldeman S, Dagenais S 2001 Cervicogenic headaches: a critical review. Spine J 1:31-46.

Henderson JM, Lad SP 2006 Motor cortex stimulation and neuropathic facial pain. Neurosurgical Focus 21(6):E6.

Kondziolka D, Lunsford LD 2005 Percutaneous retrogasserian glycerol rhizotomy for trigeminal neuralgia: technique and expectations. Neurosurgical Focus 18(5):E7.

Lifshutz JI, Johnson WD 2001 History of hydrocephalus and its treatments. Neurosurgical Focus 11(2):E1.

Lopez BC, Hamlyn PJ, Zakrzewska JM 2004 Systematic review of ablative neurosurgical techniques for the treatment of trigeminal neuralgia. Neurosurgery 54:973-982.

Osenbach RK 2004 In: Follett KA (ed) Neurosurgical pain management. Elsevier Saunders, Philadelphia.

Pearce JM 2006 Glossopharyngeal neuralgia. Eur Neurol 55:49-52.

Weiner RL 2006 Occipital Neurostimulation (ONS) for Treatment of intractable headache disorders. Pain Medicine 7(suppl 1): S137-S139.

Index

A

ablative neurosurgery, 357–8, 360
abscesses
    brain, 27, 63, 362
    dental, 121, 244
active exercise, 183
active myofascial trigger points, 302
activities of daily living (ADL)
    assessment, 160
    and treatment outcome, 154
acupoints, 321, 322
acupuncture, 321
    CNS effects, 326
    complications, 330
    deep needling, 324
    electroacupuncture, 327–8
    fMRI studies, 326
    management of headaches, 324
    mechanism, 327
acute angle closure glaucoma, 128, 129–30
acute severe new-onset headache ('First or Worst'), 15
adolescents see children/adolescents
age
    and neck movement, 173
    as 'red flag', 6
    and tinnitus, 123
    in vestibular dysfunction, 150
airflow restriction
    and pain, 62–3
    and sleep bruxism treatment, 64–5
alcohol, 226
allergic responses, 104, 225
allergists, referral to, 63
allodynia, 25, 98–100, 108
almotriptan, 28, 29
amaurosis fugax, painful, 130
amines, vasoactive, 230
amitriptyline, 29, 30, 199, 200, 293, 294
    with cognitive–behavioral therapy, 287

analgesia
    overuse, 20–1, 100
    perpetuating headache, 20–1
anesthetic in cervicogenic headache, 9, 43
aneurysm, ruptured, 17
antecedents of headache, 278, 279–80
anterior scalene, 174, 175
anti-inflammatories, 100
antibiotics, 117, 118
antiepileptics, 29, 30
anxiety
    in children/adolescents, 34
    as headache trigger, 280, 289
    management, 251
    and migraine, 26
    psychiatric assessment, 291
    sleep-related, 64
anxiolytics, 64
applied kinesiology (AK), 206
arm movement exercises, 187
arteriovenous malformation (AVM), 17
arthrodesis, surgical, 51
aspartame sensitivity, 226–7
aspirin, 28–9
assessment of headache, 240–50
    differential diagnosis guidelines, 241, 242–3
    investigations/imaging, 250
    physical, 242–3, 244–50
        cervical area, 247
        posture, 245–7
        spatula test, 249–50
        temporomandibular area, 247–9
    psychological, 280–2
    'red flags', 240–1
    subjective, 242
        aggravating factors, 241, 243–4
        pain distribution, 241
associated myofascial trigger points, 302
ataxia, 143

sleep disorders (*Continued*)
  and headache, 55–63
  respiratory, 55
sleep quality with TTH, 62
sleep-related/morning headaches, 6, 9, 59, 61–3
  assessment, 243–4
  classification, 59
  differential diagnosis, 63
  referral, 63–4
  symptoms, 63
sleep structure, 56–7
  and bruxism, 56–9
  cyclic alternating patterns (CAP), 57
  hypnogram, 56
  microarousals, 57, 58
  ultradian sleep cycles, 57
slump position, 245, 344, 345
slump test, 245
SMT *see* spinal manipulative, therapy
'snapping of the brain', 63
social support, measuring, 282
sodium valproate (valproic acid), 29, 30, 294
somatic dysfunction, 214–15
somatization disorder, 292
space-occupying lesions, cerebral
  differential diagnosis, 27
  neurosurgery, 362–3
spatula test, 249–50
spinal locking, 218
spinal manipulative (manual) therapy (SMT)
  contraindications, 200–1
  description, 195–6
  effects, 197
  and head pain, 197
  headache management, 197–200, 255
    cervicogenic headache, 109, 198, 199–200,
      254–5
    migraine, 197, 198, 199
    systematic reviews, 200
    tension-type headache, 198, 200
spinal mobilization, 49, 253
spinal muscle retraining, 109
spinal nerve stimulation, 358
spinal subluxation *see* subluxation
splenius capitis, 314–15, 318
stabbing headache, 14
standing balance, 177
Staphylococcus aureus, 117
START osteopathic diagnosis, 214, 215

Step Test, 145
stereotactic radiosurgery, 359
sternocleidomastoid, 174, 175, 311–12, 317
  in cervicogenic headache, 240
steroids, intra-articular, 49
stress
  in cervicogenic headache, 105–6
  cognitive–behavioral therapy for, 284
  diagnosis, 106
  experimentally-induced, 106
  as headache trigger, 105–6, 279, 280, 289
    mechanism, 107
  and immune system, 107
  and otalgia, 120
  and TMD, 70
stress management, 254, 264
stroke, 24, 26, 63
stylohyoid, 265
sub-occipital muscle group, 315–16, 318
subarachnoid hemorrhage (SAH)
  causes, 16
  diagnosis, 5–6, 16–17
  differential diagnosis, 27
  due to trauma, 7
  grading (Hunt and Hess scale), 16
  prevalence, 14
  sleep-related, 63
subdural hematoma, 18
subluxation, 195–6
  clinical signs, 196
  diagnosis, 196
  pain mechanisms, 197
suboccipital inhibition, 216
substance abuse, 291
  case study, 295
substance P, 96, 97
sumatriptan, 28, 29, 291
SUNCT syndrome, 19, 134
surgery
  in Ménière's disease, 148
  in trigeminal neuralgia, 133
swallowing
  normal, 269
  and orofacial dysfunctions, 269–70
  tongue teeth breathing/swallowing (TTBS)
    exercise, 268–9
'swimmer's ear', 117
sympathetic nervous system, 213, 214
synovitis, 74

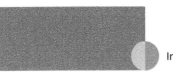

W

Z

Printed and bound by CPI Group (UK) Ltd, Croydon, CR0 4YY

03/10/2024

01040360-0018